CANCER

STEP OUTSIDE THE BOX

"I read Ty's book during the summer of 2009; I thought it would be another average get-well cancer book. Once I started, I could not stop reading. It contained page after page of well researched and documented facts. As an Herbalist and Naturopath, we know these secrets, yet because of FDA rules, we cannot publicly state them to the public at large. Please read this book ... Someone you know will be diagnosed with cancer; you may be your friend's hero with this information!"
~ *Shelton R. Hendriex, Naturopath & Herbalist, Cincinnati, Ohio, USA*

"This book truly is a reference manual to better health and a cancer free life. The author has done a great job of filtering out all the junk on the internet leaving you with the very best." ~ *Simon Jackson, Invercargill, New Zealand*

"I have read about 10 books about alternative cures for cancer. This book is superior in several ways...Personally an alternative cancer treatment has worked for me. This is an unusual book; this is a book everyone should read." ~ *Paul Leveille, California, USA*

"I have read many books on various illnesses and their causes, but this one beats them all by far." ~ *Claudine M. Gregg, Alaska, USA*

"I am a RN for almost 28 years and am currently working in a hospital setting. I found Ty Bollingers book Cancer-Step Outside the Box ... I have learned so much about cancer treatments and just good nutrition ...This is one of the best, easy to read books, with so much research done on multiple treatments with easy to use information. I can't say enough good about the book ..." ~ *R. Lowe, Cleveland, Ohio, USA*

"Every doctor should read this book...This is a great book that contains a wealth of information. But it's only for those who can think for themselves. Thank you Ty and watch your back now." ~ *V. Kravets, Pennsylvania, USA*

"I bought this for my ex-wife who had/has pancreatic cancer, and been told to 'go home and put your affairs in order.' She has found this book to be a constant source of useful information, and it is at least partly to thank for her amazing recovery and continuing good health. Highly recommended."
~ *Charles W. Dart, Jersey, Channel Islands*

"... it was easy to read and I didn't need a professor or a scientist to translate it for me. Ty is right on target with his description of the current state of affairs with the Medical establishment and Big Pharma, and their desire to keep patients as customers rather than cure them." ~ *Jessica Jordan, Nebraska, USA*

"This book is amazing. You would have to read well over 100 hand-picked books on this subject to get the information contained in this book ... The author made it simple enough for an elementary child to understand... If you are like me you will have a hard time putting the book down." ~ *Sherry, Coopersberg, Pennsylvania, USA*

"It is by far the best book in my library." ~ *Danielle Yerardi, Kentucky, USA*

"I was diagnosed with ovarian cancer over 3 years ago and have had multiple surgeries and several types of chemotherapy. When my cancer came back immediately after stopping my last chemo, I knew I needed a different approach. I found this book, immediately ordered it, & it changed my life ...I started reading the book and didn't put it down for two days until I had finished it. I now have hope to live and heal. What a great resource!"
~ *Denise L., Florida, USA*

"The recommendations in this book have helped my brother-in-law thus far in his fight with colon cancer. He was diagnosed at Stage 4 … and given 3-6 months. The colon cancer protocol … helped reduce his tumor size 50% in the first 3 weeks he used it. Very thorough and well researched." ~ *D. Hulslander, Dallas, Texas, USA*

"Not only does Ty Bollinger tell it like it is; he says it from the heart. In today's modern world, reliable information is very hard to come by. Ty you are truly a gem! Thank you." ~ *Zelko Segovic, Melbourne, Australia*

"Since being diagnosed with prostate cancer 18 months ago, I have studied alternative measures against cancer intensely. Bollinger's superb book is the best source I have found on this subject." ~ *John Memory, North Carolina, USA*

"Wow! This book is a real eye opener! Some of what I read … was enough to convince even my skeptical husband. I found this book easy to read even though Mr. Bollinger used some medical/biological terminology - even my teenagers are able to understand his writing." ~ *Jannie Bahrs, New Mexico, USA*

"This amazing book has helped me a lot with my fight with lung cancer. Keep doing what you are doing Ty." ~ *Sigthor Aegisson, Tokyo, Japan*

"As a licensed medical professional, who has witnessed countless numbers of Americans dying from conditions that are very reversible with alternate medical interventions, it is refreshing to read a book that "spills the beans" and lets the "cat out of the bag" on what is really occurring in conventional medicine, run by Big Pharma … Mr. Bollinger has compiled a "gold mine of information for you in this book." ~ *Peggy Krizan, Gillette, Wyoming, USA*

"This book is amazing! Thoroughly researched, well written and the most informative book that I have come across … since my husband was diagnosed with a brain tumour … I was in complete despair following my husband's diagnosis; this book gave me hope and inspiration and gave us back some control over our situation. The more that I read the more I learned, I cannot believe how naïve I was about conventional medical options … This book gave me strength, the old adage: knowledge is power." ~ *Diana Thomas, UK*

"I just learned of a possible problem with breast cancer and, instead of panicking, I realized after reading <u>Cancer – Step Outside the Box</u> that I actually do have some control over this disease … [this] book is extremely well-researched and very educational…a must-read…I couldn't put the book down once I started reading it." ~ *Paula Deschene, California, USA*

"I am not a journalist, that's Ty's job, so I won't drag this out … I am a cancer survivor and this book was a huge contribution to my survival (it's one of the best books on the subject). Ty is a rebel…maybe even somewhat eccentric, but you can't ignore what he's saying. Read this book if you or someone you care about has cancer…'nuff said." ~ *Brad Matznick, Michigan, USA*

"This is an unbelievable book - which opens your eyes to the brainwashing we have all been subject to. Read the book; it could be a life saver." ~ *Mrs. S.L. Coulthard, Norwich, United Kingdom*

"Time will surely prove Mr. Bollinger's important contribution to mankind via his book, <u>Cancer – Step Outside the Box</u>." ~ *B. McCoy, New Mexico, USA*

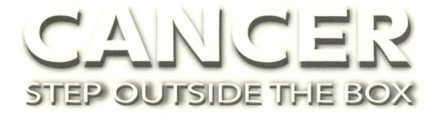

CANCER
STEP OUTSIDE THE BOX

Ty M. Bollinger

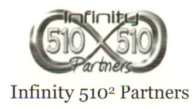

Infinity 510² Partners

Foreword by R. Webster Kehr

CANCER – STEP OUTSIDE THE BOX
6TH EDITION

To order more copies of this book,
please visit the following website:

www.CancerTruth.net

www.Infinity510Partners.com

**Before you read this book, I must give you the
following FDA mandated warning and disclaimer:**

I am not a doctor; thus, I have not been formally "miseducated." I am not certified in medicine; therefore, there is no certificate or diploma disgracing the interior of my home or office and no monument to the biggest revenue generating fraud ever perpetrated on human kind.

This book is for educational purposes only. It is not intended as a substitute for the diagnosis, treatment, or advice of a qualified, licensed medical professional. The facts presented in the following pages are offered as information only, **not** medical advice, and in **no way** should anyone infer that I am practicing medicine.

A conscious effort has been made to only present information that is both accurate and truthful. However, I assume no responsibility for inaccuracies in my source materials, nor do I assume responsibility for how this material is used. This is not a comprehensive book; thus, it does not contain information on all alternative cancer treatments, but rather those treatment protocols which I have deemed the most important and most effective.

My statements regarding alternative treatments for cancer have not been evaluated by the FDA, which I oftentimes refer to as the "Federal Death Administration."

DEDICATION

This book is dedicated to my wonderful wife, Charlene, who is my "Princess" and my best friend. She is my "dream girl" and bride of eighteen years, the mother of our four children - Brianna, Bryce, Tabitha, and Charity. She truly is my inspiration, a gift straight from God, the most shining example of His grace in my life, and my most passionate encourager. She truly is the "wind beneath my wings." As the Bible says, she is my "help meet."

Without her support and belief in me, I would never have written this book. She not only supported me and encouraged me, but she was a faithful "sounding board" for discussing which topics should (and should not) be included in the book. **Thank you Princess, for all that you are, for all that you do, and for our four beautiful children!**

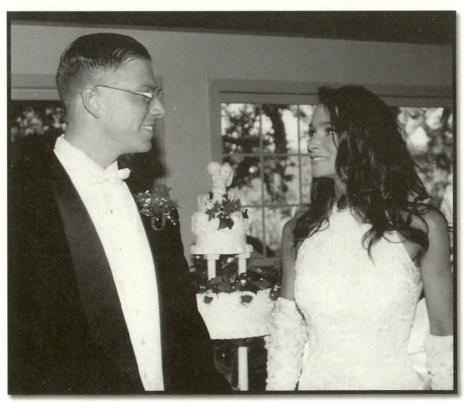

At our wedding on December 23, 1995

Bollinger family photo taken on our 17th Anniversary (December 23, 2012)

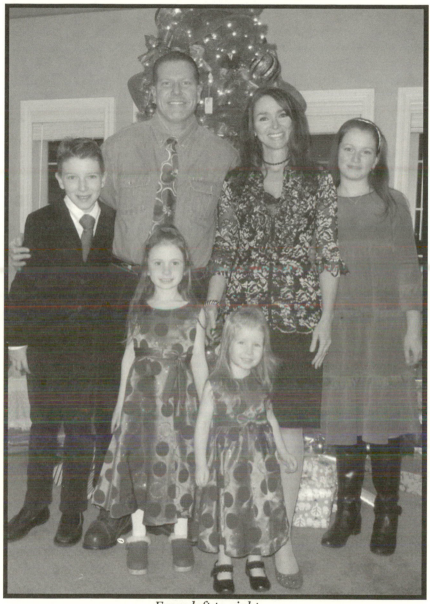

From left to right:
Bryce, Tabitha, Ty, Charlene, Charity, and Brianna

Acknowledgements

First of all, I want to give a special thanks to Webster Kehr, my friend and comrade in the fight for truth in the cancer war. Webster has compiled the most complete cancer website in the world: www.cancertutor.com. Without his research, expertise, and assistance, this book would only have been a pipe dream and would never have come to fruition.

Special thanks goes to my friend, Dr. Darrell Wolfe, for his pioneering work in the areas of cleansing and nutrition. His booklets, Spoiled Rotten, The Fungus Within Us, and Reclaim Your Inner Terrain, were especially helpful to me in the writing of this book.

Special thanks also goes to my friend, Dr. Rashid Buttar, for his wisdom and insight relating to the facts on toxicity, nutrition, and supplementation. Dr. Buttar has successfully treated thousands of cancer patients over the past decade and truly is a medical maverick. His website is www.drbuttar.com and his best-selling book is entitled The 9 Steps to Keep the Doctor Away.

Thanks to Dr. David Gregg for his insights into the causes of cancer, especially the biochemical processes which he has hypothesized and his theories on DMSO and cesium chloride. I have learned much from Dr. Gregg's work. On a side note, Dr. Gregg was also the person who "*woke me up*" to what's **really** happening behind the scenes in world events.

Thanks to Bill Henderson, author of several books on treating cancer, for his research, support, encouragement, and for his sincere care and concern for cancer patients. Bill is an amazing man and truly loves helping people. Bill's website is www.beating-cancer-gently.com.

Thanks to my friend, Mike Vrentas, developer of the Cellect Budwig protocol, for his pioneering research into one of the most effective cancer treatments available. Mike's website is www.cellectbudwig.com.

Thanks to my friend, Mike Adams, aka "the Health Ranger." With his permission, I have sprinkled several "Counterthink" comics throughout the book. Mike's website is www.naturalnews.com.

I also want to acknowledge the medical "mavericks" that did **not** settle for the status quo in cancer treatments. The courage, innovation, & dedication of these doctors, researchers, & authors have saved the lives of thousands of cancer patients. It is only because of their groundbreaking work that a book like this (by a "non-doctor" like me) is possible.

To my brother, Ron, and sister, Cherith, I want you both to know that I love you. I know it's been hard losing Mom and Dad, but I am thankful that we all have such fond memories of both of them.

To my four precious children, Brianna, Bryce, Tabitha, and Charity:
"Daddy loves you!"

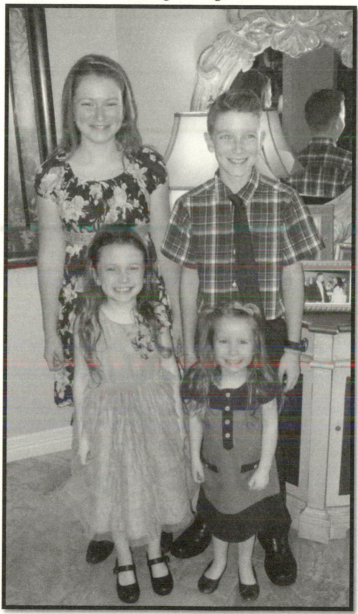

November 2013

In Memory Of

This book is in memory of my mom, Jerry Jean Bollinger Taylor, and my dad, Charles Graham Bollinger. Mom and Dad were the best parents I could have ever asked for, and they both loved me unconditionally. They were always there to support me, to love me, and to point me to the Lord.

In different ways, they were each my hero. When I look back on my life, I can honestly say that I do not have a single bad memory of Mom and Dad. Their smiles were contagious, and so was their zest for life. Now that they are both gone, there are two holes in my heart which will never be filled. But I will see them both again in Heaven. That is my hope.

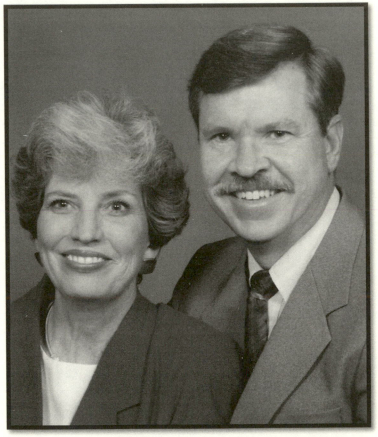

The last picture of Mom and Dad – taken in 1995

TABLE OF CONTENTS

PART III - Detox, Diet, Nutrition, Supplements, & GMO

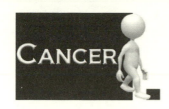
FOREWORD

One day I came home from work and my wife happened to be in one of the bedrooms. I walked into the bedroom and she looked at me and said: *"I went to the doctor today and he said I have diabetes."* As near as I can remember, these are the exact words I said to her: *"So what? The cure for type 2 diabetes is on my website, just go to my website."*

I then walked out of the room without another word being spoken. A couple of hours later I concluded I had been a bit brash, so I went to the health food store and bought the things she needed that I could buy locally, then I ordered the rest from the Internet. Within 2 months she was able to quit monitoring her blood glucose. The cure is found at www.cancertutor.com/Diabetes/Diabetes_Type_II.htm.

Had my wife told me her doctor told her she had breast cancer or pancreatic cancer or just about any other kind of cancer, my response to her would have been identical, except for substituting whatever kind of cancer she had for the term "type 2 diabetes." My website is similar to Cancer – Step Outside the Box, in that it is designed to point people in the right direction to save them months of doing their own research. Curing newly diagnosed cancer is easy; however, there are a few kinds of cancer (like squamous cell carcinoma) for which you need to pick the correct treatment the first time or you may not get a second chance.

A cancer cell is described as being "undifferentiated." What this means is that a cancer cell has no useful function. For example, a group of cancer cells cannot form muscle tissue, nor can a cancer cell become a functional part of muscle tissue. A cancer cell cannot become a functional part of a heart muscle. It cannot perform a function as part of the liver. A cancer cell can do nothing that is constructive. It just sits there. A cancer cell is like a blob of oil – you cannot integrate it into the frame of an automobile while it is still a blob of oil.

In a similar way a cancer cell cannot become part of tumor tissue, since tumor tissue must be composed entirely of healthy cells. The cancer cells just sit inside the tumor tissue, doing nothing except multiplying and refusing to die. Biopsies essentially are looking for cancer cells that are just sitting there. Because the majority of the cells in a tumor are healthy cells (all of the functional cells are healthy cells), there are not enough cancer cells inside a tumor to kill a person. In other words, no person has ever died from the cancer cells inside a tumor. This is because there cannot be enough cancer cells in a tumor to kill a person. Likewise, no one ever died from the cancer cells inside of the prostate gland. Benign tumors have grown to hundreds of pounds and still not killed the patient.

What kills cancer patients is the **spreading** of their cancer cells. When the cancer spreads enough, there are enough cancer cells to kill a person. A large number of cancer cells will literally suck the life out of a cancer patient by stealing glucose and nutrients from healthy cells by creating toxins like lactic acid. But in order to kill a person, the spreading has to go far beyond any tumor (there are rare exceptions to this rule, such as when a tumor is blocking the flow of vital fluids). Yet, in spite of these facts, oncologists continue to talk to patients about their tumors.

This quote, by the late Dr. Philip Binzel explains what I am talking about.

> *"When a patient is found to have a tumor, the only thing the doctor discusses with that patient is what he intends to do about the tumor. If a patient with a tumor is receiving radiation or chemotherapy, the only question that is asked is, 'How is the tumor doing?' No one ever asks how the patient is doing. In my medical training, I remember well seeing patients who were getting radiation and/or chemotherapy. The tumor would get smaller and smaller, but the patient would be getting sicker and sicker. At autopsy we would hear, 'Isn't that marvelous! The tumor is gone!' Yes, it was, but so was the patient. **How many millions of times are we going to have to repeat these scenarios before we realize that we are treating the wrong thing?***
>
> *In primary cancer, with only a few exceptions, the tumor is neither health-endangering nor life-threatening. I am going to repeat that statement. In primary cancer, with few exceptions, the tumor is neither health-endangering nor life-threatening. **What is health-endangering and life-threatening is the spread of that disease through the rest of the body**. There is nothing in surgery that will prevent the spread of cancer. There is nothing in radiation that will prevent the spread of the disease. There is nothing in chemotherapy that will prevent the spread of the disease. How do we know? Just look at the statistics! There is a statistic known as 'survival time.' Survival time is defined as that interval of*

time between when the diagnosis of cancer is first made in a given patient and when that patient dies from his disease.

In the past fifty years, tremendous progress has been made in the early diagnosis of cancer. In that period of time, tremendous progress had been made in the surgical ability to remove tumors. Tremendous progress has been made in the use of radiation and chemotherapy in their ability to shrink or destroy tumors. **But, the survival time of the cancer patient today is no greater than it was fifty years ago**. *What does this mean? It obviously means that we are treating the wrong thing!"* – Dr. Philip Binzel, Alive and Well, Chapter 14

In a nutshell, Dr. Binzel is saying is that nothing in orthodox medicine stops the spread of the cancer. You might think that chemotherapy is designed to stop the spread of cancer. Chemotherapy does not target cancer cells. It kills fast growing cells, whether cancerous or non-cancerous. Some cancer cells are not fast growing, thus chemotherapy may not kill them. Some cancer cells develop a resistance to synthetic drugs, so chemotherapy cannot kill them, etc.

The bottom line is that if a person took enough chemotherapy to kill all of their cancer cells, the patient would die from the toxicity of chemotherapy long before the cancer cells would all be killed.

Chemotherapy can only slow down the cancer; it cannot stop it from spreading and killing the patient.

Chemotherapy puts people in "remission," but in almost all cases the patient will come out of remission and die. Many cancer patients don't live long enough to go into remission, others go into remission several times.

Surgery certainly does not stop cancer that has already spread because in almost every case the cancer has spread far beyond what a surgeon can cut out. Radiation is like a rifle. Can you put out a carpet fire (*i.e.,* a spreading cancer) with a rifle? The only thing orthodox medicine can do is shrink tumors and slow down the cancer and temporarily put patients in remission; orthodox medicine cannot stop the spreading of cancer – **PERIOD**!

What this means is that the Food and Drug Administration (FDA) has **never** approved a chemotherapy drug that can target cancer cells or stop the spread of cancer. Every chemotherapy drug they have ever approved is virtually worthless or does more harm than good. Furthermore, the American Medical Association (AMA, which is nothing but a labor union) has **never** approved a procedure that can stop the spread of cancer.

No medical doctor (who uses the "Big 3") has ever administered a synthetic drug or done a medical procedure that stopped the spread of cancer. That is not what they do. What they do is slow down the cancer, in some cases. You might ask: do they want to stop the spread of cancer and cure the patient? While individual doctors may want to cure their patients, as far as an industry is concerned, the evidence is overwhelming that the answer to that question is "**NO!**"

This book, Cancer – Step Outside the Box, will discuss case after case of natural cancer treatments (*i.e.*, alternative cancer treatments), and even some orthodox cancer treatments, that were shut down by the authorities (usually the AMA, FDA or FTC) **because** they were too effective at curing cancer!!

There is a pattern in medicine that effective cancer treatments are shut down from public view and highly **ineffective** synthetic drugs (profitable because they can be patented) are routinely approved by the FDA. It is a scam the likes of which the world has never before seen. Future doctors will look at this generation of "doctors" in total disgust. They have had many opportunities to cure cancer, but rather than cure cancer, they bury the treatment and make it illegal to use.

The only logical motto to assign to both Big Pharma (the pharmaceutical industry) and Big Medicine (the AMA) is this: "*It is far, far more profitable to slow down the spread of cancer than to stop the spread of cancer. Everything that stops the spread of cancer MUST be shut down.*"

The long term goal of the quid pro quo marriage made in hell between the FDA, AMA and Big Pharma (*i.e.*, the core of the "Cancer Industry"), is to make cancer into a chronic disease like diabetes, whereby the patient becomes a long-term profit center. Just look at the newspapers. Almost every week some new drug is approved by the FDA that extends the life of cancer patients, compared to prior worthless drugs. That is exactly what they want to do.

You will never see a cure for a cancer unless it is an extremely rare type of cancer; such that the public relations propaganda is of more financial benefit to the Cancer Industry than the money lost to the cure. You will **never** see a cure for breast cancer, for example.

The child of the marriage made in hell is the American Cancer Society propaganda machine that is tasked to make orthodox cancer treatments look far, far more effective than they really are. They are the makeup artists for the monster. You probably think the true cure rate of orthodox medicine is 40% to 50% and growing rapidly. Nope. It has been 3% for the last 80 years and it isn't going anywhere.

Are there any natural cancer treatments (*i.e.*, alternative cancer treatments), meaning the use of molecules from Mother Nature, that have been shown to target cancer cells and stop the spread of cancer and cure a patient? You probably think the answer is "no." That would be the wrong answer. There are dozens of alternative cancer treatments that can stop the spread of cancer and even cure the cancer completely. In this excellent book, Ty Bollinger discusses the most proven of these treatments.

However, as you might suspect, the FDA has **never** approved one of these cancer treatments because the drug companies have never submitted one of them to the FDA. This is partly because Big Pharma cannot patent natural molecules (and thus make their obscene profits), and it is partly because the AMA doesn't want cancer to be cured. The AMA does not allow medical doctors to use effective cancer treatments. Since these treatments have not been submitted to the FDA by the pharmaceutical industry, the FDA labels them as "unproven," no matter how much scientific evidence there is for the treatment.

That is why accountants, housewives, farmers, engineers, etc. are leading the battle against the Cancer Industry. But these people have absolutely zero clout with the media. By the way, the FDA, National Cancer Institute (NCI), National Institutes of Health (NIH), ad nauseam, are **not** the angels in this equation. They too have sold their souls and know exactly what is going on.

Mother Nature's molecules, as a general rule, **ALWAYS** target cancer cells or do no harm to normal cells. Thus, Mother Nature's molecules can be used in much, much higher doses than Big Pharma's molecules. That is why Mother Nature has a true cure rate that is **thirty times higher** than orthodox medicine for recently diagnosed patients!!

Mother Nature (*i.e.*, God) knows a lot more about cancer than the pharmaceutical industry chemists. More importantly, Mother Nature has a lot more integrity than the executives of the pharmaceutical companies. Judgment Day will take care of them and their brothers in the tobacco industry, federal government, etc., forever, but that is probably not your immediate concern. Your immediate concern is that Mother Nature knows how to target cancer cells and stop the spreading of cancer.

So why haven't you been brainwashed into believing in alternative medicine? Why haven't you heard these things a thousand times on television or radio or in the major magazines?

Because if they told you these things, the pharmaceutical industry would pull all of their advertising money and give that advertising money to a competing station or magazine. Also, to a large degree the same people who make huge profits supplying and working with orthodox medicine also own the large television and radio networks. For example, General Electric, which makes huge profits from supplying hospitals with expensive equipment, and by selling prescription drugs, etc. owns the NBC network and at least 30 major NBC affiliates. General Electric is a member of the Cancer Industry and they own NBC!

What you know about cancer has been carefully designed and crafted by the pharmaceutical industry propaganda artists to keep you in the dark about the vast superiority of Mother Nature at treating cancer.

Unfortunately, some of the people who are on the natural side of the street (*i.e.*, the alternative medicine people) do not have any more integrity than the tobacco companies and pharmaceutical companies. The good news is that this book, Cancer – Step Outside the Box, will set the record straight. It will tell you about the alternative cancer treatments that really work and in many cases the vendors or clinics that will assist you in using the treatments. However, this book is just as important for people who don't have cancer as it is for people who do have cancer.

Consider these factual statistics:

> ➤ A true cure rate of 90% or more can easily be achieved by cancer patients who avoid orthodox medicine, go with alternative medicine first, and do their homework.
> ➤ The true cure rate of orthodox medicine is 3% or less.
> ➤ 95% of cancer patients who go with alternative cancer treatments have previously had the full orthodox treatment and have been sent home to die, meaning alternative medicine is handed a large number of cancer patients already in critical condition.
> ➤ For those who wait to go with alternative cancer treatments until after they have been sent home to die, only a handful of the 300+ alternative cancer treatments are strong enough to give them a chance of survival.
> ➤ But even for those rare people who do find one of those potent treatments (e.g. *those who read this book*), at best they only have a chance of survival of about 50%.

In other words, if you go with alternative medicine <u>first</u>, your chance of survival is 90% or more, if you do your homework.

If you go with orthodox medicine first, and then alternative medicine second, you will have years of suffering, and if you are lucky, you will then have a 50% chance of survival.

As you can see, books like <u>Cancer – Step Outside the Box</u> are critical to read. This book may save you months of research time and point you in the exact direction you need to go.

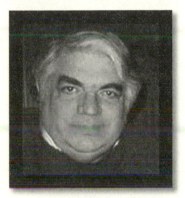

~ R. Webster Kehr
aka the "Cancer Tutor"
www.cancertutor.com
www.new-cancer-treatments.org

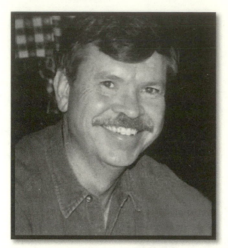
Graham Bollinger (*my dad*)

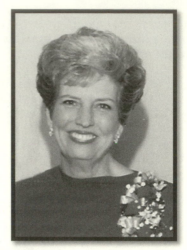
Jerry Bollinger Taylor (*my mom*)

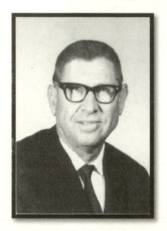
Conal Bollinger (*my granddad*)

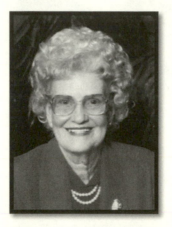
Helen Cade (*my grandmom*)

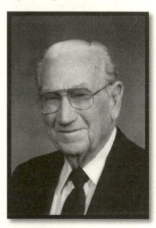
D.E. McCoy (*my granddad*)

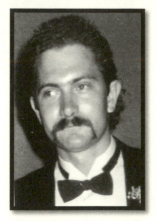
Glenn McCoy (*my cousin*)

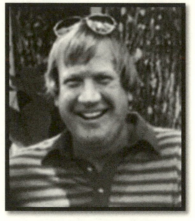
Joel Bollinger (*my uncle*)

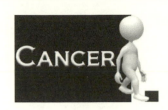
INTRODUCTION

My name is Ty Bollinger. One hundred years ago, it was estimated that only one out of eighty Americans was diagnosed with cancer. Today, approximately one in three Americans will be diagnosed with cancer during their lifetime. It is estimated that by the year 2020, one in two Americans will have the same diagnosis. Cancer fatalities account for approximately 12% of all deaths worldwide each year.

Across the globe, over ten million people are diagnosed with cancer annually and almost seven million die from cancer. According to the World Health Organization, global cancer rates could increase by 50% in the next fifteen years. The USA ranks in the top three countries with the highest cancer rate in both men and women. Sounds like a "cancer epidemic," doesn't it?

Most families have been touched by cancer. My family is no exception.

> ➤ In July 1996, my dad, Graham Bollinger, died of cancer.
> ➤ In November 1996, my granddad, Conal Bollinger, died of cancer.
> ➤ In May 1997, my cousin, Glenn McCoy, died of cancer.
> ➤ In July 1997, my uncle, Joel Bollinger, died of cancer.
> ➤ In February 1999, my grandmom, Helen Cade, died of cancer.
> ➤ In August 1999, my granddad, D.E. McCoy, died of cancer.
> ➤ In February 2004, my mom, Jerry Bollinger Taylor, died of cancer.

As you can easily see, my family has been devastated by cancer.

The first section of this book is in honor of my mom and dad, as I attempt to tell the stories of their last days, their separate battles with cancer, and the way that they both inspired and touched all of the people who visited them. During the weeks just before my Dad died in 1996, I began my "cancer journey." What I have learned on my journey has truly amazed me. Not only have I learned about the incredible effectiveness of many alternative cancer treatments and the remarkable recoveries of literally thousands of supposedly terminal cancer patients, but I have also learned about the medical industry's suppression of these treatments and persecution of the courageous and innovative medical mavericks that have stepped "outside the box" and developed these treatments. I have learned about the politics of cancer and the greed of the pharmaceutical companies. I have learned about the war between proponents of conventional and alternative cancer treatments. I am saddened that both Dad and Mom would probably be alive today if knowledge of these alternative cancer treatments had been made available to the public.

One interesting thing I have learned is that alternative cancer treatments involve much, much more than just taking a quick trip to the local health food store and buying a few bottles of vitamins and minerals. The science behind alternative cancer treatments is truly remarkable. The specific mechanisms by which certain protocols fight cancer are amazing. As a matter of fact, several alternative cancer treatments have been developed by Nobel Prize winners.

Currently, if you Google "cancer," you'll get over 250,000,000 hits. Saying that there's a *"lot of information out there"* is like saying that the ocean is *"a little bit wet."* This amount of information can easily overwhelm someone who is just beginning to research cancer. It is at this point that people can soon become lost in the cancer "jungle." At such a critical time in your life, just who do you trust?

Many websites sell all sorts of pills and potions. Some websites like quackwatch.com do nothing more than criticize alternative cancer treatments, while their willful and hypocritical inattention to accuracy is a disgrace. Other sites are overly technical and are virtually impossible to comprehend. How can you sort through it all? Who's right? Who's wrong? It's easy to become overloaded, and say *"Forget it – this is impossible – I won't even bother."*

When Sam Houston was battling Santa Anna in the 1830s and retreating daily, legend has it that he said, *"It's time to draw a line in the sand."* To which a cowhand serving under him said, *"Well Captain, you've got plenty of sand to choose from."* With so much readily accessible information on cancer and cancer treatments, choosing where to draw the line in the sand is harder than ever. It is my hope that Cancer – Step Outside the Box will be your "line in the sand" since it clearly and succinctly explains the facts and deceptions about cancer and cancer treatments.

Most people have neither the money nor the time to buy and read the numerous books that have been published on the medical, financial, and political aspects of cancer. I am optimistic that this book will serve as a concise, yet comprehensive, source of information on the intricate and reprehensible politics of cancer and help readers make informed decisions concerning nutrition, cancer prevention, and alternative cancer treatment protocols.

I am a CPA. When I was working toward my master's degree in taxation at Baylor University, one of the many valuable skills I developed was the ability to thoroughly research an extremely complex subject, come to a conclusion based upon the specific facts and circumstances, and then summarize my findings in a concise memorandum. "Deciphering" the Internal Revenue Code into layman's terms is no easy task, but I believe that this ability has enabled me to summarize and organize vast amounts of cancer research and to ultimately write this book.

In the accounting profession, we prepare financial statements for our clients. One type of financial statement is referred to as a "compilation," which is basically nothing more than compiling numbers provided by our clients. In other words, we take their information and present it in a format which is easily recognizable and understandable. In a very real sense, this book is nothing more than a compilation of information I have learned from reading dozens of books and visiting thousands of websites.

By no means is this book a scholarly work. I decided to write this book in layman's terms, with a minimum of medical jargon and without long lists of references. Now, don't get me wrong, I do cite numerous studies, I do have numerous scientific references, and I do quote numerous experts. But, I have tried to keep these references "sprinkled" throughout the book in situations where they are important and relevant. There is a glossary at the end of the book to assist you, as well as an index.

Honestly, there are dozens of outstanding books on the subjects of cancer, nutrition, and treatment protocols, but far too many of them are mired down in voluminous amounts of medical jargon and technical details, thus they are either too difficult to understand or just too boring to read. Many of these books leave you with more questions than answers. You begin reading confused; and when you finish reading, you're even more confused. Others write in a type of "cryptic gobbledygook" that can only be deciphered by other doctors, scientists, and academicians.

Unlike Emeril Lagasse, who likes to "kick it up a notch," my goal was to "bring it down a notch" and enable you to actually comprehend complex medical information as it regards to cancer, nutrition, and overall health. However, this book does contain much terminology which builds upon earlier definitions, so I strongly suggest that you read it from start to finish, without skipping sections. I hope and pray that you find this information useful in your pursuit to prevent, fight, and/or cure your cancer. May the Lord use it as a stepping stone for you to either reclaim or maintain your health.

If you are willing to be open-minded and step "outside the box," I think you will benefit from the book.

God Bless!

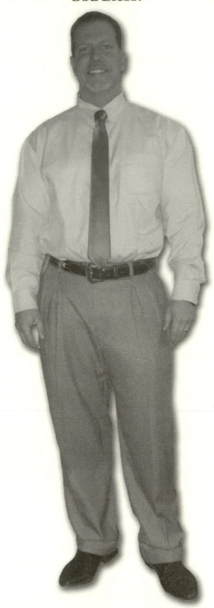

Ty M. Bollinger
Author
ty@cancertruth.net

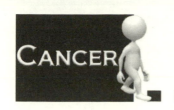

MOM & DAD

> MOM AND DAD WERE THE BEST PARENTS I COULD
> HAVE EVER ASKED FOR, AND THEY BOTH LOVED ME
> UNCONDITIONALLY. IN DIFFERENT WAYS, THEY
> WERE EACH MY HERO. NOW THAT THEY ARE BOTH
> GONE, THERE ARE TWO HOLES IN MY HEART WHICH
> WILL NEVER BE FILLED. BUT I WILL SEE THEM BOTH
> AGAIN IN HEAVEN. THAT IS MY HOPE.

CHARLES GRAHAM BOLLINGER

Around 5 PM on July 1, 1996, Charlene and I stopped by Subway and got a few sandwiches, then we headed over to my parents' house in Northwest San Antonio. My dad, Graham, had been having abdominal pains for a few weeks. He had gone to the doctor and they thought it may be a parasite in his stomach, perhaps cyclospora, which is promulgated through bad strawberries. Little did we know that this would be the last time we would all eat together. After dinner, Dad and I were upstairs talking about what may be the cause of his stomach pain when, out of the blue, he said *"I sure hope I don't have cancer."* I responded, *"Oh, don't worry Dad, I'm sure it's nothing major...you're only 52 years old."*

Later in the evening, we were all upstairs visiting. Charlene and I were getting ready to go to the gym and work out. All of a sudden, Dad doubled over in pain, grasping his abdomen. It was a pain which none of us had ever seen before. Dad was 6'2" and about 220 pounds, and he was tough. But the pain overwhelmed him, and we began to worry...really worry. Mom's face was filled with fear as she told her husband of almost thirty years that he needed to go to the hospital. He said that he would be alright and tried to go downstairs. I had to support him while he struggled down to the living room. Once downstairs, it was evident that Dad was not getting any better, and I told Dad that we needed to get to the hospital ASAP. Dad agreed.

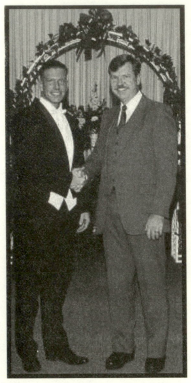

Physically, Dad was a picture of health, so we thought. He didn't drink alcohol, didn't smoke, and exercised regularly. Spiritually, he was a giant. He walked with Jesus the way few ever have, and his priorities were well defined: 1) God, 2) Wife, 3) Children & Parents, and 4) everything else.

Since Dad never engaged in behavior which would typically cause any serious medical condition, we were sure it must be a minor thing. Off to the hospital we went.

On the way, it was evident that Dad was in excruciating pain, but his only words were words of apology for the inconvenience he was causing the rest of the family. He said over and over what good nurses he had as Charlene stroked his hair and Mom cooled his forehead with a wet rag. His thoughts were, as always, focused on others rather than himself. Around 7 PM, we arrived at the hospital. Dad was admitted immediately, and the doctors began to run a series of tests to diagnose the problem.

I called my brother Ron and told him to come to the hospital. We decided not to call my sister, Cherith, who was in college at Hardin-Simmons University in Abilene, until more was known.

By 9 o'clock, the doctors had preliminarily assessed the problem to be gallstones, with the operation to remove them scheduled for the next morning. With everything seemingly alright, Charlene and I had to leave to clean a couple of small office buildings for our janitorial service. We planned on coming back to the hospital to check on everything when we finished...probably around midnight.

As we arrived back at the hospital just before midnight, much to our surprise, Mom told us that they had already taken Dad into surgery. Perhaps the gallstones were worse than originally anticipated. I called Cherith and told her that Dad was in surgery for gallstones, but not to worry. Everything was going to be fine.

One o'clock, two o'clock in the morning... still no word from the doctors. After three hours of surgery, it was apparent that the problem was a bit more serious than originally perceived. Three o'clock AM and we were really worried. Finally, about 3:30 AM, the surgeon met all of us in the waiting room - Ron, Charlene, Mom, and me. I'll never forget the look on his face when he came out of the operating room. It was one of both shock and hopelessness. Shaking his head in despair, the first words he said were *"It's just so advanced...and he's so young. It's cancer."* Mom almost collapsed and began to weep uncontrollably. We all began to weep. How could this be? It was just supposed to be a gallstone operation! Ron ran out of the room in tears. We all comforted each other with hugs and words of hope. I called Cherith again to tell her the bad news. It was 4 AM.

The doctors had to remove about a third of Dad's colon and a large part of his stomach as well. They had cut an eight inch incision running vertically down his stomach. The cancer had metastasized to his lymph nodes and pretty much all over his abdominal region. We went home to get a couple of hours of sleep and returned to the hospital around 11 AM Tuesday.

The doctors told us not to mention the cancer yet to Dad; so with all the cheer we could muster, we entered his hospital room. He looked tired and confused. He didn't know what had happened to him, remembering only coming to the hospital the night before. We all encouraged him that everything was going to be OK and that he just needed to get some rest.

One of Dad's nurses was a fine Christian man named Jeff Ronk. We attended church with Jeff, and he helped calm our fears and assured us that Dad was in good hands and that he would personally make sure that he received the highest degree of care. What a blessing for God to have placed Jeff in this situation.

Several members of our church began to arrive at the hospital. Dad and Mom had attended Believer's Fellowship since they moved to San Antonio about eight years prior, and the church members were like family to them. Around 1 PM, Charlene and I were leaving the hospital to get some sleep during the afternoon hours when we saw Jim Bryant, an elder in our church, drive up and park. As we began to inform him of Dad's condition, all I could say was *"Dad has cancer...it's real bad"* as we all began to cry and hug each other.

That afternoon, we tried to get some sleep, but it was difficult. Charlene and I didn't have any children at that time, and all I could think was that Dad wouldn't be around to see his future grandchildren. Charlene and I had only been married six months. All I could do was softly sob as I lay there.

When we arrived back at the hospital, we were amazed at the number of people who were there to see Dad. He was a man who loved to chat, was always friendly, and made others feel important because he would take the time to listen to them. He lived for Jesus and did his best to treat others the way Jesus would have treated them. The waiting room was full of people and food – fruit cakes and cookies, sodas and sandwiches, apples and bananas. Some looked despondent while others seemed joyous to be able to serve the family.

Dad still didn't know that he had cancer, and we didn't want to tell him. But I didn't feel right about Dad being in the dark, so I asked the doctor if I could tell Dad the truth. The doctor said that was a good idea. I had never been in a situation like that before, and I wasn't sure what to say to Dad, but I knew that the words would be there when I needed them. I knew that I needed to be strong for my family and my Dad, so I entered Dad's room and held his hand. *"Dad...do you know what has happened?"* I asked. Dad shook his head from side to side. *"They found cancer in your stomach last night and took it out."*

I expected Dad to look shocked, but he didn't look surprised. As a matter of fact, he looked like he suspected it and was relieved to know the truth. Being an intelligent man, he probably could tell that something must be fishy since half the church had been there to visit that day. *"It's going to be OK, Dad. They got all the cancer and you just need to rest and recover."* Although the doctors indicated that they definitely did not get all the cancer, I figured that this little fib wouldn't hurt anything and may help his spirit and mental state.

Dad stayed in recovery for the entire day as reality began to set in with the family. He had actually had a four hour surgery for stomach cancer! It was almost as if we were watching ourselves on TV, not at all reality, bewildered by the twisted turn of events in the past 24 hours. Imagine the transition from thinking that Dad had a mere parasite to the stark reality that he actually was being devoured by cancer. It was as if someone was playing a practical joke and things were going to be normal soon...**but this was no joke**.

Why had this happened? We just didn't understand. Dad was a healthy man of only 52 years. He exercised regularly, watched what he ate, and had no vices. He didn't smoke or drink, and had only taken a few aspirin in his entire life. This didn't seem fair. People like Dad weren't supposed to get cancer. Cancer was for people who were careless about what they put in their body...not someone like my dad.

The doctors discharged Dad from the hospital on Friday, July 12th. I had begun researching alternative cancer treatments and was very interested in taking Dad to the Bio-Medical Center (formerly the Hoxsey Clinic) in Tijuana, Mexico. I also had read about the healing properties in fresh carrot and beet juice, so I went to the whole foods store to get some organic vegetables.

While confined to his bed at home, Dad had written a letter to the church stating that he, like the apostle Paul, didn't know if he would live or die, but wanted to trust God and give Him the glory no matter what. Dad's exact words were, *"To live is Christ, and to die is gain."* We took it to church on Sunday and gave it to our pastor, Bruce Blakey. He read it to the congregation – many of them were in tears.

Tuesday afternoon was spent together at Dad and Mom's house. Dad and I had listened to a sermon as he rested. Charlene and Mom took some time to get Mom's nails and hair done. I was optimistic about the possibility of Dad traveling to Tijuana, Mexico to visit the Bio-Medical Center. Their alternative cancer treatments had achieved phenomenal results, and I was sure that they could help Dad. I made several calls and spoke to the doctors at the clinic. Tentative plans for the middle of August were set, and I was already thinking about the possibility of a full recovery for my Dad.

If Dad could just recover from the surgery, he could begin the herbal remedies that were available at the Bio-Medical Center. But that was a big *"IF."* As he lay napping, I began to realize just how much Dad meant to me. I began to cry softly as I realized that it was a very real possibility that he actually might not recover, but I held back the tears when I saw Mom and Charlene pull into the driveway.

They both looked radiant as they emerged from the car as they laughed and chatted. It was nice for me to see them smile, as the past two weeks had been filled with so much sadness. As Dad slept, we discussed the plans to take him to Mexico once he was physically able. We all agreed that if Dad were to recover from surgery soon, there was an excellent chance that the Bio-Medical Center would be able to cure the cancer naturally. It was our only hope...it was our fervent prayer...

Charlene and I left about 5 PM to take care of the janitorial business. We finished around 11 PM and upon arrival back at our apartment, I saw that there were twelve messages on the answering machine. I felt an immediate knot in my stomach as I realized that something bad must have happened to Dad. As we listened to the messages, our hearts began to race faster and faster. The first message was my brother Ron telling us that around 7 PM, Dad had begun to bleed out of his nose and rectum and Mom had called an ambulance. He was back in the emergency room. The stitches from the first surgery had not held, and he was bleeding internally.

The next morning, Wednesday, at around 8 AM, we were able to see Dad for the first time since he was re-admitted to the hospital. His face was swollen so badly from the blood transfusions that he was almost unrecognizable. I'll never forget Mom and Charlene as they emerged from his hospital room after seeing him. At first glance from someone who didn't know Dad, he looked very bad. Not a pretty sight, if you know what I mean. Even his voice didn't sound like him at all. As Charlene went in to visit with Mom by his side, she said she got to feed him ice chips.

Of course, Dad was pleasant and smiling with a thankful heart for the ice. Just then, Charlene in her heart knew she was beholding one of the most beautiful men in the world. Before she could even speak it, Mom said, *"He's beautiful, isn't he?"* Charlene emphatically said, *"Yes!"* with a big smile. They both saw Dad's inner beauty. As I went into his hospital room, the first thing he wanted to talk about was his life insurance policy. He said, *"Ty, take care of your mother,"* as I began to cry. I knew that Dad knew he didn't have much time left.

That Friday, I was in Dad's hospital room with John Gordon, an elder at our church. Over the past few days, he had an astonishing eighteen pints of blood transfused. They just couldn't stop the internal bleeding. He was on a morphine drip and was coming in and out of consciousness. When someone is under that much sedation, you really get a true picture of their heart, as they really have no control over what they say. And it was confirmed that Dad's heart belonged to the Lord.

I remember at one point that Dad woke up, looked up at me and said slowly as he had an oxygen mask over his face and being filled with morphine, *"I love you Ty."* Then, he looked across the room and saw John Gordon, and said *"Hello brother John."* As he wasn't able to have any water or even ice chips at this point, he said, *"I sure am thirsty. I sure could use a cold glass of water. But I sure am thankful I have the* ***'Rivers of Living Water'.****"* Then, he let go of our hands and said, *"Sleep."* And immediately, he was back asleep.

Later that evening, we spoke to the doctor who informed us that Dad's kidneys were shutting down and that we needed to make a decision as to whether or not to place him on life support. Based upon Dad's specific request, we told the doctor that we were not interested in that option. I remember staying up most of the night, faced with the stark reality that Dad was going to die soon.

The next day, Grandmom and Granddad came down from Dallas to see Dad one last time. Sunday morning, Charlene and I traveled with Ron and Uncle Tim to Ingram, Texas to purchase a grave site and a tombstone. We took Dad's car, and during the hour drive up to Ingram, we listened to one of his cassette tapes. I remember hearing one of his favorite songs and beginning to weep as I reminisced about Dad playing the song over and over.

That evening, Dad met with the entire family and spoke directly to each person, telling all of us that he loved us and that he had no regrets.

God's grace was shining through Dad, and he was a pillar of strength. After we met with Dad, the doctors said that his heart had sped up to around 180 beats per minute, and that it was only a matter of hours until he was gone.

On Monday afternoon, Dad went into a coma. He never recovered. On Thursday, July 25, 1996 at 7:10 AM, Charlene and Mom and I watched him take his last breath. Immediately after his last breath here on earth, Dad went to be with his Savior, Jesus Christ.

You can rest assured that in his final weeks and days, Dad reflected on his life and on the love that he had for each and every member of his family. And when his time came, the angels came to take him to that wonderful place where God dwells and where he will spend eternity. He is now with his Lord and Savior, Jesus Christ, learning and worshiping Him.

It has now been almost eighteen years since he died, but in "heaven time" it is as if he just arrived. In the words of that great hymn, Amazing Grace, **"When we've been there ten thousand years, bright shining as the sun, we've no less days to sing God's praise, than when we first begun."**

JERRY JEAN BOLLINGER TAYLOR

Dad's death devastated Mom. They had been married 30 years, and she was now alone for the first time in three decades. She cried constantly and seemed unhappy with life. Mom had always been the type person to light up the room when she entered, but without Dad, she must have felt empty and hopeless. Charlene and I spent countless hours with Mom, especially during the first year after Dad died, trying to console her and attempting to distract her from her deep sorrow.

In November of 2001, Mom got engaged to Jack Taylor. We never thought she would re-marry, but we underestimated God. Jack Taylor was the preacher who had married Mom and Dad some 30 years prior, and he had recently lost his wife to cancer. Mom and Jack fell in love and were to be married in May of 2002. We were thrilled for them both. In January of 2002, I flew from Pittsburgh to San Antonio to be with Mom during surgery. Two months prior, in October 2001, the doctors had discovered a small cancerous tumor in Mom's stomach, and she was to have it removed. This was a common surgery, and there was nothing to worry about. So we thought. . .

Thirty minutes into surgery, Dr. Caldarola came out of the surgery room in tears. You see, Mom taught 5th grade at Castle Hills First

Baptist School in San Antonio, and she had taught all of Dr. Caldarola's children. His wife was the school nurse. They all loved Mom. Dr. Caldarola said that her entire stomach was riddled with cancer, and the only options were to sew her up or to take out her entire stomach (a total gastrectomy). I asked him, *"If this were your mother, what would you do?"* He said that he would remove her stomach. I then said, *"Go for it."* That was our decision.

Jack Taylor is a phenomenal man. The next morning, after Mom had a total gastrectomy and with the doctors bleak about the possibility of her surviving more than a few months, Mom was adamant about not marrying Jack and putting him through this again, since he had recently lost his first wife, Barbara, to cancer. But Jack told her that he was still going to marry her and that he would take care of her. How many other men would have been that committed to their fiancé? Especially after they had just lost their wife to cancer? As I said, Jack Taylor is a phenomenal man of God!

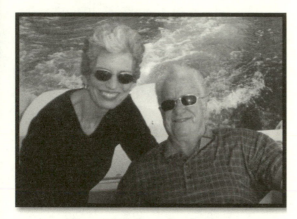

Mom and Jack – taken in 2003

Well, they **did** get married in May of 2002, just as Jack had promised Mom. Jack is an evangelist, and they traveled the world, spreading the Gospel of Jesus as well as their story of falling in love again. Mom had so much fun traveling the world with Jack. She would laugh proudly as she told us that she was the "Vice President" of Dimensions Ministries.

Her last few months were difficult as she was in constant pain, as the cancer ravaged her body, and she eventually had a massive stroke. But Jack Taylor, God bless his soul, stood by her side the entire time. **I cannot say enough good things about him.** Mom and Jack had nearly two wonderful years together before she went home to be with the Lord on February 15, 2004.

Here is mom's memorial tribute, written by my wife, Charlene:

Jerry Jean Bollinger Taylor, age 62, went to be with the Lord Jesus on February 15, 2004. She was born on July 5, 1941, in Artesia, New Mexico, to Helen and David Ernest McCoy. She now joins her first husband, Charles Graham Bollinger, her sweet mother, Helen Cade, and her father, D.E. McCoy, who are absent from the body and present with the Lord. Although we are all so thankful and happy that she is with our Savior Jesus, we will miss her greatly. She has been a lighthouse for all of us – the hands and feet of Jesus. She gave us wisdom and kindness, love and acceptance, pure goodness and beauty beyond mere words. She poured herself out every moment she lived in service to Jesus, her family, and many dear friends.

Her beautiful radiant smile would always light up the room wherever she was. All who knew her were blessed and encouraged by her. She wanted most of all to bring glory to God's name, no matter the cost to herself. The weaker she became physically, the more the Lord gave her His joy and strength. One the last Bible verses the Lord impressed on her heart was Nehemiah 8:10: *"The joy of the Lord is my strength."* His grace once again proved to be all sufficient. She died as she lived, praising our Savior Jesus.

Jerry Jean became a Christian at the tender age of seven. She attended Hardin-Simmons University where she was voted Princess on the Homecoming Court and President of the Cowgirls service organization her senior year. What a beauty! She was a youth leader at First Baptist Church of Dallas, where she met and married her sweetheart Charles Graham Bollinger. Together they raised a family and brought glory to the Lord in all that they did. She taught various ladies Bible studies through the years and helped people learn about salvation through Jesus Christ and the Christian faith. She also taught English, History, and Reading at various Christian schools.

From 1987 to 2001, she taught the 5th and 6th grades at Castle Hills First Baptist School. She lost her sweet first husband to cancer in July of 1996. It was a sad time for all. We never thought she could ever remarry. She was too happily married to Graham.

But we all underestimated our Lord...

On May 4, 2002, she married her "Resurrection Man" Jack Taylor and lived almost two glorious years together traveling the country getting to tell everyone about Jesus - their first love. She was not only proud to be Jack's wife, but also proud and beaming to stand beside him in his ministry for the Lord as Vice President of Dimensions Ministries. Her beloved husband, Jack, is the founder and President. On January 19, Jerry suffered a massive stroke while on a cruise on the South Pacific. She spent two weeks in the hospital at Papeete, Tahiti before being brought to San Antonio on February 5, 2004.

She is survived by her husband, Jack Taylor; children, Ty and Charlene Bollinger, Ron Bollinger, Cherith and Dru Moore, Tim Taylor and Michelle, Tammy Snell and Bill; grandchildren, Brianna and Bryce Bollinger, Baby Moore - due in July, Blake and Brice Taylor, Kimber

Snell, Tim Snell, Chris Snell and Clayton Snell; mother-in-law, Newell Bollinger; brothers, Tim McCoy and Susan, Ron McCoy and Cathy, John Cade and Patti; sister, Ernestine Clark and Lloyd; and numerous nieces, nephews, aunts, uncles, and cousins.

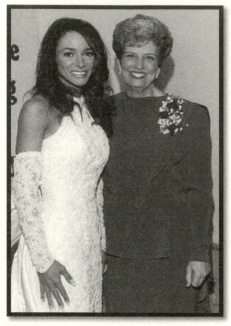

Charlene and Mom at our wedding in 1995

If she could speak to you today, she would say: *"Look to Me (Jesus), and be ye saved, all the ends of the earth"* (Isaiah 45:22). She would want to see you repent and believe and receive eternal life with the Father in heaven through Jesus our only Savior and God. *"You will seek Me and find Me when you search for Me with all of your heart."* (Jeremiah 29:19) *"Ask, and it will be given to you; seek, and you will find; knock, and it will be opened to you."* (Matthew 7:7)

She would say that Jesus will not be found anywhere but the Bible. Search the Scriptures, taste and see that the Lord is good! She wants to see you there with her in heaven. Are you ready?

Her hope is built on nothing less than Jesus' blood and righteousness. She'll dare not trust the sweetest frame, but wholly lean on Jesus name.

"Go therefore and make disciples of all the nations, baptizing them in the name of the Father and the Son and the Holy Spirit, teaching them to observe all that I commanded you; and lo, I am with you always, even to the end of the age." (Matthew 28:19-20)

PART 1

BIG MEDICINE

BIG PHARMA

BIG PROFITS

&

THE "BIG 3"

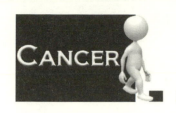

CHAPTER 1
THE CANCER INDUSTRY
& MEDICAL MAFIA

> "ANY DOCTOR IN THE UNITED STATES WHO CURES CANCER USING ALTERNATIVE METHODS WILL BE DESTROYED. YOU CANNOT NAME ME A DOCTOR DOING WELL WITH CANCER USING ALTERNATIVE THERAPIES THAT IS NOT UNDER ATTACK. AND I KNOW THESE PEOPLE; I'VE INTERVIEWED THEM."   -DR. GARY NULL

BRACE YOURSELF

What you are about to read will probably challenge everything you have heard since you were born. From the crib, we have been taught to blindly believe everything we read in the papers and on the internet, what we hear on the radio, and what we watch on TV. As a result, America is chock full of "*sheeple*" (*i.e.*, people who are meek like sheep, easily persuaded, intellectually dependent, and tend to follow the crowd).

In this book, I am going to ask you to step outside "the box" and actually think for yourself. I am going to ask you to get past the "no way" factor which is common to most Americans. Tanya Harter Pierce, author of <u>Outsmart Your Cancer</u>, calls this the "disbelief factor." When I first began to learn about successful alternative cancer treatments almost a decade ago and would share the knowledge with others, the common response was **"NO WAY!"**

You see, the "no way" factor is based on the misperception that if alternative cancer treatments really worked, then there is "no way" that oncologists everywhere would still be using conventional treatments. What most of us don't realize is that most oncologists also suffer from the "no way" factor since they believe that if alternative cancer treatments were effective, then there is simply "no way" that they would have graduated from medical school without hearing about them. Unfortunately, medical schools are largely funded by large pharmaceutical companies who have a vested interest in conventional treatments, since the main goal of all publicly traded companies (including pharmaceutical companies) is increasing shareholder profits.

The information in this book will likely shock you. At times, your natural reaction will be skepticism, doubt, and disbelief. I completely understand those reactions, as I have had them myself. We have all been brainwashed to react this way. A recent Johns Hopkins study found that television causes brain damage and an inability to exhibit critical thinking, so those of us that grew up glued to the television must overcome this brainwashing in order to free our minds. If you are able to step outside "the box" for a few hours while you read this book, I know you will be glad that you did. As a matter of fact, it may just save your life or the life of a loved one!

CONSPIRACY & THE CANCER INDUSTRY

As the saying goes, *"just because you're paranoid doesn't mean that they're not out to get you."* The truth is that conspiracy theories abound, and there are just as many websites on the internet to debunk them. Some of these conspiracy theories are nonsense, some of them are plausible, and some of them are quite likely the truth. Folks, from what I can see, the "cancer conspiracy" is alive and well.

But this is nothing new. In the introduction to his book The Healing of Cancer, Barry Lynes documents that this conspiracy has existed for over half a century: *"In 1953, a U.S. Senate Investigation reported that a conspiracy existed to suppress effective cancer treatments. The Senator in charge of the investigation conveniently died. The investigation was halted. It was neither the first nor the last of a number of strange deaths involving people in positions to do damage to those running the nation's cancer program."*

He continues, *"For many years, the American Medical Association (AMA) and the American Cancer Society (ACS) coordinated their 'hit' lists of innovative cancer researchers who were to be ostracized."* Mr. Lynes quotes one investigative reporter as referring to the AMA and the ACS as a *"network of vigilantes prepared to pounce on anyone who promotes a cancer therapy that runs against their substantial prejudices and profits."*

I used to believe that the "cancer conspiracy" was an unintentional result of the love of money and that there were really no malicious intentions at its roots. However, due to stories like the three that follow, I believe that I was a bit naïve in my initial assessment of the situation.

In 1931, Cornelius Rhoads, a pathologist from the Rockefeller Institute for Medical Research, purposely infected human test subjects in Puerto Rico with cancer cells, and thirteen of them **died**. Despite the fact that Rhoads gave a written testimony stating he believed all Puerto Ricans should be killed, he later established the U.S. Army Biological Warfare facilities in Maryland, Utah and Panama, and was named to the U.S. Atomic Energy Commission, where he began a series of radiation exposure experiments on American soldiers and civilian hospital patients.

Then, in 1963, Chester M. Southam (who injected Ohio State Prison inmates with live cancer cells in 1952) performed the same procedure on twenty-two senile, African-American female patients at the Brooklyn Jewish Chronic Disease Hospital in order to watch their immunological response. He told the patients that they were receiving "some cells," but conveniently left out the fact that they were **cancer cells**. Ironically, Southam eventually became president of the American Association for Cancer Research!

In 1981, the Seattle-based Genetic Systems Corporation began an ongoing medical experiment called "Protocol No. 126" in which cancer patients at the Fred Hutchinson Cancer Research Center in Seattle were given bone marrow transplants that contained eight experimental proteins made by Genetic Systems, rather than standard bone marrow transplants. As a result, 19 human "subjects" **died** from complications directly related to the experimental treatment.

Please note that the above are not merely isolated occurrences. There are hundreds more similar stories over the past century. You can learn more about the sordid history of human medical experimentation at the following website: http://www.naturalnews.com/019187.html.

Does this necessarily mean that **all** of the people who work in the medical field and the cancer research field are knowingly participating in human experimentation or are consciously part of a conspiracy to hold back a cure for cancer? **Of course not.** That notion is patently absurd. Most doctors, nurses, and health care professionals truly care about people and are doing what they honestly believe is best for their patients. As a matter of fact, almost everyone (including medical professionals) has been touched by cancer.

In his 1975 audio cassette "The Politics of Cancer," G. Edward Griffin explains *"let's face it, these people die from cancer like everybody else...it's obvious that these people are not consciously holding back a control [cure] for cancer. It does mean, however, that the [pharmaceutical-chemical] cartel's medical monopoly has created a climate of bias in our educational system, in which scientific truth often is sacrificed to vested interests...if the money is coming from drug companies, or indirectly from drug companies, the impetus is in the direction of drug research. That doesn't mean somebody blew the whistle and said 'hey, don't research nutrition!' It just means that nobody is financing nutrition research. So it is a bias where scientific truth often is obscured by vested interest."*

In this book, <u>Cancer-Step Outside the Box</u>, you will learn that the "emperors" parading themselves as medical "experts" concerning cancer treatment have no clothes!! I will demonstrate that for the past century, there has been a conspiracy to do the following:

➤ **Suppress** alternative cancer treatments and persecute those who advocate such treatments
➤ **Brainwash** the public to believe that chemotherapy, radiation, and surgery (the "Big 3") are the only viable options to treat cancer
➤ **Advertise** and **sell** the "Big 3," since the goal of the "Cancer Industry" is to make money.

First of all, let me define some basic terminology, nicknames, and slangs. "Big Medicine" is comprised of the National Cancer Institute (NCI), the American Cancer Society (ACS), and the American Medical Association (AMA). The multi-national pharmaceutical giants are herein referred to as "Big Pharma." The network of corporate polluters, Big Medicine, the FDA, Big Pharma, industry front groups, and political lobbying groups comprise the "Cancer Industry," whose goal is to maintain the status quo and keep the public **unaware** of alternative cancer treatments, thus insuring shareholder profits for Big Pharma. In my opinion, the deplorable tactics (of these corrupt bureaucrats and businessmen) bear a strong resem-blance to the thuggish behavior of the "Cosa Nostra," so I oftentimes use the term "Medical Mafia" as a generic (and, yes, pejorative) slang to refer to this group of criminal thugs.

THE INCEPTION OF THE "MEDICAL MAFIA"

In order to put things in perspective, let me tell you a little bit about the roots of the "Medical Mafia." Let's put on our history caps and go all the way back to the year 1910 and learn about John D. Rockefeller and the Flexner report. I'll bet you've never heard of this report, have you?

You see, Rockefeller's goal was to dominate the oil, chemical, and pharmaceutical markets, so his company (Standard Oil of New Jersey) purchased a controlling interest in a huge German drug/chemical company called I.G. Farben.

On a side note, I.G. Farben was the single largest donor to the election campaign of Adolph Hitler. One year before Hitler seized power, I.G. Farben donated 400,000 marks to Hitler, his Nazi party, and his private army (the "SS"). Accordingly, after Hitler's seizure of power, I.G. Farben was the single largest profiteer of the German conquest of the world during World War II. While millions of people were being imprisoned and murdered, I.G. Farben was profiting.

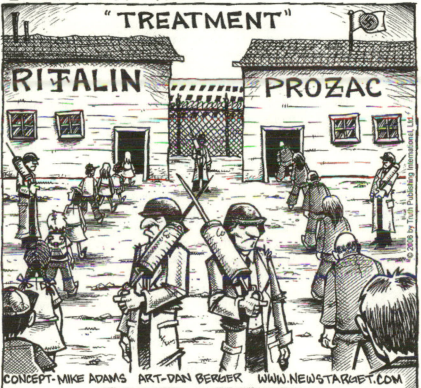

Thanks to Mike Adams and *www.NaturalNews.com* for the cartoon above.

I.G. Auschwitz, a 100% subsidiary of I.G. Farben, was the largest industrial complex of the world for manufacturing synthetic gasoline and rubber for the conquest of Europe. Auschwitz used the concentration camp prisoners as "slave labor" in their factory. But there was no "retirement plan" for the prisoners of Auschwitz. Those who were too frail or too ill to work were selected at the main gate of the Auschwitz factory and sent to the gas chambers. Even the chemical gas Zyklon-B used for the annihilation of millions of innocent people resulted from I.G. Farben's drawing boards and factories.

In 1941, Otto Armbrust (the I.G. Farben board member responsible for the Auschwitz project), stated to his colleagues, "*Our new friendship with the SS is a blessing. We have determined all measures integrating the concentration camps to benefit our company.*" The I.G. Farben cartel used the victims of the concentration camps as human guinea pigs. Tens of thousands of them died during human experiments such as the testing of new and unknown vaccinations. All in all, over 300,000 prisoners passed through the Auschwitz facility. Over 25,000 were worked to death, while countless others were murdered in the gas chambers or by human experimentation.

One would think that after the end of the war, due to their participation in the murder of millions of people at Auschwitz, I.G. Farben board members would have been "blackballed" by American pharmaceutical companies. Nothing could be further from the truth. Have you ever heard of Bayer Corporation? Of course you have. In 1956, Bayer appointed Fritz ter Meer, I.G. Farben board member and **convicted war criminal** from the Nuremberg trials, as Chairman of its board. (Joseph Borkin, The Crime and Punishment of I.G. Farben)

But I digress. Let's go back to 1910 and back to our history lesson on the Flexner report. In order to build his drug cartel, Rockefeller needed to "re-educate" the medical profession to prescribe more pharmaceutical drugs, so he hired Abraham Flexner to travel the country and assess the success of American medical schools. In reality, there was very little "assessing" going on by Flexner; the results of his study were predetermined.

Eventually, Flexner submitted a report to The Carnegie Foundation entitled "Medical Education in the United States and Canada," commonly referred to as the "Flexner report." Published in 1910, the Flexner report emphatically recommended the strengthening of courses in pharmacology and the addition of research departments at all "qualified" medical schools. In a nutshell, the gist of the report was that it was far too easy to start a medical school and that most medical schools were not teaching "sound medicine." In other words, they weren't pushing enough drugs.

With public backing secured by the publication of the Flexner report, Carnegie and Rockefeller commenced a major "upgrade" in medical education by financing only those medical schools that taught what they wanted to be taught. In other words, they began to immediately shower hundreds of millions of dollars on those medical schools that were teaching "drug intensive" medicine.

Predictably, those schools that had the financing churned out the better doctors. In return for the financing, the schools were required to continue teaching course material that was exclusively drug oriented, with no emphasis put on natural medicine. The end result of the Flexner report was that all accredited medical schools became heavily oriented toward drugs and drug research.

In 1913, the AMA went on the offensive even more strongly by their establishment of the "Propaganda Department," which was dedicated to attacking any and all unconventional medical treatments and anyone (M.D. or not) who practiced them. You see, the predetermined purpose of the Flexner Report was to label doctors who didn't prescribe drugs as "charlatans" and "quacks." Medical schools that offered courses in natural therapies and homeopathy were told to either drop these courses from their curriculum or lose their accreditation. Is it any wonder that the total number of accredited medical schools in the USA was cut in half between 1910 and 1944? The end result of the Flexner report was that all accredited medical schools became heavily oriented toward drugs and drug research.

The medical sociologist Paul Starr wrote in his Pulitzer Prize-winning book (The Social Transformation of American Medicine): "*The AMA Council became a national accrediting agency for medical schools, as an increasing number of states adopted its judgments of unacceptable institutions.*" Further, he noted: "*Even though no legislative body ever set up ... the AMA Council on Medical Education, their decisions came to have the force of law.*" So the AMA became the new doorkeeper and was empowered to determine which medical schools were properly following the standards of conventional medicine and which ones were not.

Contrary to popular notion, the AMA is not a governmental entity. It is a private organization which began in 1847, and it is basically the "physicians' union." The only difference between the AMA and the steelworkers' union is that the AMA members wear white collars, while the steelworkers wear blue collars. And much like many labor unions, at the apex of this organization are the "mafia bosses."

In the end, Rockefeller's plan was a smashing success, and conflicts of interest between Big Pharma and Big Medicine continue to this day. In his book, Cancer-Gate: How to Win The Losing Cancer War, Dr.

Samuel Epstein demonstrates that over the past century, the ACS, NCI, and AMA have all become corroded with major institutional and personal conflicts of interest with Big Pharma. As candidly admitted by a recent NCI director, the NCI has become a *"government pharmaceutical company."*

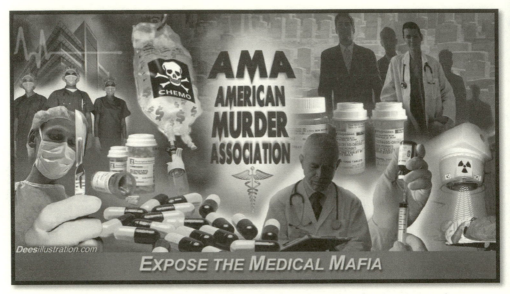

Thanks to David Dees and ***www.DeesIllustration.com*** for the picture above.

Dr. Epstein also chronicles how, for monetary reasons, the Cancer Industry is suppressing mountains of information about environmental causes of cancer rather than making this information available to the public. In his book <u>The Politics of Cancer Revisited</u>, Dr. Epstein states that *"the cancer establishment has also failed to provide the public, particularly African American and underprivileged ethnic groups, with their disproportionately higher cancer incidence rates, with information on avoidable carcinogenic exposures, thus depriving them of their right-to-know and effectively preventing them from taking action to protect themselves – a flagrant denial of environmental justice."*

It's a simple economic equation, folks. Keeping the public **ignorant** about the causes of cancer results in more cancer patients. More cancer patients results in more sales of chemotherapy drugs, more radiation, and more surgery.

You see, **money**, rather than moral ethics, is the deciding factor for the Cancer Industry and the Medical Mafia. To be honest, their goal is to provide temporary relief by treating the **symptoms** of cancer with drugs, while never addressing the **cause** of the cancer. This insures regular visits to the doctor's office and requires the patient to routinely return to the pharmacy to refill his prescriptions. This is what the game is all about folks, plain and simple. Big Pharma is nothing more than a conglomeration of companies that can best be described as glorified "**drug pushers**." Deny it or deal with it. Stick your head back in the sand if necessary. Think happy thoughts. Or keep reading and keep an open mind. It's your choice.

I have one request: Please don't disregard the facts contained in this book just because your doctor never mentioned them to you, or because some of them are hard to believe, or because the alternative cancer treatments have been labeled "quackery" or "nonsense" by the Cancer Industry, or because many of them are diametrically opposed to the propaganda you hear on the nightly news. Please try to step "outside the box" and open your mind to the possibility that you have been lied to and that there are much more effective cancer treatments than the "Big 3" (chemo, radiation, & surgery). The late Dr. Robert Atkins put it best: *"There is not one, but many cures for cancer available. But they are all being systematically suppressed by the ACS, the NCI and the major oncology centers. They have too much of an interest in the status quo."*

The survival of the Medical Mafia and Big Pharma is dependent upon the elimination (by any means) of effective natural health treatments. By making it more difficult to access natural health remedies, these "medical gangsters" are protecting their monopoly while simultaneously feeding their own megalomania. Truth be told, especially relating to cancer treatments, the Medical Mafia and their Big Pharma buddies are running a huge extortion scheme, and their tactics make Pol Pot look like a choir boy! Regardless if you are a doctor or a patient, if you cross the Medical Mafia, then you will likely be visited by one of their "leg-breakers" who will attempt to intimidate and coerce you into submission and obedience.

In the words of Dr. Henry Jones: *"Soon after the medical monopoly was formed, it began to push its agenda of destroying all competition. A well-organized and well-funded nationwide purge of all non-MD's was undertaken. Over the course of the first half of the 20ᵗʰ Century this medical monopoly managed to shut down over 40 medical schools. Their idea was to keep the number of doctors low in order to keep fees up. After WWII the medical monopoly started rigidly controlling how many of each medical specialty it would allow to be trained.The medical monopoly also managed to outlaw or margin-alize over 70 healthcare professions. 'Protection of the healthcare consumer' was, as always, the rationale for this power grab. Whether the object of destruction by the medical monopoly be homeopaths, midwives, chiropractors, or internet prescribers, the purge is conducted in the same manner. No scientific proof or research data is offered to discredit these practitioners. The entire approach is one of character assassination..."* www.thenhf.com/articles/articles_728/articles_728.htm

THE CANCER WAR

The "War on Cancer" was officially declared by the Federal Government in 1971, and enthusiastically signed into law by President Richard Nixon. Over the past almost four decades, it has in reality become a quagmire, a "medical Vietnam," an endless, calculated "no-win" war on cancer, since countless billions of dollars are being made each year by its perpetuation. Since 1971, over **$2 TRILLION** has been spent on conventional cancer research and treatments.

Nevertheless, despite (or perhaps because of) these unparalleled costs, the Cancer Industry remains largely closed to innovative ideas in the realm of alternative cancer treatments. According to Dr. John Bailer, who spent twenty years on the staff of the NCI and was editor of its journal, speaking at the Annual Meeting of the American Association for the Advancement of Science in May 1985, *"My overall assessment is that the national cancer program must be judged a qualified **failure**."*

As a matter of fact, the Cancer Industry (led by their "mafia dons") has waged another war – a war against those who advocate the use of alternative cancer treatments. At the root of this new war is the almighty **dollar.** Don't believe me? What are the top five alternative cancer treatments? Can you even name **one** alternative cancer treatment? The Medical Mafia and Big Pharma have the media in their pockets, thus the only cancer treatments known to most of us are the "Big 3." Unless you are an internet junkie, it is likely that you have not been exposed to much good information about alternative cancer treatments. The truth is that since conventional treatments **pay** the best, they are touted as the most effective treatments. It's all about the economics of cancer, not finding a cure. In his book <u>Gangsters in Medicine</u>, Thomas Smith accurately states, *"[The medical system] is not organized to heal and cure disease; it is a commercial venture organized to make money for its practitioners."*

Being a CPA, I tend to look at things from an "economic" perspective. And I must tell you that from an economic perspective, the Cancer Industry has the perfect business model. Big Pharma and the other chemical companies make **huge profits** from selling carcinogenic chemicals that are dumped (oftentimes intentionally) in our food, water, and air. Then, they make even **more profits** by manufacturing and selling expensive, ineffective, toxic drugs to treat the cancers and other diseases caused by their own products. Then, in baseball lingo, they complete the "triple play" by **selling additional drugs** to make the side-effects of the primary drugs more bearable. In business lingo, the Cancer Industry is sitting on a "cash cow." Unfortunately, this cash cow is a scam at the expense of cancer patients.

Adding insult to injury, they let John and Jane Taxpayer (*i.e.,* you and me) fund their research into more ways to **not cure** cancer while still pushing their drugs at obscene profits. To ensure that the public remains blissfully unaware of the true facts about cancer, they have set up front group cheerleaders (like the ACS) to spread disinformation in the name of cancer education, while the rest of the Medical Mafia is busy fighting a hostile turf war to make sure that alternative cancer treatments remain suppressed and the doctors that use these treatments are persecuted and run out of the county.

One of the ways that this turf war is fought is through advertising. Not only does Big Pharma make billions of dollars annually on the sale of drugs, but they also dump billions of dollars into the advertising of prescription drugs each year. And, since people in America typically make their key decisions based solely on what they see on TV and what they hear on the radio, is it any wonder that we are largely uninformed concerning alternative cancer treatments? The Medical Mafia has done everything in its power to make sure you **do not** know the truth about alternative cancer treatments. The TV stations and other media don't dare broadcast anything which may hurt one of their biggest advertisers – Big Pharma.

Back in 1996, had we been aware of the successful alternative cancer treatments available, my Dad may not have died. I am angered and disgusted that the Medical Mafia suppresses natural cancer treatments, persecutes doctors that utilize them, and makes it next to impossible to gain access to these treatments, thus causing the death of untold millions of cancer victims. This next true story will break your heart.

The Alexander Horwin Story (*in the words of his mother, Raphaele*): *"On August 10, 1998, at age two, our son Alexander Horwin was diagnosed with the most common pediatric brain tumor, medulloblastoma. After Alexander endured two brain surgeries my husband and I located the best non-toxic therapy that had proven successful in treating brain cancer. However, on September 21, 1998, **the FDA denied** Alexander access to this potentially life-saving treatment. The oncologists told us that without their "state-of-the-art" chemotherapy, the cancer would soon return. We knew nothing of the history, efficacy and actual danger of chemotherapy but instinctively knew it was a poor choice for therapy. However, now that the FDA had denied Alexander his best chance of survival using a non-toxic* *therapy that had saved other children, we had no other treatment options left. Reluctantly we started chemo on October 7, 1998. The protocol was entitled CCG 9921 which consisted of intravenous administration of four chemo drugs: vincristine, cisplatin, cyclophosphamide (also called cytoxan), and VP16 (also called etoposide). Alexander completed his third month of chemotherapy in December 1998 and died on January 31, 1999. He was just two and a half years old."* www.ouralexander.org

Yes, there is definitely a war between the Medical Mafia and advocates of alternative cancer treatments. If you believe that the Medical Mafia acts in the public's best interest, then perhaps you should read the book written by Dr. Harvey Wiley, the founder of the FDA (in 1906) and its first director. In The History of the Crime Against the Food Law, he describes the absolute corruption that occurred within just a few years of its founding. He quickly realized that its initial purpose had been subverted; he resigned and then wrote the book.

The same problems have persisted at the FDA for almost a century. The Medical Mafia has a history of corruption and conflict of interests with Big Pharma. According to former FDA commissioner, Dr. Herbert Ley, as quoted in the San Francisco Chronicle on January 1, 1970: *"the thing that bugs me is that the people think the FDA is protecting them. It isn't. What the FDA is doing and what the public thinks it is doing are as different as night and day."* In 1969, Dr. Ley testified before the Senate committee and described several cases of deliberate dishonesty in drug testing. One case involved a professor who had tested almost 100 drugs for 28 different drug companies. Dr. Ley testified, *"Patients who died, left the hospital, or dropped out of the study were replaced by other patients in the tests without notification in the records. Forty-one patients reported as participating in studies were dead or not in the hospital during the studies."* (U.S. Senate, *Competitive Problems in the Pharmaceutical Industry*, 1969)

In the early 1970s, an "internal affairs" type of FDA study revealed that one in five doctors who carry out field research of new drugs had "invented the data" they sent to the drug companies and pocketed the fees. **In other words, 20% of the doctors just made stuff up!** (*Science*, 1973, vol. 180, p. 1038) According to Dr. Judith Jones, former Director of the Division of Drug Experience at the FDA, if the data obtained by a clinician proves unsatisfactory towards the drug being investigated, it is standard operating procedure for the drug company to continue trials elsewhere until they get the satisfactory results and testimonials they desire. Unfavorable results are almost never published and clinicians are pressured into shutting up. (Arabella Melville & Colin Johnson, Cured to Death - The Effects of Prescription Drugs)

Doctors are the principal "drug researchers" for Big Pharma. Keep in mind that the incentive for clinicians to fabricate data (lie) is enormous. In exchange for "favorable research" results, these doctors are rewarded with research grants, gifts, and lavish perks. According to John Braithwaite in his book <u>Corporate Crime in the Pharmaceutical Industry</u>, Big Pharma pays up to $1,000 per subject, thus enabling many of these doctors to earn over $1 million a year from drug research alone. And don't be fooled – these doctors know very well that if they do not produce "favorable results" for Big Pharma, that their "gravy train" will soon come to a screeching halt. You see, lots of drugs **MUST** be sold. In order to achieve this, anything goes: lies, fraud, and kickbacks.

Folks, the deck is stacked in this cancer war; it's heavily stacked **against** successful alternative cancer treatments.

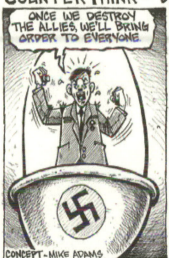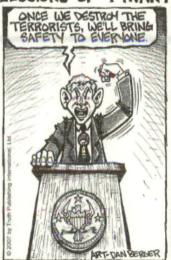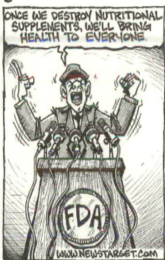

Thanks to Mike Adams and *www.NaturalNews.com* for the cartoon above.

To succeed in the cancer war, we must have people with the intestinal fortitude to speak out without fear of being labeled "politically incorrect" or a "conspiracy theorist" (which is nothing more than a derogatory name used to dismiss a critical thinker). Mike Adams (the "Health Ranger") is one such warrior. In his ever-so-candid style, he asserts: "*Western medicine has failed our people. Today, even while prescription drugs are more frequently consumed than ever before in the history of civilization, our nation has skyrocketing rates of obesity and chronic disease.*"

He continues: *"Western medicine simply does not work. It is an outmoded system of medicine dominated by the financial interests of pharmaceutical companies, power-hungry officials at the FDA, and old-school doctors whose myopic view of health prevents them from exploring the true causes of healing. Modern medical schools don't even teach healing or nutrition. **No practitioner of western medicine** has ever taught me a single thing about being healthy."* www.naturalnews.com/adamshealthstats.html

My friend Webster Kehr describes the cancer war in the following manner: *"When people hear the term 'war,' they think of guns, tanks, jet airplanes & soldiers. They think about mindless tyrants shaking their fists on television. But the war in medicine is very different. The tyrants in this war hide their real intentions. This is a 'war' where the weapons are information. Welcome to the 21st century, the century where America's most dangerous and deadly enemies are within."* www.cancertutor.com/WarBetween/War_Believe.html

No matter how many people shave their heads or run for the cure or cycle all over the place, as long as the Medical Mafia is in control, the "cancer war" will never be won. According to Dr. Linus Pauling, (*two-time Nobel Prize winner*), "M*ost cancer research is largely a fraud and the major cancer research organizations are derelict in their duties to the people who support them.*"

This cancer war is one of the most costly **frauds** (*in terms of money and human suffering*) that have ever been perpetrated on the American public. Staggering amounts of money have been spent in its pursuit, but the "cancer emperor" is naked.

According to C.S. Lewis in <u>The Screwtape Letters</u>: *"The greatest evil is not now done in those sordid 'dens of crime' that Dickens loved to paint. It is not done even in concentration camps and labour camps. In those we see its final result. But it is conceived and ordered (moved, seconded, carried and minuted) in clean, carpeted, warmed and well-lighted offices, by quiet men with white collars and cut fingernails, and smooth-shaven cheeks who do not need to raise their voices. Hence, naturally enough, my symbol for Hell is something like...the offices of a thoroughly nasty business concern."*

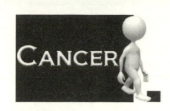

CHAPTER 2
LIES, PROPAGANDA, & GREED

> "EVERYONE SHOULD KNOW THAT MOST CANCER RESEARCH IS LARGELY A FRAUD AND THAT THE MAJOR CANCER RESEARCH ORGANIZATIONS ARE DERELICT IN THEIR DUTIES TO THE PEOPLE WHO SUPPORT THEM."   -DR. LINUS PAULING

SMOKE & MIRRORS

I used to fear being diagnosed with cancer, and just recently have I begun to understand why I was so fearful. I, along with 99% of Americans, had been snookered and brainwashed into believing the lies propagated by Big Pharma's propaganda machine which instills deceit upon our schools, books, professional journals, magazines, radio shows, TV shows, and of course, the vast majority of conventional doctors, nurses, and other health professionals.

Deliberate misrepresentation of facts has always been the standard operating procedure of the directors of mass media. They cannot afford objective journalism interpreting events as they actually occur. That would be too dangerous. You see, we are spoon fed our opinions since the day we were born. Daily events always are "spun" to favor a certain side's position. Those that disagree with the spin and actually think for themselves are frequently labeled "radicals" and "kooks." Reality becomes fiction and fiction becomes reality. This is all part of the "smoke and mirrors" that are so prominent in our "American Idol - Reality TV" generation.

According to American journalist Russel Wayne Baker, *"An educated person is one who has learned that information almost always turns out to be at best incomplete and very often false, misleading, fictitious, mendacious - just dead wrong."*

But this smoke and mirrors is nothing new. It began almost a century ago, when, due to his uncanny ability to reframe an issue, Edwin L. Bernays earned the nickname "the Father of Spin." From his 1928 chronicle <u>Propaganda</u>, we learn how Bernays took the ideas of his famous uncle (Sigmund Freud) and applied them to the emerging science of mass persuasion. The only difference was that rather than using these principles the way Freudian psychology does (to discover the unconscious mind), Bernays used his uncle's techniques for marketing purposes in order to create illusions, deceive, mask agendas, and brainwash the general public. In a telling quote, Bernays once described the general public as a *"herd that needed to be led."* Bernays never deviated from his fundamental axiom to *"control the masses without their knowing it."*

How did Bernays do it? His techniques were simple: create the illusion that there is some favorable research by using phrases like *"numerous studies have shown…"* or *"research has proven…"* or *"scientific investigators have found…"* but then never really cite anything. If anyone doubts or questions you, attack their character and/or their intellect. According to Adolph Hitler, *"If you tell a lie long enough, eventually it will be believed as truth…The greater the lie, the more likely that people will believe it."* These techniques are still being utilized today by most advertisers, including Big Pharma.

For instance, Big Pharma regularly develops newer and better prescription drugs, with their main goal being to increase shareholder profits, despite the fact that many of these drugs are toxic and deadly. The drugs are advertised over and over and over again, on TV, radio, magazines, medical journals, and in promotional literature. Despite the lack of scientific evidence to support the use of these drugs, we are conditioned to believe that they are the answer to our medical problems. If anyone dares to disagree, their character is attacked, and their intellect is challenged.

A recent study carried out by the Institute for Evidence-Based Medicine in Germany has found that 94% of the information contained in promotional literature sent to doctors by Big Pharma has absolutely **no** scientific basis. That's utterly amazing, if you really think about it. Mike Adams, the "Health Ranger," pulls no punches: *"Pharmaceutical companies engage in mass scientific fraud in order to distort their studies and get drugs approved based on rather shaky science, but what surprises me about this new research is the extent of it: 94% of the marketing claims are unsubstantiated and unsupported by scientific evidence. That's an alarming number - it means **19 of 20** statements made by drug companies in their marketing literature are* ***false****."* <u>www.naturalnews.com/001895.html</u>

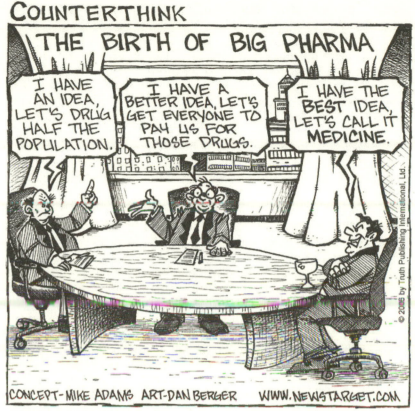

Thanks to Mike Adams and *www.NaturalNews.com* for the cartoon above.

As it relates to cancer treatments, brainwashing and deception is essential, since the goal of the Cancer Industry is to continually convince us that alternative cancer treatments do **not** work (despite evidence to the contrary), while simultaneously telling us that the "Big 3" cancer treatments **do** work (despite evidence to the contrary). The smoke and mirrors utilized to accomplish this monumental deception make David Copperfield look like a rank amateur! Most issues of conventional cancer "wisdom" are scientifically implanted in the public consciousness by a thousand sound bites and commercials each day. **This is called brainwashing**.

We are brainwashed into believing that prescription drugs are the answer for cancer (and all other ailments as well). Are you sick? Just watch TV for half an hour, write down the name of the latest prescription drug, and call your doctor. I'm sure that he'll be glad to prescribe it for you. You see, your doctor has likely been brainwashed, too. Big Pharma pays for over 90% of the advertising space in medical journals. I will cite some mind-boggling statistics relating to medical journals later in the book.

What is the last time you saw a commercial about proper nutrition as it relates to our health? What about all of those nutrition "geeks" telling you to eat raw, live, whole foods? Many conventional doctors will tell you not to listen to that nonsense, that there is no evidence to support the correlation between diet and degenerative diseases such as cancer. They will tell you that physicians who believe that cancer can be cured with a change in diet are just a bunch of medical "quacks." Please be aware that this is another characteristic of a successful propaganda campaign: dehumanize the opposition by **labeling** and **name calling**.

We are conditioned to believe almost anything, as long as the information comes from a "trusted source." In his article entitled "The Doors of Perception: Why Americans Will Believe Almost Anything," Dr. Tim O'Shea tells the story of how leaded gas was introduced to the USA: *"In 1922, General Motors discovered that adding lead to gasoline gave cars more horsepower. When there was some concern about safety, GM paid the Bureau of Mines to do some fake "testing" and publish spurious research that 'proved' that inhalation of lead was harmless. Enter Charles Kettering. Founder of the world famous Sloan-Kettering Memorial Institute for medical research, Charles Kettering also happened to be an executive with General Motors. By some strange coincidence, we soon have Sloan-Kettering issuing reports stating that lead occurs naturally in the body and that the body has a way of eliminating low level exposure. Through its association with The Industrial Hygiene Foundation and PR giant Hill & Knowlton, Sloane-Kettering opposed all anti-lead research for years. Without organized scientific opposition, for the next 60 years more and more gasoline became leaded, until by the 1970s, 90% or our gasoline was leaded. Finally it became too obvious to hide that lead was a major carcinogen, which they knew all along, and leaded gas was phased out in the late 1980s. But during those 60 years, it is estimated that some 30 million tons of lead were released in vapor form onto American streets and highways – 30 million tons. **That is PR, my friends**."* www.thedoctorwithin.com

THE CANCER PROPAGANDA MACHINE & BRAINWASHING

The Medical Mafia and Big Pharma have essentially obtained complete control over politicians and the media. You see, people can't be brainwashed without a massive propaganda campaign. And rest assured, the cancer propaganda machine (*i.e.,* TV, newspapers, professional journals, radio, etc) is alive and well. Media executives and publishers are careful not to publish anything which offends their biggest advertisers (Big Pharma) and to shape their content in such a manner as to please them. In less polite terms, this is called "media whoring."

A recent survey of network TV newscasts found that nearly 25% of all the commercials were for prescription drugs: Viagra, Claritin, Celebrex, Allegra, Levitra, Zoloft, Cialas, Nexium, and the list goes on and on. Big Pharma spends hundreds of millions of dollars each year on television and print ads for prescription drugs. This is how we are **brainwashed.** They are constantly bombarding us with the mantra that newer and better drugs are the only answer to the disease epidemic. Eventually, most of us just believe what we see on TV and what we are told by our doctor.

This is the key to propaganda: people must **not** be taught how to think for themselves. They must be conditioned to trust those in power and believe what they hear on TV and the radio. As a result, we have lost the ability to think logically for ourselves. We have become "dumb and dumber." Interestingly, when we watch TV, activity in the higher brain regions (such as the neo-cortex) is diminished, while activity in the lower brain regions (such as the limbic system) increases. This basically means that we become "zombies" when we watch TV and are open to manipulation.

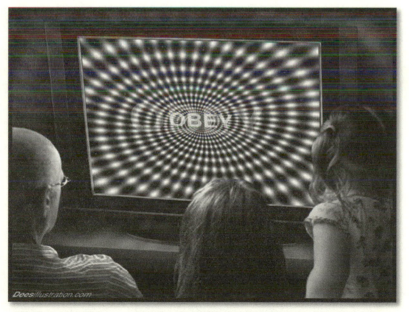

Thanks to David Dees and ***www.DeesIllustration.com*** for the picture above.

Have you ever noticed that we are continuously being warned **against** obtaining information on cancer prevention and treatments from the internet? Headlines read that alternative cancer websites pose a health risk! We regularly see quotes from physicians (many of whom have sold their souls) similar to this one: *"There is no good evidence that any alternative treatment can prevent cancer."* In order to make a statement like that, a physician must either be outright lying or utterly unaware of the last century of cancer research.

What is clear is that the Cancer Industry is conducting a pervasive propaganda campaign, based on fear and ignorance, in order to prevent people from learning about alternative treatments for cancer. Frankly, the Cancer Industry would rather people remain ignorant. They do **not** want people to be informed about anything other than the treatments that they promote and control. Ideally, what the Cancer Industry wants is a form of censorship. Ultimately, they want websites to be flagged to indicate which ones are "official" cancer websites. Of course, only the websites publishing content that agrees 100% with the corrupt Cancer Industry would be qualified to receive such an emblem.

So, in light of the above facts, always keep in mind that what you hear about conventional cancer treatments from your doctors, in medical journals, on TV, on the radio, and in magazines is a labyrinth of lies and frauds, aimed at convincing us that the cure to cancer is newer, better, chemotherapy drugs and funding more drug research. And always remember that even the editors of the medical journals have prostituted themselves to Big Pharma. As Albert Einstein once said, *"The ruling class has the schools and press under its thumb. This enables it to sway the emotions of the masses."*

In addition to censorship, another tool commonly used to brainwash and mislead is the element of disguise. You have seen those insects that are able to disguise themselves as twigs or leaves, when in reality they are nothing more than a chameleon. This is what the Cancer Industry does. They pretend to be acting in the cancer patient's best interest, while they are actually acting in their own best interest. Don't be deceived into believing that the Cancer Industry is comprised of altruistic folks who desperately want to find a cure for cancer. They are concerned with one thing and one thing only: **MONEY**.

Without a doubt, my favorite alternative cancer website is Webster Kehr's www.cancertutor.com. I quote him throughout this book, due largely to the fact that he grasps this issue and has more insight than anyone I have ever met. He is a brilliant man. Here is his opinion of the media and its relationship to Big Pharma: *"The media has many different techniques they routinely use to brainwash the general public. They can all be summarized in two words: 'whited sepulcher.'*

They lie, withhold information, deceive you, tell half-truths, and so on . . . The media are nothing but worthless whores. They sell-out to the highest bidder, which is always the corrupt pharmaceutical industry. Everything they say is aimed to please those that pay the most."

In his book, <u>The War Between Orthodox Medicine and Alternative Medicine</u>, Mr. Kehr uses an excellent example to illustrate brainwashing. He uses the theory of evolution, which is the only theory of origins which is taught in our public schools. In his book, the illustration is quite long, so I have summarized it here. To make it simple, let's assume that there are only 2 groups of people: 1) those who believe in evolution and 2) those who believe in Creation. The evolutionists represent the "Establishment" while the Creationists represent the "Renegades" who disagree with the "Establishment."

You have the choice of siding with the Establishment or the Renegades. In some cases this choice could affect your job. For example, if you are a Christian teaching biology in a public high school and you teach Creationism in your classroom, then you might lose your job. If you are looking for a promotion, then there is no question as to which theory you will teach. The evolution side of the fence has virtually all the benefits. But let's just suppose you are one of those rare people who are more interested in truth than benefits.

Suppose you want to know the truth about which theory is actually based on the evidence. You first interview the evolutionists, since you learned in school that evolution has been proven to be true. The person tells you about the Big Bang, he elaborates on microevolution, macroevolution, explains why there are no missing links, and so on. As you are walking away, the evolutionist stops you and begins to tell you why Creation is not a valid position and continues to tell you that Christians are nothing but idiots and buffoons.

After this conversation, you feel that you understand both sides of the origins issue. You decide it is not necessary to talk to a Creationist because you already think you understand their views and why their views are wrong. Now, if you made such a decision, then you would be making a common mistake: you would have heard both sides of the issue, but you would have only heard them from one person on one side of the fence. But you haven't heard the arguments of the Creationists, from a Creationist, nor have you heard why the Creationists think that the evolutionists are wrong.

Do you really know both sides of the issue? No you don't! Until you learn about the pro-Creationist views from a Creationist, and you hear the anti-evolution views from a Creationist, you don't have a basis for making an objective decision. Now, our entire lives, we have been taught that the Creationists are all a bunch of religious nuts, haven't we? We have been taught <u>not</u> to listen to the "renegades." We have been conditioned to believe that we already have all the answers and that there are no open issues up for debate. We have been taught <u>not</u> to listen to the people on both sides of the fence.

However, one day, just for the heck of it, you decide to talk to a Creationist. As he begins to speak, you are instantly amazed at the fact that he can talk, since the evolutionists had always told you that the Creationists had the IQ of a rodent and wore beenie caps with rotors. Not only can he speak, but he waxes eloquent about DNA, cell membranes, nucleotide chains, and protein chains. He states that the complexity of the Universe mandates a Creator since it is absurd that a 300,000 nucleotide chain can randomly form. And even if it did, the statistical probability that the first DNA had a permutation of nucleotides, such that 300 viable proteins could be created by this DNA genome, has a probability that is far less than $10^{-30,000}$.

He proves the necessity of a Creator due to the complexity of one nucleotide chain, which is a component of DNA. You quickly do some math in your head. You remember from science class that there are 10^{80} atoms in our universe. Then, you imagine there are $10^{29,920}$ universes just like ours in a cluster (that is a one followed by 29,920 zeros). All of these universes combined would have $10^{30,000}$ atoms. WOW! Finally, you come out of your daydreaming and realize that he was still talking while you were doing the math in your head.

Then he tells you about the ridiculous probability of the first cell membrane forming by accident. He articulates about how incredibly complex a eukaryotic cell is, so complex that even the exobiologists admit that one could not form by accident from a prebiotic pool. Then you learn that the first DNA and first cell membrane could <u>not</u> have formed in the same prebiotic pool, and thus you are told it was virtually impossible that they could ever get together. He talks about irreducible complexity, and then he begins to tell you about the problems with the evolutionist's views.

You learn about the mathematical absurdities which must be accepted in order to have faith in the theory of evolution. You then hear how "punctuated equilibrium" is really a super irreducibly complex protein system, and how absurd it is to claim that it was not necessary for irreducibly complex protein systems to have mutated all at once, but at the same time to believe in punctuated equilibrium. You hear why the phylogenetic tree is really a cover-up for the gaps in transitional species. You also learn about the massive assumptions evolutionists make with regards to carbon dating bones. You also hear the totally unproven assumptions and very shallow logic evolutionists make with respect to mitochondrial DNA and nuclear DNA. And so on...

Ten hours pass and you realize that the Creationist is still talking. You also realize it has been several hours since you had a clue what he was talking about. **This is not what you expected**. You expected some wild and crazy theories. But now you realize that Creationists are not stupid, they are not buffoons, and they really do have some very strong arguments. You also realize that the evolutionists had no idea what the Creationists actually believed. You finally go home, very confused.

According to Mr. Kehr, *"This simple story demonstrates the very sad state of affairs in America and throughout the world. Neither schools, nor corporations, nor governments want anyone to hear both sides of any issue from [the people on] both sides of the fence. They would rather have a brainwashed student than a thinking student. Schools act as if they have all of the answers and that it is not necessary to teach students to think for themselves. Students are graded on how well they regurgitate "facts," not on how well they think. Students learn very early on that all of the benefits are on one side of the fence and that they should spend their life gathering up the benefits."*

He continues, *"People are taught from birth to assume and expect that those in the "establishment" (such as the schools, the news broadcasters and newspapers): 1) Have no vested interests or conflicts of interest, 2) Have perfect intelligence, 3) Have all the facts for both sides of the fence, 4) Are totally neutral and unbiased, 5) Have perfect integrity, 6) Have your best interests in mind, and 7) Are truly open-minded. And above all, you are never, never allowed to think that money or power could possibly influence what the establishment teaches you. Dream on, this is the real world we are talking about."*

This story is a perfect example of the propaganda we constantly hear about alternative cancer treatments. Many cancer patients who were pronounced "terminal" by their conventional doctors went on to use alternative therapies, recovered fully, and are alive and well 10, 15, 20 or more years after their "terminal" diagnoses. However, the Cancer Industry **ignores** the existence of these cancer survivors or dismisses them as "anecdotal evidence." I recently did a radio interview, and one of the callers used that exact phrase. When I told him of four people that I know personally who have recovered from terminal cancer by using natural cancer treatments, he said *"I don't want to hear about your anecdotal evidence."* What a buffoon.

One trick from the Cancer Industry is to claim that people who got well through alternative therapies somehow magically recovered due to a delayed reaction from the "Big 3." How absurd! Another popular ploy is to claim that cancer patients who were cured through alternative therapies simply underwent "spontaneous remission." This is medical lingo for "unexplained recovery;" a fig leaf to cloak doctors' ignorance of what actually happened. The most comprehensive study ever undertaken on the spontaneous remission of advanced cancers turned up only 176 such cases in the world from 1900 to 1965.

Statistically speaking, it almost **never** happens. So, when you hear conventional doctors attributing the miraculous, sudden recovery of an alternative cancer patient to "spontaneous remission," have pity on them. They are merely hallucinating in a dream world matrix created by the Cancer Industry.

MONEY & GREED

In the Bible, 1 Timothy 6:10 says, *"The love of money is the root of all kinds of evil."* The economics of cancer treatment are astonishing! In the year 2010, over **$75 BILLION** was spent on cancer treatments in the USA alone! It's easy to see why the Medical Mafia goes to such lengths to destroy "quacks." Those who profit from toxic therapies like chemotherapy and radiation might be out of business and have to find another way to send their kids to Harvard or Yale if an effective, natural, non-toxic alternative were made available.

The marketing of expensive, toxic drugs lies at the heart of Big Pharma. The pharmaceutical companies not only make billions of dollars in profits from toxic chemotherapy drugs every year, but they also make millions of dollars in profits every year for developing drugs to treat the problems **caused** by the chemotherapy drugs! *"There is nothing else in the health-care field that can do what a good prescription drug can do--on the money side. It is a business to be envied by all."* - *New York Times*, July 28, 1989.

In his book, The Story of the Medical Conspiracy Against America, Eustace Mullins quotes Patrick McGrady, Sr., who was science editor of the ACS and its principal "spin doctor" in the media for over two decades. In 1978, McGrady made an interesting statement: *"Nobody in the science and medical departments (at the ACS) is capable of doing real science. They are wonderful pros who know how to raise money. They don't know how to prevent cancer or cure patients."*

Have you ever wondered why, despite the billions of dollars spent on cancer research over many decades, and the constant promise of a cure which is always *"just around the corner,"* cancer continues to increase?

Do you think that Big Pharma **really** wants somebody to come along with an inexpensive, natural, non-toxic, effective cancer cure? Or do you think that Big Pharma will do whatever it takes to retain their profits? Do you really think that the Cancer Industry is looking for a "magic bullet" to wipe out cancer?

A magic bullet would result in the termination of research programs, the obsolescence of skills, and an end to extravagant lifestyles of Big Pharma's executives. A magic bullet would kink the "money hose" of the Cancer Industry and render obsolete the "Big 3" treatments which are essential to maintain the flow of cash. Sadly, the fact of the matter is that many of those in the medical community have absolutely no interest in discovering a magic bullet to cure cancer, since it would cost Big Pharma billions of dollars.

It is interesting to note that written into the charter of the ACS is the clause that states that if a cure for cancer is ever found, on that day, the Society will **disband**. So think about it, is this an organization that is truly going to be motivated to find a cure for cancer? What do you think? To ask the ACS to find a cancer cure is to say, "*Now go and be successful. And then, once you have achieved your goal, promptly commit suicide.*"

The fact is that the eradication of cancer is by its very nature opposed to the interests of Big Pharma, as it would destroy their investment. In my opinion, Big Pharma's main goal is to **perpetuate disease**, not eradicate it. You see, they will do anything to keep the cash cow alive and well. Their survival is dependent on the elimination, by any means, of successful alternative cancer treatments. No profitable business will ever try to eliminate itself. Period. That is why a cure for cancer will **never** come from the Cancer Industry. It is a colossal act of political expediency and greed that has turned what should have been an easy-to-solve medical puzzle into the fraud that we now call the Cancer Industry.

Have you heard of Parkinson's Second Law? "*Expenditures rise to meet income.*" Every year, the cancer collection plates go out, to industry, foundations, and private individuals. The mantra - "*Give us your money, because we are making progress every day and we can't stop now. We are just too close!*" Revenues rise, so therefore, expenditures must be created to justify the revenues. This anathematizes the search for cancer cures that are natural and inexpensive. This is why the entire apparatus of the Cancer Industry is set up to **suppress** and **censor** any information that does not support their widespread need for expensive, man-made cancer treatments.

COUNTERTHINK

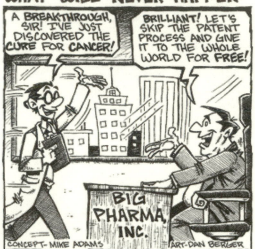
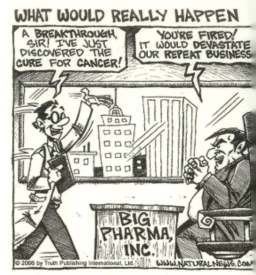

Thanks to Mike Adams and *www.NaturalNews.com* for the cartoon above.

In order to protect the profits of Big Pharma, any and all potentially successful alternative cancer therapy must be disbelieved, denied, discouraged, and disallowed at all costs. The Cancer Industry is prepared to do whatever it takes to suppress and censor **all** alternative cancer treatments. **This includes bribery.** One major reason that the healthcare system is in such a mess today is that Big Medicine has allowed itself to be bought off by Big Pharma.

In his book, <u>Dissent in Medicine - Nine Doctors Speak Out</u>, Dr. Alan Levin writes, "*Young physicians are offered research grants by drug companies. Medical schools are given large sums of money for clinical trials and basic pharmaceutical research. Drug companies regularly host lavish dinner and cocktail parties for groups of physicians. They provide funding for the establishment of hospital buildings, medical school buildings, and 'independent' research institutes...practicing physicians are intimidated into using treatment regimes which they know do not work. One glaring example is cancer chemotherapy.*"

According to Mike Adams, "*It's not an exaggeration to call this a **medical holocaust**. These drug companies seem determined to dose the entire population with as many simultaneous prescriptions as possible, as long as it generates profits for their shareholders. Business ethics are nowhere to be found in the pharmaceutical* industry these days: **it's all about money, profits, power and control**." www.naturalnews.com/001298.html

In her book, The Medical Mafia, Dr. Guylaine Lanctot states, "*The medical establishment works closely with the drug multinationals whose main objective is profits, and whose worst nightmare would be an epidemic of good health. Lots of drugs MUST be sold. In order to achieve this, anything goes: lies, fraud, and kickbacks. Doctors are the principal salespeople of the drug companies. They are rewarded with research grants, gifts, and lavish perks. The principal buyers are the public - from infants to the elderly - who MUST be thoroughly medicated and vaccinated...at any cost! Why do the authorities forbid alternative medicine? Because they are serving the industry, and the industry cannot make money with herbs, vitamins, and homeopathy. They cannot patent natural remedies. That is why they push synthetics. They control medicine, and that is why they are able to tell medical schools what they can and cannot teach.*"

In July 2004, Dr. Marcia Angell wrote an article entitled "The Truth About The Drug Companies." For over twenty years, Dr. Angell was editor of the *New England Journal of Medicine*, one of the most esteemed medical journals in the world. She asserts: "*Over the past two decades the pharmaceutical industry has moved very far from its original high purpose of discovering and producing useful new drugs. Now primarily a marketing machine to sell drugs of dubious benefit, this industry uses its wealth and power to co-opt every institution that might stand in its way, including the U.S. Congress, the FDA, academic medical centers, and the medical profession itself. People need to know that there are some checks and balances on this industry, so that its quest for profits doesn't push every other consideration aside. But there aren't such checks and balances ... The most startling fact about 2002 is that the combined profits for the ten drug companies in the Fortune 500 ($35.9 billion) were more than the profits for all the other 490 businesses put together ($33.7 billion).*" www.nybooks.com/articles/17244

What is the heart of conventional medicine? According to Webster Kehr: "*Find a natural substance that cures something, bury this fact, then fabricate, synthesize, and mutate the key natural substance, then patent the mutation, and make huge profits.*" In his book, World Without Cancer-The Story of Vitamin B17, Edward Griffin writes, "*With billions of dollars spent each year in research, with additional billions taken in from the cancer-related sale of drugs, and with vote-hungry politicians promising ever-increasing government programs, we find that, today, there are more people making a living from cancer than dying from it. If the riddle were to be solved by a simple vitamin, this gigantic commercial and political industry could be wiped out overnight. The result is that the science of cancer therapy is not nearly as complicated as the politics of cancer therapy."*

The Cancer Industry survives and thrives by perpetually searching for "the cure" but never finding it. This multi-billion dollar juggernaut is simply not interested in finding a cure, unless that cure consists of patented drugs that can be sold at a premium and need to be taken for the rest of the patient's life, thus creating a perpetual "revenue stream." So, in all actuality, the Cancer Industry is perpetuating lies and fraud. This fraud is of unspeakable magnitude, it has spanned more than a century, and it has unnecessarily caused the premature deaths of tens of millions of people, including both of my parents.

Dr. Matthias Rath hits the nail on the head when he states, *"the pharmaceutical industry is an investment industry driven by the profits of its shareholders. Improving human health is not the driving force of this industry...never before in the history of mankind was a greater crime committed than the genocide organized by the pharmaceutical drug cartel in the interest of the multi-billion dollar investment business with disease."* www4.dr-rath-foundation.org

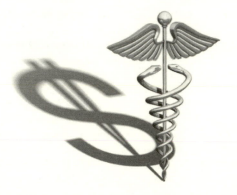

DOCTORS, MEDICAL JOURNALS, CONFLICTS OF INTEREST & FRAUD

Before Mom died, she was cared for by some of the finest doctors in America. Dr. Tim Shepherd is one of the finest doctors I know. He and his wife, Virginia Shepherd, are two of the most wonderful Christians I've ever met. They opened their own home to my mother and cared for her as if she were their own parent. Their eleven children "adopted" Mom as their very own grandmom and each one of them held a special place in mom's heart. I am eternally grateful to the entire Shepherd family; they will always hold a special place in my heart.

If I had a medical crisis, I would trust most doctors to give me the finest care possible. If I were involved in a car accident and needed a limb to be reconnected, I would definitely head for a hospital. My good friend, Dr. Irvin Sahni, MD, is one of the finest orthopedic spine surgeons in the world. The procedures he has developed are nothing less than extraordinary. Many medical conditions which would have been a death sentence 50 years ago are now easily cured with amazing advancements in medical technology. A few years ago, I saw a medical TV special where doctors cured a small girl of Turret's Syndrome through placing an electrode in her brain. It was truly amazing. I saw another special where surgeons reconstructed the face of a lady whose facial skin had been eaten by parasites. I was astounded! These are just a couple examples of the enormous advancements in medical technology and procedures over the past half century.

However, while incredible advancements have been made in many areas of medicine, the view of most doctors concerning the **treatment of cancer** has been obscured by the disinformation of the cancer propaganda machine. The bottom line is that most doctors do exactly what the Medical Mafia tells them to do and have not learned to think for themselves. Most doctors are still thinking "inside the box" when it comes to cancer. The problem is that the cancer "box" is largely the creation of Big Pharma attempting to peddle their poisons (such as chemotherapy) in an effort to increase profits for their shareholders at the expense of the cancer patient.

The Cancer Industry is built on the foundation of treating the **symptoms** of cancer, while doing virtually nothing to treat the actual **cause** of cancer or **prevent** it. It reminds me of an old Chinese proverb: *"The superior doctor prevents sickness; the mediocre doctor attends to impending sickness; the inferior doctor treats actual sickness."* However, the problem is not the doctors...it is **the system.**

I want to make it clear that I firmly believe that most doctors are altruistic champions for their patients and sincerely want what is best for them. Make no mistake, I wholeheartedly believe that most physicians make decisions based upon what they **think** is best for the patient. "**Think**" being the key word. Unfortunately, most oncologists (cancer doctors) do not even consider cancer treatments that they were not taught in medical school. As I mentioned, doctors also suffer from the "no way" factor. They believe that if alternative treatments really worked, there is no way that they would have graduated from medical school without learning these protocols.

In other words, most doctors have a tendency to believe that not only what they were taught **must** be true, but they also believe that what they were **not** taught **must not** be important! So you can rest assured that your doctor has likely been brainwashed into believing that the only viable treatments for cancer are chemo, surgery, and radiation. "Poison, slash, and burn" ... the "Big 3." It is also likely that your doctor knows next to nothing about nutrition or alternative cancer treatments and fully believes that alternative practitioners are nothing but "quacks." Go ahead, ask your doctor about amino acid therapy, or enzyme therapy, or ozone therapy. Be prepared to be chastised and/or ridiculed for your "naïveté."

Where does your doctor get his continuing education? From those "prestigious" medical journals; you know, the ones so prominently displayed on the cabinets. *"It would be nice to think of medical journals as these bastions of truth and light that have no bias, but in fact, they're businesses, and they make their money, in many cases, from drug company advertisement, and also from sales of the glossy reprints of the drug favorable articles to industry. And interestingly, several former editors and chiefs of major medical journals, Richard Smith of the BMJ (British Medical Journal), Richard Horton of the Lancet, and also a couple of former editors-in-chief of the New England Journal of Medicine have written books and opined heavily on the favorable impact of drug company influence on medical publishing. There are strong conflicts by the journal to publish drug company favorable articles in order to reap those hundred thousand dollars or so in reprint sales for the favorable articles, and also to keep the drug companies happy so that they continue to get drug company advertising."*- Dr. Beatrice Golomb (in an interview with Dr. Joseph Mercola 6/12/2010)

Medical journals are in all probability your doctor's **only** sources to keep abreast of the new developments in the medical field. These journals pretend to be so objective and scientific and incorruptible, but the reality is that they don't want to alienate their advertisers – Big Pharma. Those full-page drug ads in the top medical journals cost millions of dollars! In 2004, Dr. Richard Horton, editor of *the Lancet*, wrote, *"Journals have devolved into information-laundering operations for the pharmaceutical industry."* I agree 100% with Dr. Golumb. Think about it. The editors of these medical journals may lack character, but they aren't stupid. **They know who "butters their bread**." According to Dr. Golomb's data, Big Pharma now spends $18.5 billion per year promoting their drugs to physicians. That amounts to $30,000 per year for every physician in the USA!

But one might say, *"Aren't the medical journals peer-reviewed?"* The fact is that fraud and deception in peer-reviewed medical journals is common-place. For example, in 1987, the *New England Journal of Medicine* (*NEJM*) ran an article that followed the research of Dr. R. Slutsky over a seven year period. During that time, Slutsky had published 137 articles in several peer-reviewed medical journals. The *NEJM* uncovered evidence that in 60 of these 137 articles (that's 44%), there was either "misrepresentation of fact" or "outright fraud." http://content.nejm.org/cgi/content/abstract/317/22/1383

Then you have the "domino effect" which takes place when scientific fraud in peer-reviewed journals is quoted by other researchers, who are re-quoted, and so on, and so on. A prime example of this was uncovered in 2010 with a story that has been called the *"largest research fraud in medical history."* Dr. Scott Reuben, a former member of Pfizer's speakers' bureau, agreed to plead guilty to **faking** dozens of research studies that were published in medical journals. Reuben accepted a $75,000 grant from Pfizer to study Celebrex in 2005 and published his "research" in a medical journal. Then, the domino effect began to occur when hundreds of doctors and researchers began to quote his research as "proof" that Celebrex helped reduce pain during post-surgical recovery. There's only one problem with all this: **No patients were ever enrolled in the study!** That's right ... he faked the **entire study** and got it published anyway.

According to the *Wall Street Journal*, Reuben also faked study data on Vioxx, a drug which the FDA admits has caused over 50,000 deaths! All in all, Reuben totally falsified 10 "scientific" papers and 21 articles published in medical journals. It turns out that Reuben had been faking research data for over 13 years.

But Reuben is just the tipe of the iceberg. Have you heard of Dr. Hwang Woo-suk? This once celebrated (but now disgraced) Korean scientist saw his shining reputation quickly dulled when a peer review panel discovered that his published research claims on stem cell cloning, thought to be groundbreaking, were, in reality, fraudulent.

In Norway, Jon Sudbo, a researcher at Norway's Comprehensive Cancer Center, reportedly admitted to fabricating research results to show that common OTC painkillers (like ibuprofen) lowered the risk of oral cancer. As it turns out, Sudbo's study, published in the prestigious British medical journal *The Lancet*, was completely fictitious. Apparently, Sudbo just "made up" patients for his supposed review of 454 people with oral cancer.

Another recent incidence of medical fraud, this one in the United States, involved Eric T. Poehlman, a top obesity researcher who apparently fabricated data in medical journals and on federal grant applications while working at the University of Vermont. According to the *Boston Globe*, Poehlman altered and "invented" research results between 1992 and 2002, during which period he published more than 200 articles.

Ten years ago I would have been shocked by this story, but not now. From thousands of hours of research, I have learned that this is standard operating procedure for the Medical Mafia. Research fraud has been occurring for decades. One popular example from the past is that of Sloan-Kettering Cancer Institute researcher Dr. William Summerlin, who, in 1974, colored patches of fur on white mice with a black marker in an attempt to prove that his new skin graft treatment was working.

Did you know that there is a formal requirement for all medical journals that any financial ties between an author and a product manufacturer be disclosed in the article? That's right. However, we live in the real world, where this almost never happens. For example, in 1998, Dr. Henry T. Stelfox revealed that 23 of 24 authors (that's 96%) defending the safety of calcium channel antagonists had financial ties with the Big Pharma companies that manufactured those exact same drugs! www.pubmedcentral.nih.gov/articlerender.fcgi?artid=35347

An eye-opening article in the May 2, 2006, issue of *PLoS Medicine* (relating to drug advertising in medical journals) concluded: *"The scholarly nature of journals confers credibility on both articles and advertisements within their pages. By exclusively featuring advertisements for drugs and devices, medical journals implicitly endorse corporate promotion of the most profitable products. Advertisements and other financial arrangements with pharmaceutical companies compromise the objectivity of journals. The primary obligation of industry is to make money for its stockholders. The primary obligation of journals should be to physicians and their patients, who depend on the accuracy of information within these publications. Medical journals should not accept advertisements from pharmaceutical companies, medical device companies, or other industries 'relevant to medicine.'"* www.plosmedicine.org/article/info:doi/10.1371/journal.pmed.0030130

A stunning report published in the June 2010 *British Medical Journal (BMJ)* revealed that top scientists who persuaded the World Health Organization (WHO) to declare H_1N_1 (aka "swine flu") a global pandemic held close financial ties to the Big Pharma companies that profited from the sale of those vaccines. This report, authored by Deborah Cohen (*BMJ* editor) and Philip Carter (journalist with London's *Bureau of Investigative Journalism*), exposed the hidden ties that drove WHO to declare a pandemic, resulting in billions of dollars in profits for the Big Pharma vaccine manufacturers.

While all the H_1N_1 "hype" was happening, the WHO refused to disclose any conflicts of interests between its top advisors and the Big Pharma companies who would make billions based on its decisions. In other words, all the kickbacks were "swept under the table." Unbelievably, in response to the *BMJ* report, WHO secretary-general (Dr. Margaret Chan) had the audacity to defend the secrecy, saying that WHO intentionally kept the financial ties a secret in order to *"...protect the integrity and independence of the members while doing this critical work... [and] also to ensure **transparency**."* So let me get this straight – they are "keeping secrets" to "ensure transparency?" Isn't that a contradiction in terms? I believe George Orwell would have called that "double speak."

Do you remember the study I mentioned earlier which concluded that the promotional literature sent to doctors from pharmaceutical companies has absolutely **no basis** in scientific fact? The study showed that virtually all of the data in Big Pharma's promotional brochures is either imprecise or has been overstated. In other words, they all contain **lies**. Now here's the scary thing: most doctors rely on the information in these brochures when making a decision about what drugs to prescribe to patients. They have blind, unsubstantiated faith that Big Pharma is engaged in rigorous scientific studies and clinical trials, they read the brochures, believe the lies, and then prescribe the drugs to their patients. The *Journal of the American Medical Association* reported in February 2002 that 87% of the physicians involved in the establishment of national guidelines on disease have financial ties to Big Pharma. Talk about conflicts of interests!

In the July 26, 2000, issue of the *JAMA,* Dr. Barbara Starfield documented that over 225,000 deaths each year are due to medical errors, which is considered to be an "iatrogenic" cause of death. What does *"iatrogenic"* mean? The term "iatrogenic" means *"caused by medical treatment."* The first part of the word, *"iatro,"* comes from the Greek word *"iatros"* for medical or medicinal, while *"genic"* comes from *"genesis,"* which means origin. A study by Harvard University professor Lucian Leape found that one million patients are injured by errors during hospital treatment annually, with some **120,000 deaths**. One out of every 200 patients in hospitals in New York State had an iatrogenic death. Remember that less than 10% of medical mistakes are reported to hospital authorities. http://www.progress.org/fold107.htm

The Nutrition Institute of America funded an independent review of "government-approved" medicine that was published in 2006. Professors Gary Null and Dorothy Smith, along with doctors Carolyn Dean, Martin Feldman and Debora Rasio titled the report "Death by Medicine." In this report, the researchers found that America's leading cause of death isn't heart disease or cancer – **it's conventional medicine.** They found that the iatrogenic death rate in the USA (death caused by doctors and/or medical treatments) is **783,936** a year! In comparison, there are only 31,940 deaths by firearms each year, 19,766 of which are suicides.

Deaths Per Year	Cause
106,000	Non-error, negative effects of drugs
88,000	Hospital infections
98,000	Medical error
115,000	Bedsores
37,136	Unnecessary procedures
108,800	Malnutrition
199,000	Outpatients
32,000	Surgery-Related
783,936	**Total deaths per year from iatrogenic causes**

So what's behind these "iatrogenic" deaths from adverse events?

Profit and politics – plain and simple.

In the words of Robert Scott Bell, modern medicine has become nothing more than the *"Church of Biological Mysticism."* I couldn't agree more. And the deadly nature of this pseudoscientific "church" is made crystal clear whenever there is a doctor's strike. In 1976 in Bogota, Columbia, there was a 52 day period in which doctors disappeared altogether except for emergency care. The death rate went down 35%. There was another doctor's strike during 1976 in Los Angeles. The death rate dropped 18%. During 1973, there was a doctor's strike in Israel. According to statistics from the *Jerusalem Burial Society*, the death rate dropped 50%.

A 2008 review published in the prestigious journal, *Social Science & Medicine,* analyzed five separate incidents in which doctor strikes led to decreased mortality. Awkwardly, they also attempted to blame the lack of elective surgeries, but in the end, they were forced to admit that *"the literature suggests that reductions in mortality may result from these strikes."*

In the 1966 *Annals of Internal Medicine*, Doctors Beaty and Petersdorf wrote: *"Iatrogenic problems are cumulative, and in an effort to extricate himself from complications of diagnosis and therapy, the physician may compound the problem by having to employ manoeuvres that are in themselves risky."* **Translation:** Doctors oftentimes perform risky procedures or prescribe toxic drugs to cover their tracks from problems caused by previously prescribed toxic drugs and risky procedures. Are you getting the picture? Doctors are dangerous! It looks like the best way to reduce deaths may be to fire the doctors.

Again, let me repeat, I am **not** saying that individual doctors are the problem. Most doctors that I know are charitable people who really want to help their patients. The problem is the **system**. Most medical students have no reason to question the information which they are being taught and are ridiculed if they do ask uncomfortable questions. Young doctors who wish to succeed know that they must remain unquestioningly faithful to the "established truths." A doctor who rocks the boat will soon find himself floundering in deep water and likely struggling to survive! To be successful, a doctor must respect the errors of his elders, hold fast to the dogma of his teachers, and close his mind to theories which are "outside the box."

Ironically, medicine is a field which demands conformity, and there is little tolerance for opinions opposing the status quo. Doctors cannot warn you about what they themselves do not know, and with little time for further education once they begin "practicing" medicine, they are, in a sense, held captive by a system which discourages them from acquiring information independently and forming their own opinions. To put it bluntly, most doctors are brainwashed into thinking "inside the box" and peer pressure keeps them there.

Unlike many other countries, the USA supports only one kind of medicine: **conventional**. Because of this, many Americans, including both of my parents, have been denied many vital health choices. According to Dr. Alan Levin, MD: *"Your family doctor is no longer free to choose the treatment he or she feels is best for you, but must follow the dictates established by physicians whose motives and alliances are such that their decisions may not be in your best interests."*

Those few doctors that dare to question the status quo are frequently ostracized and blackballed. You should know that a physician risks jail time and having his medical license revoked for recommending or using alternative cancer treatments, despite the fact that there is overwhelming scientific evidence to support their efficacy. Doctors who dare to offer patients new hope and new treatments are scorned, abused, persecuted, vilified, forced to go into hiding, and/or threatened with imprisonment.

For instance, Dr. Stanislaw Burzynski of Houston, Texas uses non-toxic antineoplastons to successfully treat brain cancer, non-Hodgkin's lymphoma, and many common cancers. The FDA's lawyers have spent tens of millions of dollars and almost two decades trying to put Dr. Burzynski in jail. The FDA has a track record of raiding the offices of alternative practitioners, destroying their medical records, and even putting them in jail. In addition, many doctors are afraid of expensive, time-consuming lawsuits, and their insurance carrier may drop them if they use alternative treatments. Their state medical boards may fine them and revoke their license. And remember, doctors are human. Due to the fact that other doctors will publicly ridicule them if they use alternative treatments, many doctors succumb to prescribing the "Big 3" as a result of peer pressure.

Disturbingly, the truth is that a bureaucratic tangle of politicians, attorneys, CEOs, and huge international corporations has taken control over our health care system, and it is they who dictate which cancer treatments are allowed and which ones are not. Doctors are basically left out in the dark when it comes to policy making decisions concerning cancer treatments. Sadly, the fact is that our sincere, dedicated, doctors, and nurses who genuinely care about their patients have very little input concerning the type of cancer therapies they are allowed to prescribe.

Bottom line: Don't expect a doctor thinking "inside the box" to buck the system. The risks are too great.

PRESCRIPTION DRUGS

Did you know that prescription drugs kill over 100,000 Americans each and every year? That's a figure from the FDA's own website.

Assuming that the figure of 100,000 per year is relatively constant and not rapidly increasing or declining, since September 11, 2001 there have been **over one million** deaths from adverse drug reactions! Yet we have never-ending crusades against firearms (*while accidental firearms deaths are down to around 600 per year*) and spend multiple **billions** of dollars inconveniencing, irradiating, and sexually molesting people at airports (*while there have been essentially zero deaths since 9/11 and only trumped-up, false flag "terrorism" events*). All the while, the FDA and Big Pharma continue to bring more toxic, deadly drugs on the market.

According to Ethan Huff, writer for NaturalNews.com, *"If al-Qaeda operatives were caught dispensing toxic chemicals disguised as medicine to innocent civilians, they would be sent off to Guantanamo Bay without trial, and locked away indefinitely. But when the FDA does the very same thing on a much more massive scale, nobody bats an eye. And yet the number of people that the FDA has killed with its drugs is far more than the number killed during 9/11 or the Oklahoma City bombing. The organized crime ring that is the federal government today is the real terrorist threat that we all face on a daily basis. And until the American people collectively wake up to this reality, we will continue to watch our friends, our families, and our children, which are the casualties of this ongoing terrorist attack, lay waste at the hands of Big Pharma and the FDA.*" I would have to concur with Ethan.

Did you know that prescription drugs injure over two million Americans each and every year? That figure is also posted on the FDA's website as well as in the *Journal of the American Medical Association*.

This is remarkable!

When you visit your doctor and take even a single prescription, you are playing "pharmaceutical roulette" and walking into the "Big Pharma Trap."

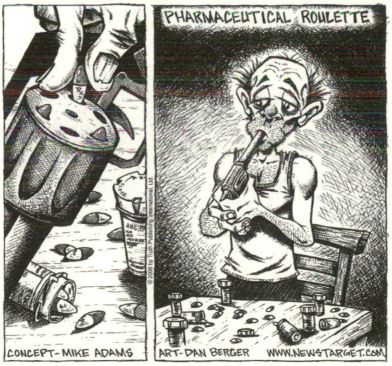

Thanks to Mike Adams and www.NaturalNews.com for the cartoon above.

The only way to win this game of roulette and actually restore your health is to give up all prescription drugs and make essential changes to your diet and lifestyle.

"But don't prescription drugs perform miracles for people's health? Don't they make us healthier?"

Well, if you watch thirty minutes of TV during prime time, you will likely see several commercials that proclaim the "gospel" of prescription drugs, loudly proclaiming that they can do wonders for people, such as helping with depression, lowering cholesterol, increasing libido, eliminating allergies, calming children, and reversing osteoporosis, just to name a few. If prescription drugs are so good for us, then let me ask you one question: ***"Where are all the 'healthy' people on drugs?"***

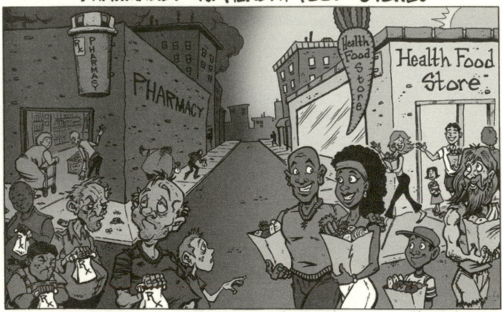

Thanks to Mike Adams and *www.NaturalNews.com* for the cartoon above.

There really aren't any, are there? If prescription drugs were good for us, then shouldn't there be hundreds of millions of Americans who are on prescription drugs who are also mentally sharp, physically fit, bursting with energy, and emotionally healthy? Well, where are these people? Typically, when you meet someone who is taking multiple prescription drugs, they are mentally fuzzy, sickly in appearance, chronically fatigued, and emotionally unstable and depressed. If you head down to your local organic market and approach the healthiest people you find, why don't you ask which prescription drugs are responsible for their health? After looking a bit dazed and confused, they will likely tell you that they do <u>not</u> take prescription drugs! The bottom line is that prescription drugs make people sicker.

Here's why: During development, prescription drugs are designed to target a single measurable marker, such as cholesterol level. Let's examine statin drugs for an example. Now, while statin drugs do lower LDL cholesterol, their mechanism of accomplishing this is the problem. They lower cholesterol by inhibiting the liver's ability to create *all types* of cholesterol, including HDL cholesterol. So, while statin drugs may positively affect *one* marker, they disrupt the body's physiology in many other ways. There are over 900 studies proving the adverse effects of statin drugs, including anemia, cancer, chronic fatigue, acidosis, liver dysfunction, thyroid disruption, Parkinson's, Alzheimer's, and even diabetes!

Of course, the entire statin drug "house of cards" begins to crumble quickly once you realize that a scientifically naïve public has been conned into a fraudulent correlation between elevated "bad" cholesterol (LDL) and cardiovascular disease. You see, the cholesterol itself, whether being transported by low-density lipoproteins (LDL) or high-density lipoproteins (HDL), is **exactly** the same. Cholesterol is simply a necessary ingredient that is required to be regularly delivered around the body for the efficient healthy development, maintenance, and functioning of our cells. It is vital for good health. Perhaps most importantly, cholesterol is an essential component in the machinery that triggers the release of neurotransmitters in the brain. That's right. Cholesterol is **not** the "bad guy" that the Medical Mafia claims. And elevated cholesterol is **not** the cause of heart disease!

According to recent research at Harvard, the primary causes of atherosclerosis (*hardening of the arteries which leads to heart disease*) are lesions and plaque in the arteries caused by **sugar** which causes insulin to be released. Insulin causes lesions in the endothelium of the arteries that become clogged with cholesterol. So, cholesterol gets the blame, but the real culprit is sugar. Cholesterol is actually your body's "repair mechanism" to correct the arterial damage resulting from excess sugar in the diet. Remove refined sugar from your diet, and you shouldn't have any issue with heart disease. Enough of my cholesterol rant ... back to prescription drugs ...

When patients begin to have additional problems which are *caused* by prescription drugs, what do they do? They head back to the doctor's office where their doctor diagnoses them with *another* disease or disorder. And then, they give them another prescription drug to help "fix" the problems caused by the first drug. I used to wait tables, and when you convince a person to order a dessert with their meal, it is called "upselling." This is exactly what Big Pharma loves – doctors who upsell their patients with more expensive prescription drugs! It's the "Big Pharma trap." It's "pharmaceutical roulette." What's the result? Higher earnings per share! Of course! And the cycle continues...one prescription after another, like boxcars on a train. Finally, the patient is broke and suffering (or dead) from chemical toxicity resulting from prescription drugs.

When you take prescription drugs on a long-term basis, it is certain that you will end up worse than you began. Now, I'm not saying that prescription drugs are totally useless. There may be certain situations where prescription drugs are helpful on a short-term basis. However, this is not the way they're being promoted today. Thanks to the culture of greed at Big Pharma and their prevalent lack of ethics, prescription drugs are being "pushed" as lifetime medications.

Big Pharma is able to obtain the FDA's "blessing" for their latest miracle drug since the clinical trials focus only on one marker while basically ignoring the other detrimental systemic effects of the drug. Their goal is to positively impact one particular marker, thus gaining FDA approval as fast as possible. There are literally thousands of markers to target, and if a prescription drug can positively alter just one of these markers (*without killing too many people during clinical trials*), then the FDA will likely approve the drug, despite the lack of evidence on the systemic effect of the drug on other body functions. This is just one of many problems with prescription drugs, since they all have a **systemic** effect.

The numerous other deleterious effects that the drug may have on the human body are largely ignored. And since prescription drugs have a systemic effect, they all have harmful side effects. When clinical trial participants start showing these side effects, they are frequently excused from the trial to make sure that trial results spin the newest wonder drug in a positive light. For example, during clinical trials for Vioxx, patients who suffered heart attacks from the drug were selectively omitted from the trial results and this fact was concealed from the general public. This is the standard operating procedure for the Medical Mafia, and is the only way that extremely toxic drugs are approved and considered to be "safe."

My friend, Mike Adams, the "Health Ranger," has reported that some prescription drugs are marked up an astounding 500,000% from the cost of their raw ingredients (no, that's **not** a typo), and a big chunk of that money goes right back into the big propaganda machine. Big Pharma claims that they need those exorbitant prices to invest in R&D,

but in reality, they spend far more on advertising than they spend on R&D. In a study by New York University researchers and published in the January 3, 2008, issue of *PLoS Medicine*, it was revealed that Big Pharma spends twice as much on advertising as it does on R&D.

According to Adams, "*Our system of modern medicine is a* **sham**, *folks. It is* **legalized drug pushing** *dominated by Big Pharma. The science is largely distorted (and often outright fraudulent), the ethics have all but disappeared, and the long-term price of all this is going to be enormous. We have an unprecedented problem on our hands that's sickening an entire generation and creating stratospheric long-term health care costs for the next round of working taxpayers unlucky enough to stumble onto all this.*" www.naturalnews.com/001352.html

Mike is dead on accurate. Here are a few stories that will knock your socks off.

- In August of 2012, Eli Lilly admitted to more than $200 million dollars worth of doctor payoffs
- In the first quarter of 2012, Eli Lilly agreed to pay $1.4 billion to settle criminal and civil allegations of promoting drugs for unapproved uses.
- Since Eli Lilly knew that Zyprexa caused diabetes and didn't let patients know this, they have already settled numerous "failure to warn" lawsuits totaling 1.2 billion dollars.
- In 2012, Eli Lilly agreed to another 1.42 billion, $615 million to settle the Justice Department's criminal investigation and approximately $800 million to settle the civil investigations brought by the states for Medicaid fraud.
- In June of 2012, an Italian Court ruled that Merck's MMR vaccine caused autism in a now 10-year old boy. As a result, a court in Rimini, Italy recently awarded the family a 15-year annuity totaling 174,000 Euros (just under $220,000).
- In July of 2012, two virologists filed a federal lawsuit against Merck (their former employer) alleging that Merck had falsified test data to fabricate a vaccine efficacy rate of 95% or higher, spiked the blood test with animal antibodies in order to artificially inflate the appearance of immune system antibodies, pressured the two virologists to "*participate in the fraud and subsequent cover-up*," used the falsified trial results to swindle the U.S. government out of "*hundreds of millions of dollars for a vaccine that does not provide adequate immunization*," and intimidated the scientists, threatening them with going to jail unless they stayed silent.
- In July of 2012, in what is now the largest criminal fraud settlement ever to come out of the pharmaceutical industry, GlaxoSmithKline plead guilty to bribery, fraud and other crimes and agreed to pay $1 billion in criminal fines and $2 billion in civil fines following a nine-

year federal investigation into its activities. According to U.S. federal investigators, GlaxoSmithKline (GSK) routinely bribed doctors with luxury vacations and paid speaking gigs, and "fabricated" drug safety data and lied to the FDA.

➢ GSK had a "bribery network" of 49,000 doctors who received financial kickbacks to prescribe more Glaxo pharmaceuticals to patients.

➢ In 2012, Pfizer agreed to pay $2.3 billion to settle criminal and civil liability due to its illegal off-label promotion of Bextra (*a painkiller already pulled from the market*), Geodon (*like Zyprexa, an atypical anti-psychotic that injures children*), Zyvox (*an antibiotic*), and Lyrica (*an epilepsy drug*).

AN ALLEGORY

"WELCOME TO THE TOWN OF ALLOPATH"
by Mike Adams

There once was a town called Allopath. It had many people, streets and cars, but due to budget limitations, there were no stop signs or traffic lights anywhere in Allopath. Not surprisingly, traffic accidents were common. Cars would crash into each other at nearly every intersection. But business was booming for the auto repair shops and local hospitals, which dominated the economy of Allopath.

As the population of Allopath grew, traffic accidents increased to an alarming level. Out of desperation, the city council hired Doctor West, a doctor of the Motor Division (M.D.) to find a solution.

Dr. West spent days examining traffic accidents. He carried an assortment of technical gear – microscopes, chemical analysis equipment, lab gear – and put them all to work as part of his investigation. The townspeople of Allopath watched on with great curiosity while Dr. West went about his work, meticulously documenting and analyzing each traffic accident, and they awaited his final report with great interest.

After weeks of investigation, Dr. West called the people of Allopath to a town meeting for the release of his report. There, in front of the city council and most of the residents of Allopath, he announced his findings: "***Traffic accidents are caused by skid marks.***"

As Dr. West explained, he found and documented a near-100% correlation between traffic accidents and skid marks. "*Wherever we find these cars colliding,*" he explained, "*we also find these skid marks.*" The town had "Skid Marks Disease," the doctor explained, and the answer to the town's epidemic of traffic accidents would, "*...require* *nothing more than treating Skid Marks Disease by making the streets skid-proof,"* Dr. West exclaimed, to great applause from the townspeople.

The city paid Dr. West his consulting fee, and then asked the good doctor to propose a method for treating this Skid Marks Disease. As chance would have it, Dr. West had recently been on a trip to Hawaii paid for by a chemical company that manufactured roadaceuticals: special chemicals used to treat roads for situations just like this one. He recommended a particular chemical coating to the city council: teflon.

"We can treat this Skid Marks Disease by coating the roads with teflon," Dr. West explained. *"The streets will then be skid-proof, and all the traffic accidents will cease!"* He went on to describe the physical properties of teflon and how its near-frictionless coating would deter nearly all vehicle skids.

The city council heartily agreed with Dr. West, and they issued new public bonds to raise the money required to buy enough teflon to coat all the city's streets. Within weeks, the streets were completely coated, and the skid marks all but disappeared. The city council paid Dr. West another consulting fee and thanked him for his expertise. The problem of traffic accidents in Allopath was solved, they thought. Although the cure was expensive, they were convinced it was worth it.

But things weren't well in Allopath. Traffic accidents quadrupled. Hospital beds were overflowing with injured residents. Auto repair businesses were booming so much that most of the city council members decided to either open their own car repair shops or invest in existing ones.

Week after week, more and more residents of Allopath were injured, and their cars were repeatedly damaged. Money piled into the pockets of the car repair shops, hospitals, tow truck companies and car parts retailers. The town economic advisor, observing this sharp increase in economic activity, announced that Allopath was booming. Its economy was healthier than ever, and Allopath could look forward to a great year of economic prosperity!

There were jobs to be had at the car repair shops. There were more nurses needed at the hospital. *"Help wanted"* signs appeared all over town at the paramedic station, the tow truck shops, and the auto glass businesses. Unemployment dropped to near zero.

But the traffic accidents continued to increase. And yet there were no skid marks. The city council was baffled. They thought they had solved this problem. Skid Marks Disease had been eradicated by the teflon treatment. Why were traffic accidents still happening? They called a town meeting to discuss the problem, and following a short discussion of the problem, an old hermit, who lived in the forest just outside of Allopath, addressed the townspeople.

"There is no such thing as Skid Marks Disease," he explained. *"This disease was invented by the roadaceuticals company to sell you teflon coatings."* The townspeople were horrified to hear such a statement. They knew Skid Marks Disease existed. The doctor had told them so. How could this hermit, who had no Motor Division (M.D.) degree, dare tell them otherwise? How could he question their collective town wisdom in such a way?

"This is a simple problem," the hermit continued. *"All we need to do is build stop signs and traffic lights. Then the traffic accidents will cease."* Without pause, one city council member remarked, *"But how can we afford stop signs? We've spent all our money on teflon treatments!"* The townspeople agreed. They had no money to buy stop signs.

Another council member added, *"And how can we stop anyway? The streets are all coated with teflon. If we build stop signs, we'll waste all the money we've spent on teflon!"* The townspeople agreed, again. What use were stop signs if they couldn't stop their cars anyway?

The hermit replied, *"But the stop signs will eliminate the need for teflon. People will be able to stop their cars, and accidents will cease. The solution is simple."*

But what might happen if stop signs actually worked, the townspeople wondered. How would it affect the booming economy of Allopath? Realizing the consequences, a burly old man who owned a local repair shop jumped to his feet and said, *"If we build these stop signs, and traffic accidents go down, I'll have to fire most of my workers!"*

It was at that moment that most of the townspeople realized their own jobs were at stake. If stop signs were built, nearly everyone would be unemployed. They all had jobs in emergency response services, car repair shops, hospitals and teflon coating maintenance. Some were now sales representatives of the roadaceuticals company. Others were importers of glass, tires, steel and other parts for cars. A few clever people were making a fortune selling wheelchairs and crutches to accident victims.

One enterprising young gentleman started a scientific journal that published research papers describing all the different kind of Skid

Marks Diseases that had been observed and documented. Another person, a fitness enthusiast, organized an annual run to raise funds to find the cure for Skid Marks Disease. It was a popular event, and all the townspeople participated as best they could: jogging, walking, or just pushing themselves along in their wheelchairs.

One way or another, nearly everyone in Allopath was economically tied to Skid Marks Disease. Out of fear of losing this economic prosperity, the townspeople voted to create a new public safety agency: the Frequent Drivers Association (FDA). This FDA would be responsible for approving or rejecting all signage, technology and chemical coatings related to the town's roads.

The FDA's board members were chosen from among the business leaders of the community: the owner of the car shop, the owner of the ambulance company, and of course, Dr. West. Soon after its inception, the FDA announced that Skid Marks Disease was, indeed, very real, as it had been carefully documented by a doctor and recently published in the town Skid Marks Disease journal.

Since there were no studies whatsoever showing stop signs to be effective for reducing traffic accidents, the FDA announced that stop signs were to be outlawed and that any person attempting to sell stop signs would be charged with fraud and locked up in the town jail. This pleased the townspeople of Allopath. With the FDA, they knew their jobs were safe. They could go on living their lives of economic prosperity, with secure jobs, knowing that the FDA would outlaw any attempt to take away their livelihood. They still had a lot of traffic accidents, but at least their jobs were secure.

And so life continued in Allopath, for a short while, at least. As traffic accidents continued at a devastating rate, more and more residents of Allopath were injured or killed. Many were left bed-ridden, unable to work, due to their injuries.

In time, the population dwindled. The once-booming town of Allopath eventually became little more than a ghost town. The hospital closed its doors, the FDA was disbanded, and the Skid Marks Disease journal stopped printing.

The few residents remaining eventually realized nothing good had come of Skid Marks Disease, the teflon coatings and the FDA. No one was any better off, as all the town's money had been spent on the disease: the teflon coatings, car parts and emergency services.

No one was any healthier, or happier, or longer-lived. Most, in fact, had lost their entire families to Skid Marks Disease.

And the hermit?

He continued to live just outside of town, at the end of a winding country road, where he lived a simple life with no cars, no roads, no teflon coatings and no FDA.

He outlived every single resident of Allopath. He gardened, took long walks through the forest, and gathered roots, leaves and berries to feed himself. In his spare time, he constructed stop signs, waiting for the next population to come along, and hoping they might listen to an old hermit with a crazy idea:

... THAT PREVENTION IS THE ANSWER, NOT THE TREATMENT OF SYMPTOMS.

~ Thanks to Mike Adams, the "Health Ranger," who authored this allegory. It can be found here: www.naturalnews.com/008674.html

~ Video of this allegory can be seen on Dr. Joseph Mercola's website: www.mercola.com/townofallopath/index.htm

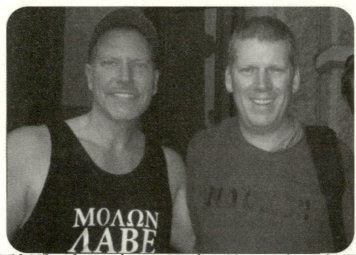

With Mike Adams at the 2013 March vs. Monsanto in Austin, TX

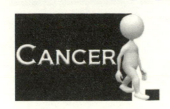

CHAPTER 3
PERSECUTION & SUPPRESSION

> "THERE IS WIDESPREAD SUPPRESSION OF NATURAL CANCER THERAPIES, & PERSECUTION OF SUCCESSFUL THERAPISTS. THE UNDISPUTED LEADER IN THIS FIELD IS THE USA."
> — WALTER LAST

IT'S A FACT FOLKS

That widespread suppression and persecution of natural medicine does exist and has existed for almost a century is a **fact**. Anyone who disputes this is either not paying attention or deliberately lying. History is chock full of examples of original thinkers who have been scorned, mocked, ruined, and imprisoned for daring to think outside the box and for displaying the audacity to threaten the status and authority of the Medical Mafia.

Daniel Haley has written a fabulous book entitled Politics in Healing: The Suppression and Manipulation of American Medicine in which he clearly demonstrates that government agencies including the FDA, NCI, and FTC have **systematically suppressed** cancer cures that worked and are continuing this suppression to this day. A former New York State Assemblyman who has spent a lifetime studying health and healing in America, Mr. Haley is a man uniquely able to tell the story of the damage greed and political influence that has been wrought on our nation's healthcare alternatives. The twelve documented cases Mr. Haley describes are not unique. However, what makes them special is that public records exist which show both the efficacy of the cancer treatments and the active suppression that makes it difficult for cancer patients to find and use these options.

Over the past century, hundreds of caring, concerned, and conscientious alternative doctors and herbalists have been treated like common criminals for the "crime" of curing people of terminal diseases in an unapproved manner by heavy-handed government agents who swoop down on clinics with machine guns and body armor. All the while, these same agencies posture themselves before TV cameras and the public under the ludicrous pretense of being servants of the people and protectors of the common good.

According to the late Dr. Robert Atkins, *"There have been many cancer cures, and all have been ruthlessly and systematically suppressed with a Gestapo-like thoroughness by the cancer establishment. The cancer establishment is the not-too-shadowy association of the American Cancer Society, the leading cancer hospitals, the National Cancer Institute and the FDA. The shadowy part is the fact that these respected institutions are very much dominated by members and friends of members of the pharmaceutical industry, which profits so incredibly much from our profession-wide obsession with chemotherapy."*

One book I have already mentioned, which I highly recommend, is a book by the famous medical historian, Hans Ruesch, entitled <u>Naked Empress or the Great Medical Fraud</u>. In this book, Ruesch exposes massive corruption and fraud in medicine, media, science, government, and industry.   Ruesch quotes J.W. Hodge, M.D. on page 75, *"The medical monopoly or medical trust, euphemistically called the American Medical Association, is not merely the meanest monopoly ever organized, but the most arrogant, dangerous and despotic organization which ever managed a free people in this or any other age. Any and all methods of healing the sick by means of safe, simple and natural remedies are sure to be assailed and denounced by the arrogant leaders of the AMA doctors' trust as 'fakes, frauds and humbugs.'"*

He continues, *"Every practitioner of the healing art who does not ally himself with the medical trust is denounced as a 'dangerous quack' and impostor by the predatory trust doctors. Every sanitarian who attempts to restore the sick to a state of health by natural means without resorting to the knife or poisonous drugs, disease imparting serums, deadly toxins or vaccines, is at once pounced upon by these medical tyrants and fanatics, bitterly denounced, vilified and persecuted to the fullest extent."* Medical mavericks with innovative cancer ideas are slandered, labeled as "quacks" or "charlatans," and persecuted, while their treatment protocols are bastardized and suppressed.

But Why? Big Medicine tells us that they are protecting us from the alternative cancer treatments since they have not been scientifically proven to be effective and they may delay the more effective conventional cancer treatments from doing their job. *"More effective* *conventional cancer treatments?*" You've got to be kidding! Is that what they call a **3%** cure rate with chemotherapy? This argument would be laughable if it were not so heartbreaking for millions of cancer victims. They aren't protecting us; they are protecting their own cash cow! And what exactly does it mean to be "*scientifically proven to be effective*" by the FDA anyway? Snickers, Twinkies, Cupcakes, Coca Cola, and thousands of other junk food products are "approved" by the FDA, but if you offer an alternative cancer treatment, then you are liable to end up in jail. Think I'm making this stuff up? **Read on**...

HARRY HOXSEY

Harry Hoxsey was born in 1901. Around 1840, Harry's grandfather, John Hoxsey, a horse breeder, had a stallion that developed cancer. When the horse was pastured, John noticed that the horse grazed primarily on a particular shrub and flowering plants. Over the course of a few months, eventually the horse was cancer free. John eventually developed an herbal tonic derived from these "wonder plants" and began to treat sick horses. John passed down the formula to his son, Harry's father, who quietly began to use the tonic to help humans with cancer. When Harry was only 10 years old, he began to help his father administer the tonic to terminal cancer victims. They had tremendous success, and eventually, when his father died, Harry was responsible for carrying on the Hoxsey healing tradition.

In 1924, at the age of only twenty-three, Harry opened the Hoxsey Cancer Clinic in Dallas. For over thirty years, he treated (and cured) many cancer patients using the Hoxsey tonic. By the 1950s, the Hoxsey Cancer Clinic in Dallas was the world's largest private cancer center, with branches in seventeen states. At that time, the head of the AMA was Morris Fishbein, who was also the editor of the *Journal of the American Medical Association (JAMA)*. Fishbein tried to purchase the rights to the tonic from Hoxsey, but when he refused, Fishbein conducted a personal vendetta against him, using the JAMA as his primary means to discredit him.

Over the course of several years, Fishbein published numerous articles in the JAMA which claimed that the Hoxsey tonic was nothing more than a "*worthless bottle of colored water*" made of "*backyard weeds.*" And due to the fact that he gave these weeds to cancer patients, Hoxsey, who was not a doctor, was arrested **over 200 times** for practicing medicine without a license! Perhaps his biggest adversary was District Attorney, Al Templeton, who had him arrested over 100 times. Al's brother, Mike, developed terminal cancer and went through the "Big 3" conventional treatments. After the doctors sent him home to die, Mike visited the Hoxsey Cancer Clinic and was eventually cured. When Al learned about his brother's miraculous recovery from terminal cancer, he quit his job and became Hoxsey's defense attorney.

Unfortunately, this was during the period that the "Big 3" conventional cancer treatments, due largely to their profitability to the entire Cancer Industry, were gaining a foothold in conventional cancer therapy. The inexpensive Hoxsey tonic posed a real threat to the profits which were

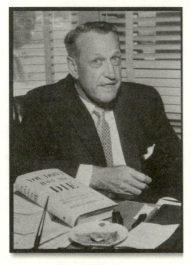

being realized from the "Big 3," so it's not hard to guess what happened next: **a huge smear campaign**. Through their subversive network of cronies and through a series of slanderous articles, the Cancer Industry effectively labeled Hoxsey *"the worst cancer quack of the century."*

However, if Hoxsey was a quack, then he sure wasn't a very good quack, since quacks are in it for the money, and the Hoxsey Cancer Clinics would treat 100% of the patients who came for treatment, even if they couldn't afford to pay for treatment. But the Medical Mafia didn't stop at slander. FDA officials would actually break into his patients' houses, intimidate them, tell them they were being duped by a quack, and steal their medicine.

Harry Hoxsey

However, in 1954, an independent team of ten physicians from around the USA made a two-day inspection of the Hoxsey Cancer Clinic in Dallas, examining case histories and speaking to patients. They then issued a remarkable statement. They declared that the clinic was *"successfully treating pathologically proven cases of cancer, both internal and external, without the use of surgery, radium or x-ray."* Of course, the results of this investigation were ignored by the Cancer Industry. Then in 1953, the Fitzgerald Report, which was commissioned by a United States Senate committee, concluded that organized medicine had *"**conspired to suppress**"* the Hoxsey therapy.

Due to a slanderous article published by Fishbein, Hoxsey sued him for libel and slander, and Hoxsey won. Fishbein was forced to resign from the AMA. **But it was too little, too late**. Hoxsey's name, along with his tonic, had already been trashed and would never recover. All of Hoxsey's clinics were eventually shut down. The Dallas clinic closed in 1960, and three years later, to escape the mounting pressure, Mildred Nelson R.N. (his long time chief nurse whose mother had been cured from terminal cancer by the Hoxsey tonic) moved the operation to Tijuana, Mexico. Harry Hoxsey died in 1974, but the Bio-Medical

Center, as the clinic is now called, continues to treat all types of cancer. Before she died, Nelson appointed her younger sister, Liz Jonas, as the administrator of the Bio-Medical Center.

As I mentioned earlier in the book, we had planned to take Dad to this clinic, but unfortunately he never recovered from the surgery. Their medical records indicate that many patients (some arriving with advanced stages of cancer) have been helped and even completely healed of cancer by the Hoxsey tonic. I personally know several folks who have been healed using this treatment, which is yet another instance of a successful alternative cancer treatment which was dismissed as "quackery" by the Cancer Industry.

ROYAL RAYMOND RIFE

Royal Raymond Rife was a brilliant scientist born in 1888. Rife developed technology which is still commonly used today in the fields of optics, electronics, radiochemistry, and biochemistry. In the 1920s, Rife invented the world's first virus microscope. On November 3, 1929, the *San Diego Union* newspaper featured a front-page article about his microscope, and many other articles followed. In 1931 he announced his results to doctors and university medical departments. A stream of eminent doctors and researchers eagerly endorsed his work. Among them was Dr. Milbank Johnson, president of the Southern California branch of the AMA and member of the board of directors of Pasadena Hospital.

By 1933, Rife had perfected that technology and had constructed the Rife Universal Microscope, which was capable of magnifying objects 60,000 times their normal size. Unlike electron microscopes which can only observe dead specimens due to the lethal chemical stains applied to them, Rife's microscope enabled him to view living organisms via a process he called "staining with light."

Like so many other pivotal discoveries in science, the principles behind Rife's super-microscopes were simple yet ingenious. For example, the microscopes never crossed light beams, as according to Rife, light diffraction is responsible for the lower resolutions seen in standard research microscopes. Through his advanced microscopes, Rife was able to show "pleomorphism," meaning that growing an organism in a different type of culture may yield a different organism entirely.

Rife was able to observe tiny living microorganisms that dwell in the human body, organisms which he felt caused cancer. He observed the reactions of various microbes as he bombarded them with infinite combinations of radio and audio frequencies. He soon discovered that certain frequencies, which he called "mortal oscillatory frequencies," would destroy the pleomorphic microbes which are active in cancers.

In early 1934, Dr. Milbank Johnson, who had become Rife's friend and supporter, arranged formal clinical trials of the Rife Beam Ray device. The medical team included a "Who's Who" of doctors and pathologists. Sixteen "terminal" cancer patients from Pasadena County Hospital volunteered to be treated with Rife's machine, which was able to kill the pleomorphic microbes inside the cancer cells. After three months, all sixteen patients were still alive. The doctors were amazed that fourteen of them literally showed **no** signs of cancer and were pronounced clinically "cured." One month later, the other two patients were also pronounced "cancer-free." Rife's "cure rate" with these sixteen terminal patients was 100%. **This was a major breakthrough**! Below is an article from the May 6, 1938, edition of the *San Diego Evening Tribune*.

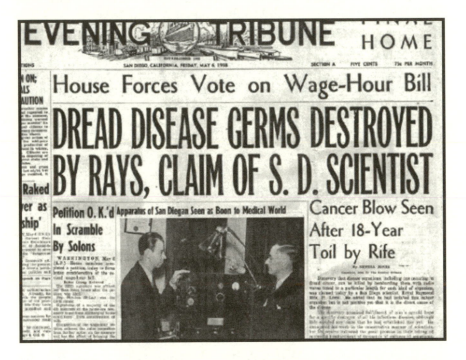

Along comes the Medical Mafia. The head of the AMA during that era was...you guessed it...the infamous Morris Fishbein. Just like he did with Harry Hoxsey, Fishbein wanted a piece of the action from the sales of these devices, so he proposed an arrangement whereby he (and the AMA) would give Rife their official blessing and then he would get his pals at the FDA to fast track their approval of Rife's device. In exchange, Fishbein would receive a huge share of the profits from the sales. **Rife refused.**

Similar to what he did to Harry Hoxsey, Fishbein and his cronies set out to destroy Rife. Rife's lab was vandalized and photographs, film, and records were stolen. His microscope was stolen, his lab was burned down, and some of his supporters died under suspicious circumstances. In 1940, two doctors who supported Rife were raided by federal officers who confiscated their equipment and notes. They were both later found dead, supposedly having committed suicide by poison.

Fast forward to 1944 ...

Dr. Milbank Johnson arranged a press conference to announce a cure for cancer using Rife's machine. There were rumors that Dr. Johnson had been approached by Big Pharma representatives with offers of money to suppress information about Rife's work. Mysteriously, the night before the press conference, Dr. Johnson suddenly died and all his notes were pronounced "lost" by executors of his estate. Although this was initially believed to be an accidental death, several years later investigators exhumed Johnson's body and detected poison.

Then the knockout blow – the police illegally confiscated the remainder of his fifty years of research. To finish the job, the medical journals, supported almost entirely by drug company revenues and controlled by the AMA, refused to publish anything about Rife's treatment. In 1971, at the age of eighty-three, Rife died from an overdose of valium and alcohol. For more information on Royal Raymond Rife, I recommend that you read The Cancer Cure That Worked by Barry Lynes.

THE RALPH MOSS STORY (in his own words)

excerpted from www.cancerdecisions.com

"In 1974, I began working at Memorial Sloan-Kettering Cancer Center, the world's leading cancer treatment hospital. I was an idealistic and eager young science writer, sincerely proud to be part of Sloan Kettering and Nixon's "War On Cancer." Ever since I was a kid, my main heroes were scientists (with the Brooklyn Dodgers running a close second!) The job at Sloan-Kettering seemed like a dream come true for me. I wanted to be part of the winning team that finally beat cancer.

Within three years, I had risen to the position of Assistant Director of Public Affairs at the Hospital. At the time, I was 34 years old, married to my high-school sweetheart, and we had a daughter and son, then nine and seven years old. We had dreams of buying a house and saving for the kids' education, so you can imagine how thrilled we were when I was promoted, with a huge raise, glowing feedback from my bosses, and was told that perks of the job would eventually include reduced tuition for the kids at New York University. Needless to say, we all were really counting on my "bright future" at Memorial Sloan-Kettering. But something soon happened that changed the course of my life forever.

A big part of my job as Assistant Director of Public Affairs was to write press releases for the media about cancer news and to write the in-hospital newsletter. I also handled calls from the press and public about cancer issues. So I was just doing a normal day's work (or so I thought) when I began interviewing an esteemed scientist at the Hospital for a newsletter article I was working on. It turned out that the scientist, Dr. Kanematsu Sugiura, had repeatedly gotten positive results shrinking tumors in mice studies with a natural substance called amygdalin (You may have heard of it as "laetrile".) Excitedly (and naively!) I told my "discovery" of Sugiura's work to the Public Affairs Director and other superiors, and laid out my plans for an article about it. Then I got the shock of my life.

They insisted that I stop working on this story immediately and never pick it up again. Why? They said that Dr. Sugiura's work was invalid and totally meaningless. But I had seen the results with my own eyes! And I knew Dr. Sugiura was a true scientist and an ethical person. Then my bosses gave me the order that I'll never forget: They told me to lie. Instead of the story I had been planning to write, they ordered me to write an article and press releases for all the major news stations emphatically stating that all amygdalin studies were negative and that the substance was worthless for cancer treatment. I protested and tried to reason with them, but it fell on deaf ears.

I will never forget how I felt on the subway ride home that day. My head was spinning with a mixture of strong feelings- confusion, shock, disappointment, fear for my own livelihood and my family's future, and behind it all, an intense need to know why this cover-up was happening. After long talks with my wife and parents (who were stunned, as you can imagine) I decided to put off writing any amygdalin press releases as long as I could while I discreetly looked into the whole thing some more on my own time. Everyone at the office seemed happy just to drop the whole thing, and we got busy with other less controversial projects.

So in the next few months, I was able to do my own investigating to answer the big question I couldn't let go of: Who were these people I *worked for and why would they want to suppress positive results in cancer research? My files grew thick as I uncovered more and more fascinating - and disturbing - facts. I had never given any thought to the politics of cancer before. Now I was putting together the pieces as I learned that:*

> *The people on Sloan-Kettering's Board of Directors were a "Who's Who" of investors in petrochemical and other polluting industries. In other words, the hospital was being run by people who made their wealth by investing in the worst cancer-causing things on the planet.*
> *CEOs of top pharmaceutical companies that produced cancer drugs also dominated the Board. They had an obvious vested interest in promoting chemotherapy and undermining natural therapies.*
> *The Chairman and the President of Bristol-Myers Squibb, the world's leading producer of chemotherapy, held high positions on MSKCC's Board.*
> *Of the nine members of the Hospital's powerful Institutional Policy Committee, seven had ties to the pharmaceutical industry.*
> *The Hospital itself invested in the stock of these same drug companies.*
> *Directors of the biggest tobacco companies in the U.S., Phillip Morris and RJR Nabisco held places of honor on the Board.*
> *Six Board Directors also served on the Boards of the New York Times, CBS, Warner Communications, Readers Digest, and other media giants.*

Not surprisingly, profits from chemotherapy drugs were skyrocketing, and the media glowingly promoted every new drug as a "breakthrough" in cancer. I kept all my notes in my filing cabinet at work. I had no idea what I would ever do with them. I just knew that I had to get to the bottom of it, for myself.

Meanwhile, the public's interest in laetrile refused to go away. A lot of people were going across the border to Mexican clinics to get the stuff, and my secretary's phone was ringing off the hook with people wanting to know what Sloan-Kettering thought of its value. I was once again told to give out the news that the studies had all been negative.

At home, I called my family together for a meeting. With their support, I decided I couldn't lie on behalf of the Hospital. In November of 1977, I stood up at a press conference and blew the whistle on Memorial Sloan Kettering Cancer Center's suppression of positive results with amygdalin. It felt like jumping off the highest diving board, but I had no doubt I was doing the right thing. I was fired the next day for "failing to carry out his most basic responsibilities" as the Hospital described it to the New York Times - in other words, failing to lie to the American people.

When I tried to pick up my things in my office, I found my files had been padlocked and two armed hospital guards escorted me from the premises.

Luckily for all of us, I have a very smart wife who all along had been making copies of my research notes and had put a complete extra set of files in a safe place. Those notes turned into my first book, The Cancer Industry, which is still in print (in an updated version) and available in bookstores. That dramatic day, when I stood up in front of the packed press conference and told the truth, was the beginning of a journey I never could have predicted. I was launched on a mission that I'm still on today – helping cancer patients find the truth about the best cancer treatments.

Well, we weren't able to buy a home until years later, the kids went to colleges on scholarships and loans, and my wife took on a demanding full-time job to help us get by. But in retrospect, my experiences as an insider in "the cancer industry" were among the best things ever to happen to me. My values were put to the test and I had to really examine what was important in my life. It is because of this difficult experience at Sloan-Kettering that I found a truly meaningful direction for my professional life, rather than just climbing Sloan-Kettering's career ladder and losing my soul in the process."

MORE PERSECUTION & SUPPRESSION

Dr. Jonathan Wright was a highly regarded nutrition specialist, but his cardinal sin was promoting natural treatments which hadn't received the FDA's blessing. In the summer of 1992, *The Civil Abolitionist* carried an article titled "FDA: The American Gestapo Prosecutor or Persecutor?" which told the story. On May 6, 1992, in what must have resembled a military invasion, Dr. Wright's clinic was assaulted by over 20 armed men who kicked open the door, pointed guns at both patients and staff, and confiscated business records, patient records, supplies, and equipment. The FDA "Gestapo" agents spent 14 hours at the clinic, searching through everything. At that point, he had not even been charged with a crime!

Why did they need to kick in the door and draw their guns? Well, police spokesman Rob Barnette explained that officers *"need to be prepared for the worst.*" But Dr. Wright hardly fit the bill of a dangerous criminal. A graduate of Harvard and the University of Michigan Medical School, he was nutrition editor of Prevention Magazine for over a decade. But he committed **the unforgivable sin** – he failed to prescribe drugs to treat illness. Rather he chose to use nutritional therapy and vitamin therapy. It is interesting to note that one of his favorite treatments was using L-Tryptophan to treat depression, but the FDA had outlawed this amino acid. Curiously, it was outlawed just a few months before the FDA put a big push on Prozac as a treatment for depression.

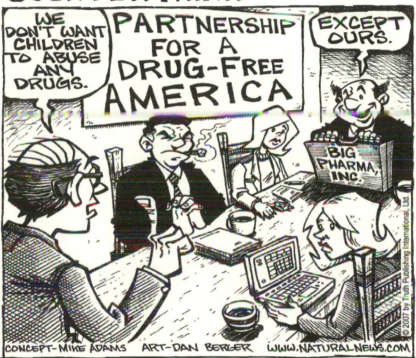

Thanks to Mike Adams and *www.NaturalNews.com* for the cartoon above.

My friend, Jason Vale, was handed a death sentence by his doctors in the mid 1990s when it was discovered that he had terminal cancer. Through extensive research, he discovered that people who once had cancer found healing properties in something as simple as the seeds of apples and apricots. It turned out that these seeds contain natural substances that kill cancer cells (Vitamin B$_{17}$). Jason immediately began to feel better by eating apple seeds as a part of his daily diet. Within a short period of time, Jason's cancer literally disappeared. When <u>Extra</u> aired Jason's story on national TV, it turned out to be the program's highest rated show to date so they chose to run that same episode the following week. The viewer response was so great that Jason was inundated with thousands of telephone calls from people all over the country.

Since then, Jason has inspired and helped thousands of people to naturally treat their own cancer. Through proper diet, nutrition, and the introduction of apple and apricot seeds into their daily diets, they have one-by-one created their own success stories that fortunately they will live to tell. In November of 2001, Jason was coerced by the FDA into signing a Consent Decree that would prevent him from sharing his story. Despite the fact that he had **not** broken any law, the FDA brought criminal charges against Jason for distributing apricot seeds.

Jason was sentenced on June 18, 2004, to sixty-three months in prison and three years of supervised release by a United States District Court in the Eastern District of New York. After serving almost four years in prison, Jason was released from jail in early 2008. Thank God! See Appendix 4 for more information on Jason and to learn a little bit more about his fascinating story.

Dr. Max Gerson developed a successful protocol to treat cancer patients using a strict regimen of nutrition, fresh juicing, and pancreatic enzymes. The medical community had an outstanding opportunity to appropriately examine alternative cancer treatments when a United States Senate Committee moved to grant extensive funds for research of his treatment, and Senators were very impressed with his results.

However, the AMA lobbied so strongly against research into alternative cancer treatments that the move was narrowly defeated in the Senate. Then the Medical Mafia used their influence to suppress Gerson's success and branded him as a "quack." Using the techniques of Edwin Bernays and Adolph Hitler, they said it loud enough and long enough that it became "common knowledge" that Gerson was a quack, despite the fact that his treatment protocol was curing terminal patients of cancer.

Standard operating procedure for the Medical Mafia and the Cancer Industry is to quickly suppress any discovery of an alternative cancer treatment and to create the public perception that a physician who discovers an alternative treatment is incompetent or "a quack." And they are quite effective – they even have websites (like quackwatch) set up for this very purpose. The truth is that Dr. Gerson's treatment was very effective; in Dr. Albert Schweitzer's words, *"I see in him (Dr. Gerson) as a medical genius who walked among us."*

Neal Deoul financed alternative cancer treatment research in the 1990s. In 1998, Maryland Attorney General Joseph Curran charged him with distributing deceptive promotional literature. Deoul had financed T-UP, Inc. which distributed cesium and T-UP (an aloe vera concentrate) to battle cancer and AIDS, despite the fact that there was not a single consumer complaint and that there were hundreds of testimonials from consumers who claimed life changing results. Ironically, as the case against Deoul unfolded in court, Deoul himself was diagnosed with an aggressive form of prostate cancer. He quietly and confidently turned to cesium and T-UP for treatment of his prostate cancer.

Of course, the Medical Mafia's physicians protested loudly and predicted the worst if he continued to refuse radiation and chemotherapy, but his condition improved as a result of taking his own medicines...**no other therapies were used**. Unfortunately, his successful treatment in the real world was not mirrored in the courtroom. A Maryland Judge found Deoul and T-UP, Inc. guilty of violating Maryland's consumer protection statutes. The critical question of whether the products actually fight cancer was never addressed in the judge's findings.

Jimmy Keller operated an alternative cancer clinic in Baton Rouge, but was forced out of the country to Tijuana, Mexico. Keller had founded the clinic after using natural methods to cure himself of terminal cancer. His own cancer had been unsuccessfully treated over two decades earlier by orthodox cancer specialists who amputated his ear and mutilated his face. As is typical with the "Big 3" orthodox treatments, Keller's cancer returned with a vengeance. He investigated natural healing methods, cured himself, and then began helping others to do so. He thought he was safe from the Medical Mafia since he was in Mexico. He was wrong.

In March 1991, Keller was abducted at gunpoint by four bounty hunters working for the U.S. Justice Department, at the command of the FDA, and forced to cross the American border. There, Keller was arrested by the FBI on twelve counts of wire fraud. What was his crime? Keller had made telephone calls across interstate lines to attract people to his Mexican clinic. Following the illegal kidnapping of Keller from Mexican soil, without extradition, he was jailed in Texas. Amazingly, his bond was set at $5 million. He was later convicted and sent to prison for two years. Keller's case was part of a trend of United States government kidnappings abroad, in full defiance of international law.

Dr. Joe Di Stefano (*a licensed nutritionist*) and Dr. Daniel Mayer (*an osteopath*) owned two Florida clinics in which they administered a product called Albarin, an extract of aloe vera, to cancer patients. Albarin was developed by Dr. Ivan Danhoff, a retired professor of medicine known as the *"father of aloe vera."* Dr. Di Stefano and Dr. Mayer had used Albarin on 100 cancer victims assigned to hospice. Amazingly, 94 of them survived with no side effects from the treatments. Overall, the clinics' recovery rate was 80%. In early October of 2001, Dr. Di Stefano exited his medical clinic at midnight after a long day's work, and was startled to hear strange noises coming from the dumpster in the back. Trash was scattered all over the ground. He peered over the top of the dumpster and saw two strangers probing in the trash. It turns out that the "trash divers" were actually FDA agents.

Then, one week later, exactly one month following the alleged "terrorist" attacks of 9/11, another "terrorist" attack occurred. And resembling 9/11, the **real terrorists** in this attack were our very own government. On October 11, 2001, one hundred twenty (120) agents from the FDA, DEA, US Customs, and various state and local law enforcement agencies raided and "seized" equipment from the clinics in Tampa and St. Petersburg. During the raids, law enforcement agents asked the patients if they wanted to be unhooked from their IVs, but not a single one said *"yes."* One of the patients complained, *"We're all adults here of our own free will. Why don't you get out of here and leave us alone?"* An FDA agent replied, *"This will be your last treatment!"* Simultaneous raids occurred against Dr. Danhoff in Grand Prairie, Texas and Jerry W. Jackson of Allied Pharmacy Services in Arlington, Texas. Jackson is the pharmacist who prepared the aloe vera extract. In this Medical Mafia atrocity, the FDA was satisfied with closing the clinics down and disallowing the aloe vera extract's use. No one went to jail. But there was the "collateral damage" of patients unable to receive more treatments and at least eight dying within a year.

Why did the government attack medical practitioners for using aloe vera extract? They were responding to complaints from **local oncologists** who were losing business! Realizing that these doctors are part of the monolithic Medical Mafia, the FDA acted with lightning speed in this Gestapo-like raid to eliminate this competitive threat. After all, if the effects of this aloe vera extract were to become widely known, it could inhibit sales of highly profitable chemo drugs. Could it be any clearer that the "war on cancer" is really a war **against** natural cancer cures? www.lef.org/magazine/mag2002/apr2002_report_clinic_01.html

In his book entitled Politics in Healing: The Suppression and Manipulation of American Medicine, Daniel Haley has documented 11 case studies of systematic suppression of proven cancer cures with substances like hydrazine sulfate, DMSO, cesium chloride, and aloe vera. Haley's conclusion: *"In a free market, where non-toxic therapies can openly compete with toxic therapies and information is not suppressed, consumers will make informed choices. This is exactly what the pharmaceutical companies don't want. Dancing to their tune, the FDA ferociously keeps off the market effective, nontoxic therapies that might provide formidable competition for patented, and often toxic, pharmaceutical drugs. By keeping these therapies off the market, the FDA is not protecting the public from harm. It is protecting the pharmaceutical companies from effective competition."*

The fact is that many successful alternative cancer treatments have been created in the past century and then lost again due to suppression and persecution. The barrier of **scientific bigotry** that separates conventional cancer research from reality remains intact. There are countless true life stories of persecution and suppression. If I were to list them all, it would take ten more books. But I'll let you do the research yourself.

Just type in these names in any search engine: Dr. Sam Chachoua, Dr. Hulda Clark, Dr. A. Keith Brewer, Dr. William Kelley, Dr. Gaston Naessens, Dr. Patrick Flanagan, Dr. Hans Nieper, J.H. Tilden, Dr. Kurt Donsbach, Dr. Stanislaw Burzynski, Dr. William Koch, Dr. F.M. Eugene Blass, Dr. Otto Warburg, Dr. Virginia Livingston, Dr. Günther Enderlein, Dr. Ernst T. Krebs, Dr. Philip E. Binzel, Jr. and the list goes on and on. Many names have been lost ...others have been crushed out of existence forever.

What do all these honorable doctors have in common? They all developed **successful alternative methods** of treating cancer for thousands of patients. And they all were persecuted by the Cancer Industry since they used "unapproved" treatments. These examples are only the tip of a huge iceberg. The Medical Mafia has an almost 100 year history of vast corruption, incompetence, persecution, and organized suppression of cancer therapies which actually work. Millions of people have suffered terribly and even died because those in charge took bribes, closed their minds to innovation, and refused to do what was morally right.

But what is going on in medicine today should not surprise us if we take a quick look at the past. Did you know that many of the world's greatest discoveries were initially rejected by the scientific community? Those who pioneered these discoveries often were ridiculed and condemned as quacks or charlatans.

According to Arthur Shopenaur, 19th century philosopher, *"Every truth passes through three stages before it is accepted. In the first it is ridiculed; in the second it is opposed; in the third, it is regarded as self-evident."*

Here are just a few examples:

> ➢ Ignaz Semmelwies was expelled from the medical society and run out of Vienna for asking surgeons to wash their hands before operating.
> ➢ Galileo was scorned for his belief that the sun is the center of the universe.
> ➢ Wilbur and Orville Wright were dismissed as "hoaxsters" by the Scientific American, the U.S. Army, and most American scientists.
> ➢ William Harvey was ridiculed for his belief that blood was pumped from the heart and moved around the body through arteries.
> ➢ Jacques Cartier discovered the cure to scurvy: tree bark and needles from the white pine (both rich in Vitamin C) stirred into a drink. He reported this to doctors when he returned to Europe, but they laughed at him. It took over 200 years before the medical experts "discovered" that scurvy is caused by a deficiency of vitamin C.
> ➢ The inventors of turbine power, the electric telegraph, the electric light, television, and space travel were all laughed at or ignored by the scientific establishment.

The irony about science (which is **supposedly** a search for new truths) is that most members of any scientific establishment seem dedicated to **opposing** real progress and suppressing original thought. Ironically, most scientific establishments seem dedicated to opposing real progress and discovery and to suppressing true science, which is supposed to be searching for new truths.

This includes the medical field. One can attack political or economic theories with some freedom, although that freedom has been greatly diminished with the advent of the "Patriot Act" and subsequent unconstitutional U.S. government "power grabs." However, there is even less freedom in the areas of science and medicine. Any scientist or physician with a new and original idea is likely to be regarded as a dangerous "hoaxster" or "quack" rather than an innovator whose ideas are worth evaluation.

The most repressive, most prejudiced, and most obscenely intolerant branch of Big Medicine is undoubtedly that part of it which claims to deal with cancer. As a matter of fact, the Cancer Industry has a list of "cancer quacks" which they publish on numerous websites. What do these so-called cancer quacks have in common? They utilize "unproven methods" for treating cancer. Let's look at this, shall we? "Unproven methods?" What exactly does this mean? Are these methods really **unproven**, or is the proof of their success being **suppressed**?

You should be aware that the Cancer Industry goes to great lengths to bury and suppress successful alternative cancer treatments. They also suppress alternative cancer treatments that do not work; thus, it appears that **all** of the treatments which they suppress do **not** work and that they are just "*doing their job to protect us.*" However, the fact is that hundreds of alternative cancer treatments **do** work, and it is unfortunate that the few snake oil salesmen do their worst damage by giving the Cancer Industry the ammunition they need to make **all** alternative cancer treatments (including the effective treatments) look like quackery.

The truth be told, most of the everyday practices of conventional medicine are unproven if we go by the government's own standards. In 1978, the Office of Technology Assessment (an arm of Congress) issued a major research report that concluded "*only 10 to 20 percent of all procedures currently used in medical practices have been shown to be efficacious by controlled trial.*" This means that between 80% and 90% of what doctors do to you is **scientifically unproven guesswork.** By the government's own definition, the majority of conventional medicine is **"quackery."** ("Assessing the Efficacy & Safety of Medical Technologies," U.S. Congress, OTA, PB 286-929, 1978)

According to Webster Kehr, "*The scientific evidence for alternative treatments can be compared to a ship the size of the Queen Mary II. The scientific evidence for orthodox treatments, by comparison, would be compared to a ship that could fit in a bathtub. I am not exaggerating. Yet the FDA says chemotherapy and orthodox medicine 'has' scientific evidence and there is 'no scientific evidence' for alternative treatments. It is nothing but pure corruption; it is nothing but lies. So how does the FDA, NIH, NCI, AMA, ACS, etc. suppress the statistically overwhelming evidence for alternative treatments for cancer? By ignoring it (i.e., blacklisting it) and babbling about their concepts of 'spontaneous remission' and what I call 'psychological remission'.*"

Interestingly, all of the alternative cancer treatments on Big Medicine's "quackery" list have the following common denominators: they are all natural, non-drugs, non-toxic, and non-patentable. Most importantly, they all successfully cure cancer! Even though chemo and radiation are completely unproven therapies and oftentimes will **kill** a cancer patient, they are not on the list. Why? Because they both are very expensive and are patentable. Let me explain.

Let's just suppose that I discovered a vitamin that cured cancer. Let's just call it Vitamin Z. In order for me to be able to tell you what Vitamin Z does and sell it to you, I would need to get Vitamin Z approved as a drug by the FDA. This would cost me between $200 and

$500 million and several years to get it approved. However, since Vitamin Z is natural and is found in most vegetables, I can't patent it. So, even after spending half a billion bucks to classify Vitamin Z as a "drug," it would still be a non-patentable drug, and anyone could sell it without my permission. I just wasted half a billion bucks and several years. As a CPA, I can tell you that it makes no business sense to try to get Vitamin Z approved by the FDA to sell as a drug.

So, even though Vitamin Z is a natural vitamin, cures cancer, and is free from harmful side effects, I cannot **tell you** that it cures cancer because it has not passed FDA scrutiny. But why would Big Medicine withhold information about something as important as the cure for cancer? Aren't they concerned with our well being? Don't they want what is best for us? Sadly, the answer to each of these questions, plain and simple, is "**no**." Since Big Medicine is beholden to Big Pharma, their treatment protocols will always include the most expensive, profitable drugs, regardless of whether or not this is in the patient's best interest.

FDA "GESTAPO" GOES NUTS ... AGAIN!

Just in case you actually thought the FDA supports freedom of speech ... think again. In yet another absurd example of the modern day Gestapo's bully tactics, in early 2010 the FDA sent a warning letter to the CEO of Diamond Foods informing him that the company's packages of walnuts were "*in violation of the Federal Food, Drug, and Cosmetic Act.*"

"*How exactly is Diamond Foods in violation?*" you might ask. Well, they had the audacity to tell the truth about some of the health benefits of walnuts on their website, such as the fact that walnuts protect against heart disease and ease joint pain. How dare they! Now, for those of you, who don't believe in miracles, please read on. According to the FDA, the exact moment that Diamond Foods listed the health benefits of walnuts on their website, the walnuts (which we all so foolishly thought to be a food) were **miraculously** transformed into a "drug," thus Diamond Foods was guilty of selling unapproved drugs!

Despite the **fact** that the health benefits of walnuts have been scientifically documented for decades, and there are over 30 peer-reviewed papers which show that walnuts reduce the risk of heart attack and improve cardiovascular health, the Federal Death Administration (FDA) claimed that the walnuts magically became "drugs" and were therefore "misbranded" while Diamond Foods was guilty of making "unauthorized" health claims.

OK, now I **really** believe that we are living in the Matrix! Let me get this straight. The FDA approved Vioxx which has killed over 50,000 people, but they have a problem with walnuts. **Give me a break!** It is crystal clear that the FDA is more concerned about protecting the profits of Big Pharma than the health of the American public.

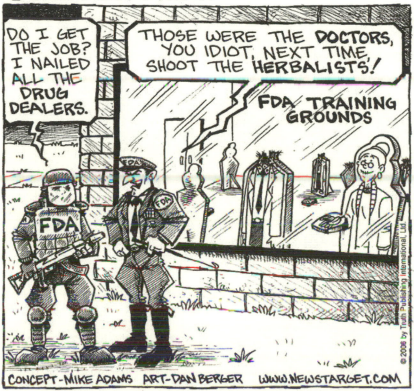

Thanks to Mike Adams and *www.NaturalNews.com* for the cartoon above.

This absurd case transports me back about a decade ago when the FDA Gestapo and the Medical Mafia set their sights on the "dangerous" cherry growing industry. You see, the cherry growers had links on their websites to some excellent scientific research (from places like Harvard) indicating that cherries reduce inflammation and pain. The FDA promptly sent them injunction letters with the usual threats (including prison) if they did not immediately remove the truth about cherries from their websites. What were those cherry growers thinking?

Didn't they know you're not supposed to put links on your website to support your health claims?

If you're **not** a drug company, then you can **not** make any health claims about your product, even if those claims are supported by thousands of peer-reviewed studies. However, if you **are** a drug company, you **can** simply pay off your researchers to fabricate data, as we saw in the last chapter in the disgusting case of Dr. Scott Reuben. Get it straight. The FDA is nothing more than the "leg-breakers" for the Medical Mafia, and they are **not** concerned with the truth and they are **not** concerned with our health. This modern day medical "hit squad" is only concerned with protecting the profits of the drug companies.

Let's imagine that there were an herb that helped to ease the chronic pain associated with terminal cancer. We'll just call it "Mary Jane." As a result of this miracle herb, cancer patients everywhere were living pain-free lives, without vomiting, actually had appetites, and weren't suffering from cachexia (wasting away). You would think that Mary Jane would be given to every cancer patient, right? Well, you would be sadly mistaken. Most likely, since Mary Jane cannot be patented, it would be outlawed as an "illegal drug" and those who used Mary Jane to treat their cancer and ease their pain would be criminalized. You see, only the "legal drugs" are allowed, despite the fact that many of the legal drugs are **lethal,** while many of the "illegal drugs" (*i.e.,* natural plants and herbs) are completely **harmless** and actually have **many** health benefits.

The Medical Mafia relentlessly persecutes those doctors that offer new, effective, non-toxic cancer therapies, and they ignore the wishes of patients who wish to try those therapies. Meanwhile they condone, support, and protect by law the "Big 3" treatments, which have been **proven** to be ineffective and toxic. The deciding issue is not whether alternative cancer treatments work better than the "Big 3." This fact is evident. The deciding issue, unfortunately, is which protocol will result in the largest profits to the drug pushers (Big Pharma).

And the winners are ... **the Medical Mafia and Big Pharma.**

And the losers are ... **the cancer patients**!

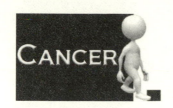

CHAPTER 4
TOXIC TREATMENTS

> "SUCCESS OF MOST CHEMOTHERAPIES IS APPALLING. THERE IS NO SCIENTIFIC EVIDENCE FOR ITS ABILITY TO EXTEND IN ANY APPRECIABLE WAY THE LIVES OF PATIENTS SUFFERING FROM THE MOST COMMON ORGANIC CANCER. CHEMOTHERAPY IS A SCIENTIFIC WASTELAND."
> -DR. ULRICH ABEL

THE "BIG 3"

If you have cancer, then it is very likely your doctor has already or will soon advise you that the only viable treatments are surgery, chemotherapy, and/or radiation. If you have a tumor, then the doctor will try to cut or "*slash*" it out via surgery. After they cut you, then they typically recommend chemo to try to kill any remaining cancer cells with toxic "*poisons*." And they will finish off with radiation, to "*burn*" whatever cancer cells remain. This is why I, and many others, refer to the "Big 3" protocol as "***Slash, Poison, and Burn***." This is the toxic protocol that we have all been misled to believe is the best way to treat cancer.

Now, with modern advancements in medicine, one would think that the "Big 3" have improved the prognosis for cancer, right? Aren't we curing a greater percentage of people with cancer now as compared to 1950? The answer is a resounding "**NO!**" As a matter of fact, the track record of the "Big 3" is so pathetic that the Cancer Industry considers it a "success" if the survival rate of patients who take the "Big 3" actually matches the survival rate of patients who do nothing at all! Each of these treatments is invasive, has devastating side effects, and treats only **symptoms**, not the **causes** of the cancer.

The fact is that the "Big 3" causes the spreading and recurrence of cancer! According to the September 21, 1989, isue of the *New England Journal of Medicine*, "*Secondary cancers are known complications of chemo therapy and irradiation used to treat Hodgkin's and non-Hodgkin's lymphomas and other primary cancers.*" Dr. Lucian Israel, a well-known oncologist, noted in his book, Conquering Cancer, that several studies have shown that cancer patients who undergo radiation therapy are more likely to have their cancer metastasize to other sites in their bodies. The radioactivity used to kill cancer cells also triggers the process of DNA mutation that creates new cancer cells of other types.

In his book, The Cancer Industry, Dr. Ralph Moss states: "*In 1902, a German doctor recorded the first case of human cancer caused by radiation: the tumor had appeared on the site of a chronic ulceration caused by X-ray exposure. Experimental studies performed in 1906 suggest that leukemia (cancer of the blood) could be caused by exposure to the radioactive element radium. By 1911, 94 cases of radiation-induced cancer had been reported, more than half of them (54) in doctors or technicians. By 1922, over 100 radiologists had died from X-ray-induced cancer . . . I had a brain cancer specialist sit in my living room and tell me that he would **never** take radiation if he had a brain tumor. And I asked him, 'But, do you send people for radiation?' and he said, 'Of course. I'd be drummed out of the hospital if I didn't'.*"

"*Complications following high-dose radiotherapy for breast cancer are: fibrous, shrunken breasts, rib fractures, pleural and/or lung scarring, nerve damage, scarring around the heart... suppression of all blood cells, immune suppression,*" according to Dr. Robert F. Jones, writing in the *Seattle Times* on July 27, 1980. He continues, "*...Many radiation complications do not occur for several years after treatment, giving the therapist and the patient a false sense of security for a year or two following therapy. The bone marrow, in which blood cells are made, is largely obliterated in the field of irradiation...This is an irreversible effect.*" In his book, Understanding Cancer, Dr. John Laszlo (a former VP of research for the ACS) indicates that when chemotherapy and radiation are given together, secondary tumors are **25 times** more likely to occur than the normal rate.

According to a study published in the *Archives of Internal Medicine (2009)*, computed tomography (CT) scans cause at least 29,000 cases of cancer and 14,500 deaths in the USA every year. In the study, researchers found that people may be exposed to four times as much radiation as estimated by earlier studies. Based on those higher measurements, a patient could get as much radiation from one CT scan as 74 mammograms or 442 chest x-rays!

Virtually all cancer surgery is unnecessary. According to Dr. Patrick McGrady, "*Even though it's been proven conclusively that lymph node excision after radiation does not prevent the spread of cervical cancer, you will still see lymphadenectomies performed all over the country routinely. This despite the fact that lymphadenectomies make women feel so bad they wish they were dead-and are a proven useless procedure.*" (*Townsend Letter for Doctors*, June 1984, p. 99)

Surgery is oftentimes responsible for the spread of the cancer, since a minute miscue or careless handling of tumor tissue by the surgeon can literally spill millions of cancer cells into the cancer patient's bloodstream. Biopsies can also result in the spread of cancer. According to Dr. William Donald Kelley in his book <u>One Answer to Cancer</u>, "*Often while making a biopsy the malignant tumor is cut across, which tends to spread or accelerate the growth. Needle biopsies can accomplish the same tragic results.*"

A 1986 report in the *New England Journal of Medicine* assessed progress against cancer in the United States during the years 1950 to 1982. Despite progress against some rare forms of cancer, which account for one to two percent of total deaths caused by the disease, the report found that the overall death rate had increased substantially since 1950. "*The main conclusion we draw is that some 35 years of intense effort focused largely on improving treatment must be judged a qualified **failure**.*" The report further concluded, "*We are **losing the war** against cancer.*"

You see, when President Nixon declared the "war on cancer," researchers were given access to billions of dollars of research money earmarked for cancer drug research. So, if you are a medical doctor who makes money through publishing cancer research, you better not challenge the status quo (*i.e.*, the "Big 3"), because if you do, then you are likely to have your funding pulled. For example, in 1966, Dr. Irwin D. Bross and four colleagues published a series of groundbreaking articles entitled "*Is Toxicity Really Necessary.*" In these articles, they merely questioned whether it was possible to find an alternative to chemotherapy and radiation, since chemo and radiation are both so toxic. The result: they promptly lost their government support for drug testing studies.

Chemotherapy is toxic, carcinogenic (causes cancer), destroys red blood cells, devastates the immune system, and kills vital organs. How toxic is chemotherapy? Think about it...your hair falls out, your immune system is destroyed, you are constantly nauseated, you get sick and vomit, you are frequently dizzy, and you have severe headaches. Are these signs that maybe this stuff is poison and doesn't belong in your body? I'm no doctor, but this sure does seem like a very strange way to "heal" someone.

One of the problems is that we're being duped by the Medical Mafia and the Cancer Industry with phony statistics, bad science, and fraudulent studies. According to Webster Kehr at www.cancertutor.com, "*The uselessness of surgery, chemotherapy and radiation is hidden behind a maze of very sophisticated false and misleading statistics, misleading definitions, meaningless concepts and many other techniques.*"

Once you "slice and dice" the phony statistics of the Cancer Industry, you will learn that the true cure rate (*i.e.,* 5-year survival) for chemotherapy is barely over 2%. As a matter of fact, according to a study conducted by the Department of Radiation Oncology at Northern Sydney Cancer Centre and published in the December 2004 issue of *Clinical Oncology*, the actual impact of chemotherapy on a 5-year survival rate in American adults is a paltry **2.1%.** See the chart below. www.ncbi.nlm.nih.gov/pubmed/15630849

Malignancy	ICD-9	Number of cancer in people aged > 20 yrs	Absolute Number of 5-year survivors due to chemotherapy	Percentage 5-year survivors due to chemotherapy
Head and neck	140–149, 160, 161	5139	97	1.9
Oesophagus	150	1521	82	4.9
Stomach	151	3001	20	0.7
Colon	153	13936	146	1.0
Rectum	154	5533	189	3.4
Pancreas	157	3567	–	–
Lung	162	20741	410	2.0
Soft tissue sarcoma	171	858	–	–
Melanoma	172	8646	–	–
Breast	174	31133	446	1.4
Uterus	179–182	4611	–	–
Cervix	180	1825	219	12
Ovary	183	3032	269	8.9
Prostate	185	23242	–	–
Testis	186	989	373	37.7
Bladder	188	6667	–	–
Kidney	189	3722	–	–
Brain	191	1824	68	3.7
Unknown primary site	195–199	6200	–	–
Non-Hodgkin's lymphoma	200 + 202	6217	653	10.5
Hodgkin's disease	201	846	341	40.3
Multiple myeloma	203	1721	–	–
Total		154971	3313	**2.1%**

Sadly, the truth is that many people who "die from cancer" really die from the conventional treatments long before they would have actually died from the cancer itself. To put it plainly, **the treatment kills them before the cancer kills them.** As a matter of fact, the chemotherapy drug "5FU" is sometimes referred to by doctors as "5 feet under" because of its deadly side effects. For most adult cancers, the typical **best case** scenario is that the "Big 3" buys a little time. In a **worst case** scenario, you will die from the treatment rather than the disease.

Thanks to Mike Adams and *www.NaturalNews.com* for the cartoon above.

But don't take it from me, here's what Dr. Allen Levin says about this topic: *"Most cancer patients in this country die of chemotherapy. Chemotherapy does not eliminate breast, colon, or lung cancers. This fact has been documented for over a decade, yet doctors still use chemotherapy for these tumors."* That's right, the "Big 3" have actually been shown to shorten life in many instances.

In his book, <u>The Topic of Cancer: When the Killing Has to Stop</u>, Dick Richards cites a number of autopsy studies which have shown that cancer patients actually died from conventional treatments before the tumor had a chance to kill them. Just think about it. Chemotherapy has always been developed from toxic poisonous chemicals, right? So, there has always been a fine line between administering a "therapeutic dose" and killing the cancer patient. Many doctors step over that line. In his book, <u>When Healing Becomes a Crime</u>, Kenny Ausubel notes that in a trial on a chemotherapy drug tested for leukemia, a whopping 42% of the patients died directly from the toxicity of the chemotherapy drug!

It's interesting to note that chemotherapy drugs were initially derived from the nitrogen mustard gas experiments during World War I and World War II. It was noticed that exposure to mustard gas caused destruction of fast growing tissues, thus it was surmised that since cancer grew quickly, these poisons could kill cancer tissue. Well, they were right...exposure to these gases did kill cancerous tissue. Make no mistake about it, chemotherapy and radiation **do** shrink the size of tumors and they kill cancer cells. But is shrinking a tumor equivalent to curing cancer? Is there a direct correlation? The answer is "**no**."

According to Dr. Ralph Moss, *"If you can shrink the tumour 50% or more for 28 days you have got the FDA's definition of an active drug. That is called a response rate, so you have a response...(but) when you look to see if there is any life prolongation from taking this treatment what you find is all kinds of **hocus pocus** and song and dance about the disease free survival, and this and that. In the end there is no proof that chemotherapy in the vast majority of cases actually extends life, and this is the **great lie** about chemotherapy, that somehow there is a correlation between shrinking a tumour and extending the life of the patient."*

Here are the facts. In 1942, Memorial Sloan-Kettering Cancer Center quietly began to treat breast cancer with these mustard gas derivatives. **No one was cured**. Chemotherapy trials were also conducted at Yale around 1943 where 160 patients were treated. Again, **no one was cured.** But, since the chemotherapy did shrink tumors, researchers were so excited that they proclaimed the chemotherapy trials to be a "success." I suppose that we need to define exactly what "success" means, don't we?

In a courageous letter to Dr. Frank Rauscher (his boss at the NCI), Dr. Dean Burk condemned the Institute's policy of continuing to endorse chemo-therapy drugs when everyone knew that they caused cancer. He argued: *"Ironically, virtually all of the chemotherapeutic anti-cancer agents now approved by the Food and Drug Administration for use or testing in human cancer patients are (1) highly or variously **toxic** at applied dosages; (2) markedly **immuno-suppressive**, that is, destructive of the patient's native resistance to a variety of diseases, including cancer; and (3) usually highly **carcinogenic**...These now well established facts have been reported in numerous publications from the National Cancer Institute itself, as well as from throughout the United States and, indeed, the world."* (4/20/73 *Letter to Frank Rauscher*, Griffin, "Private Papers")

In his book, Questioning Chemotherapy, Dr. Ralph Moss writes, "*The amount of toxic chemicals needed to kill every last cancer cell was found to kill the patient long before it eliminated the tumor...I remembered the story of a celebrated Sloan Kettering chemotherapist who, when he found out that he had advanced cancer, told his colleagues, 'Do anything you want -* **but no chemotherapy**.*' It was an open secret that an official of Sloan Kettering sent his mother to Germany for alternative treatment...Perhaps the strangest thing about chemotherapy is that many of these drugs themselves are carcinogenic. This may seem astonishing to the average reader – that cancer-fighting drugs themselves cause cancer. Yet this is an undeniable fact.*"

According to Dr. John Diamond, "*A study of over 10,000 patients shows clearly that chemo's supposedly strong track record with Hodgkin's disease (lymphoma) is actually a lie. Patients who underwent chemo were 14 times more likely to develop leukemia and 6 times more likely to develop cancers of the bones, joints, and soft tissues than those patients who did not undergo chemotherapy.*" (*NCI Journal* 87:10) The March 21, 1996, issue of the *New England Journal of Medicine* reported that "*children who are successfully treated for Hodgkin's disease are 18 times more likely later to develop secondary malignant tumours. Girls face a 35% chance of developing breast cancer by the time they are 40 – which is 75 times greater than the average. The risk of leukemia increased markedly four years after the ending of successful treatment, and reached a plateau after 14 years, but the risk of developing solid tumours remained high and approached 30% at 30 years.*"

Do you think that your oncologist would submit himself to chemo if he were diagnosed with cancer? The McGill Cancer Center in Montreal, one of the largest and most esteemed cancer treatment centers in the world, surveyed 64 oncologists to see how they would respond to a diagnosis of cancer. The results will blow your mind. Are you sitting down? Fifty-eight (58) said that chemotherapy was unacceptable to them and their family members due to the fact that the drugs don't work and are toxic to one's system. (Philip Day, Cancer: Why We're Still Dying to Know the Truth) That means 91% of the oncologists would **not** take chemo themselves! Do you think they know something they are not telling the general public?

In the addendum to the 2nd edition of his book, The Persecution and Trial of Gaston Naessens, Christopher Bird describes his personal encounters with several physicians who were well aware they were treating patients with protocols that did **not** work. "*Thirteen of the doctors who called me were eager to know how they could get access to treatments such as those devised by Gaston Naessens for* *themselves, their wives, or their relatives to treat grave cases of cancer with which they had become afflicted. In each case, I interjected my own question: 'Doctor, how come you're not advising yourself (or those close to you) to go the same prescription route you've been recommending for so long to your patients? Chemotherapy, or radiation, or the like?' And each time, though phrased slightly differently, the answer came back:* **'Because we know it doesn't work!'** *When I heard this answer, sometimes voiced late at night, I wondered if I were living in a world gone medically mad."* www.hbci.com/~wenonah/new/naessens.htm

Cancer is a disease which always results from a compromised immune system. Chemotherapy is known to devastate the immune system. Herein lies the conundrum: **How can you cure a disease which results from a compromised immune system with a drug which further compromises the immune system?** Think about that. It makes no sense whatsoever!

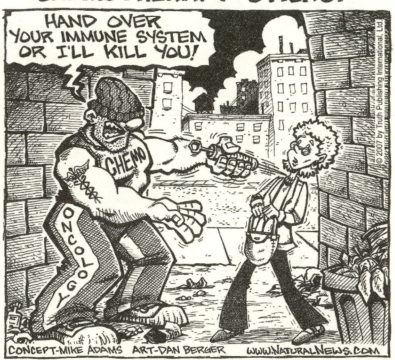

Thanks to Mike Adams and *www.NaturalNews.com* for the cartoon above.

In the 1980s, Dr. Ulrich Abel, a German epidemiologist, did a compreh-ensive analysis of every major study and clinical trial of chemotherapy that has ever been done. To insure that he didn't leave anyone out, he contacted over 350 medical centers worldwide requesting them to furnish him with anything they had published on the subject of cancer. By the time he published his report, it is likely that he knew more about chemotherapy than any person in the world. The results were amazing! In his report, published in *The Lancet*, August of 1991, Dr. Abel stated, *"Success of most chemotherapies is appalling...There is **no scientific evidence** for its ability to extend in any appreciable way the lives of patients suffering from the most common organic cancer...Chemotherapy for malignancies too advanced for surgery, which accounts for 80% of all cancers, is a **scientific wasteland**."* Of course, the Medical Mafia immediately attacked Dr. Abel's character since they couldn't attack his science. This is standard operating procedure. Not surprisingly, no main-stream media outlet ever mentioned Abel's comprehensive study: **it was totally buried.**

Dr. Glenn Warner, who died in 2000, was one of the most highly qualified cancer specialists in the United States. He used alternative treatments on his cancer patients with great success. On the treatment of cancer in this country he said: *"We have a multi-billion dollar industry that is killing people, right and left, just for financial gain. Their idea of research is to see whether two doses of this poison is better than three doses of that poison."* Dr. Alan C. Nixon, past president of the American Chemical Society asserts, *"As a chemist trained to interpret data, it is incomprehensible to me that physicians can ignore the clear evidence that chemotherapy does much, much more harm than good."* According to Dr. Charles Mathe, French cancer specialist, *"If I contracted cancer, I would never go to a standard cancer treatment centre. Only cancer victims who live far from such centres have a chance."*

Yet, day after day, year after year, the Cancer Industry continues to put these toxic chemicals into the bodies of cancer patients. And the patients let them do it, even volunteering for new "guinea pig" studies, simply because someone with a degree from a school of disease (also known as medical school) told them it was their *"only option."* It costs lots of money for them to poison the body of cancer patients, and the patients gladly pay it. Sadly, some people will spend six figures a year poisoning their bodies because their *"doctor told them to do it."*

I wasn't surprised to learn that recent research indicates that pharmacists who dispense chemotherapy are in danger of "second hand chemo." The July 10, 2010, edition of the *Seattle Times* reported: *"Danish epidemiologists used cancer-registry data from the 1940s through the late 1980s to first report a significantly increased risk of leukemia among oncology nurses and, later, physicians. Last year, another Danish study of more than 92,000 nurses found an elevated risk for breast, thyroid, nervous-system and brain cancers. ...A just-completed study from the U.S. Centers for Disease Control (CDC) – 10 years in the making and the largest to date – confirms that chemo continues to contaminate the work spaces where it's used and in some cases is still being found in the urine of those who handle it."*

People who live in glass houses should never throw stones, they say. And you might similarly say that pharmacists who deal in chemical poison shouldn't be surprised to one day discover they are killing themselves with it.

In the words of Mike Adams, *"Treating cancer with chemotherapy is like treating alcoholism with vodka. It's like treating heart disease with cheese, or like treating diabetes with high-fructose corn syrup. Cancer cannot be cured by the very thing that causes it. Don't let some cancer doctor talk you into chemotherapy using his fear tactics. They're good at that. So next time he insists that you take some chemotherapy, **ask him to drink some first**. If your oncologist isn't willing to drink chemotherapy in front of you to prove it's safe, why on earth would you agree to have it injected in your body?"* www.naturalnews.com/029191_secondhand_chemotherapy_cancer.html

MANIPULATING THE TERMS

Is the media lying when they say that we are winning the war on cancer? In a word, "**yes**," but only because the Cancer Industry has been lying to the media. The Cancer Industry tells us that due to advancements in chemotherapy, people are living longer. **This is a lie.** They have been able to perpetuate this myth by manipulating the data and the terms.

Dr. John Bailer, who spent 20 years on the staff of the NCI and was editor of its journal, sheds some light on this subject: *"The five year survival statistics of the American Cancer Society are very misleading. They now count things that are not cancer, and, because we are able to diagnose at an earlier stage of the disease, patients falsely appear to live longer. Our whole cancer research in the past 20 years has been a total failure. More people over 30 are dying from cancer than ever before... More women with mild or benign diseases are being included in statistics and reported as being 'cured.' When government officials point to survival figures and say they are winning the war against cancer they are using those survival rates improperly."* www.ghchealth.com/chemotherapy-quotes.html

Here is how G. Edward Griffin puts it in his book <u>World Without Cancer</u>: "*It is clear that the American Cancer Society – or at least someone very high within it—is trying to give the American people a good old-fashioned* **snow job**. *The truth of the matter is – ACS statistics notwithstanding – orthodox medicine does not have 'proven cancer cures,' and what it does have is pitifully inadequate considering the prestige it enjoys, the money it collects, and the snobbish scorn it heaps upon those who do not wish to subscribe to its treatments.*"

The Cancer Industry uses snobbery, bigotry, intimidation, and manipulation to keep cancer patients completely ignorant of the truth concerning the toxic "Big 3" treatments and the non-toxic alternative cancer treatments. As the old saying goes, "*He who defines the terms wins the argument.*" Here is how the Cancer Industry has been manipulating the data and re-defining the terms (*i.e.*, lying to us) about the effects of the "Big 3":

➢ The Cancer Industry has defined the term "cure" to apply to a cancer patient who survives over five years from the date of diagnosis. It does not mean "healed" nor does it mean "free of cancer." Due to improve-ments in cancer diagnosis, we are now able to see a tumor months if not years earlier than we could previously with sophisticated blood tests and imaging equipment. As a result, patients are now living longer from the point of diagnosis, since diagnosis happens earlier. However, if a patient develops the same cancer again after the period is up, or if they are disfigured by the disease or treatment, or if they drop dead two days after the period is up, they are still deemed to be "cured."

➢ The Cancer Industry typically omits certain groups of people from their statistics and includes certain groups based upon what will make their statistics look more favorable for the "Big 3." That's right. They choose the sample. For example, lung cancer patients are typically excluded from their statistics, despite the fact that lung cancer is the leading cause of cancer death. And certain cancers like non-melanoma skin cancers are **always** included in their samples, since 99% of non-melanoma skin cancer patients live over five years, so they increase the "cure" percentage. Fishy, huh?

➢ The Cancer Industry typically will remove a patient who dies during a "Big 3" treatment protocol from the population of the sample. What does this mean? It means that if there are ten patients on a chemotherapy protocol which is to last sixty days, and nine of them die before the sixtieth day while only one patient makes it to the end of the treatment, then the nine are removed and the treatment is said to have a 100% cure rate!

➢ Another trick the Cancer Industry uses in their statistics is to ignore counting people who die from the effects of the "Big 3." In other words, let's say you have chosen chemotherapy, and as a result of your newly compromised immune system, you catch pneumonia and die. Well, did you know that your death will likely **not** be counted as a death from cancer? That's exactly what happened to my mom. The cancer "treatment" caused her to have a massive stroke, and her death certificate indicates "death from stroke." So, in the warped perspective of the Cancer Industry, despite the fact that she is now dead, my mom's cancer treatments were a success. How twisted is that?

➢ Also, the Cancer Industry tells us that if a chemotherapy drug shrinks the size of a tumor, then it must be considered effective. But what does effective mean? Does it mean that the patient will live longer? **No**. It has been well documented that shrinkage of a tumor has little to do with a longer survival rate.

TUMOR TIZZY

The Cancer Industry is in a "tumor tizzy." Most oncologists are so obsessed with shrinking the size of a tumor that they miss the mark completely. You see, chemotherapy does shrink tumors; that is true. However, despite the fact that oncologists are successfully able to shrink tumors, oftentimes the cancer patient still dies. But why? The reason is the tumor size has nothing do to with curing cancer. A tumor is like the "check engine" light in your car. It appears only after a problem has developed, but the light itself is not the problem. Do you smash the light, or do you attempt to fix the underlying problem? A tumor is just a signal that something has gone terribly wrong in the body. It is just the tip of the iceberg.

According to Webster Kehr: *"Orthodox medicine, with its focus on the highly profitable tumor, has brainwashed the public into thinking that the tumor is the cancer. I have actually seen orthodox web sites that say that tumors are made exclusively of cancer cells. All of this is* **hogwash**. *A tumor cannot be made exclusively of cancer cells any more than a house can be made exclusively out of crude oil. Cancer cells* **cannot** *form tissue. There is* **no way** *a tumor can be made exclusively out of cancer cells. Cancer cells reside in the tissue of the tumor. That is why they do biopsies. Thus, if you kill the cancer cells in the tumor, the tumor is nothing but a harmless piece of tissue! With alternative cancer treatments, little, if any, attention is paid to the size of the tumor. If the tumor gets a little bigger, for many types of cancer that is no big deal. It is the* **cancer cells in the tissue of the tumor** *that are important, not the tissue itself. But it is not even the cancer cells in the tissue of a tumor that threatens the life of the patient ... it is the* **spreading** *of cancer that kills cancer patients. Nothing in orthodox medicine deals with the spreading of the cancer."*

In his book, <u>Alive and Well,</u> Dr. Binzel states that in primary cancer (with only a few exceptions) the tumor is neither health endangering nor life threatening. What is health endangering and life threatening is the spread of cancer through the rest of the body. **There is nothing in surgery** today that will prevent the spread of cancer. **There is nothing in chemotherapy or radiation** that will prevent the spread of cancer. How do we know? Just look at the statistics. The survival time of a cancer patient today is no different to what it was half a century ago. The only advancement in the last 50 years has been the improvement on ways to kill tumors via chemo and radiation.

By focusing only on the tumor and not the real cause of the cancer (*i.e.*, a weakened immune system), mainstream cancer treatments have left the *"fox in the henhouse"*...and he will most certainly strike again! According to Binzel: *"The problem with many (not all) Doctors and Oncologists in today's society is that they have been trained to be 'tumor orientated' ... For example, when a patient is found to have a tumor, the only thing the doctor discusses with that patient is what he intends to do about the tumor...no one ever asks how the patient is doing. In my medical training, I remember well seeing patients who were getting radiation and/or chemotherapy. The tumor would get smaller and smaller, but the patient would be getting sicker and sicker. At autopsy we would hear, 'Isn't that marvelous! The tumor is gone!' Yes, it was, but so was the patient. How many millions of times are we going to have to repeat these scenarios before we realize that we are treating the **wrong thing**?"*

IS YOUR HOUSE ON FIRE?

Suppose you own a nice, comfortable, $300,000 house in the country, but near a small city. While you have gone to the store, your house catches on fire. As you return home, you see that two rooms of your house are in flames and the fire is spreading. You immediately call the fire department. Twenty minutes later three fire trucks show up. The men and women in the first fire truck pull out heavy suits and axes and run to the house and start cutting down parts of the house that have already burned. They furiously cut; when they have cut out about 10% of the parts of the house that have already burned, they quit and go back to their fire truck.

You note that they did absolutely nothing to stop the spreading of the fire. What they cut out wasn't even burning and it certainly had nothing to do with stopping the raging fire. You watch the men and women in the second fire truck pull out a fire hose and started spraying a powder on the fire. The amount of powder they were spraying did not seem to you to be enough to put out the fire. But you notice that while the powder is slowing down the spreading of the fire, it is also severely damaging the parts of the house that are not on fire.

Puzzled, you ask the fireman what the powder is. They say it is a very toxic acid that is capable of putting the fire out, but they can't spray very much of it on the fire because if they did, the entire house would be reduced to a pile of rubble by the acid. Thus, all they can do is slow down the spreading of the fire, but they can't stop the spreading of the fire. Even more puzzled, you ask them why they did not bring water in their fire truck. They said that using water on a house fire is an old "wives tale" and water is not effective. They state the government regulatory agency, the Fire Development Administration (FDA) has researched water and has declared that water is an "unproven" method to put out house fires.

You silently mumble to yourself that there must be a huge underground connection between the FDA and the chemical companies. While you have been talking to the men and women in the second truck, five men have jumped out of the third fire truck. They ask you where the couch is in the living room. You point in the general direction of the couch in the living room, which you assume by now is on fire. Each of them immediately pulls out a 30-06 caliber rifle and starts shooting at the couch from where they are standing next to their fire truck. You scream at them and ask them what they are doing. They respond that they have been taught that couches are very bad to have in a house during a fire, so they are trying to shoot the couch to pieces. They comment: "*We think we are doing some good.*" You say that even if the couch is helping spread the fire, that they are blowing holes in the front and back of the house trying to shoot the couch to pieces from outside the house.

While the spreading of the house fire did slow down because of the toxic acids, within two hours you no longer have a house. The fire men and women are quite proud that they slowed down the fire. They tell you that your house lasted an extra hour because of their work. They give each other "high fives," get in their fire trucks, and head back to the fire station. Between the fire, the acid and the bullets, your house has been reduced to rubble. The cutting out of the wood that had already burned, by the first fire truck, had absolutely no effect on stopping the fire. In fact, nothing stopped the spreading of the fire, it only slowed it down. You are astonished at what you have seen. You ponder why the "investigative journalists" have not jumped on this situation. Then you realize how much the chemical companies advertise on television, and you realize why the "investigative journalists" have kept their mouths shut. A week later, as you drive by the fire department, you notice that all of the cars in the parking lot are very expensive cars. A month later you know why they are driving very expensive cars. They have sent you a bill for their services: $100,000. But they note in the bill that the house insurance company will pay most of the bill. You are puzzled when you look at your house insurance policy and realize the insurance company will not pay the bill if the fire department uses water.

"Is Your House on Fire?" was written by Webster Kehr and it brilliantly illustrates the sheer inadequacy of the "Big 3." Of course, the first fire truck represents surgery, the second fire truck represents chemotherapy, and the third fire truck represents radiation. ***Slash, Poison, and Burn.***

Despite the fact that the "Big 3" conventional cancer treatments are toxic, immunosuppressive, and carcinogenic, oncologists continue to prescribe this treatment protocol. But why? **Follow the money trail.** The "Big 3" treatments are the foundation of a multi-**billion** dollar business. Sadly, if you have cancer and choose the "Big 3," the odds indicate that you will die from complications of the treatment before you have time to die from your cancer. Ironically, in a demented kind of way, I guess you could say that the "Big 3" cancer treatments **do** prevent many cancer patients from dying from **cancer** ... They die from the **"treatments"** instead.

THE KATIE WERNECKE STORY

Katie Wernecke was diagnosed with Hodgkin's lymphoma (cancer of the lymph nodes) in January 2005 when she was only 12 years old. Her parents took her to the emergency room with what they believed was pneumonia, but it turned out to be much worse. Doctors persuaded them that Katie needed chemotherapy, and they acquiesced. However, doctors recommended radiation as well, but the Werneckes refused. Katie is quoted as saying, *"I don't need radiation treatment. And nobody asked me what I wanted. It's my body."*

In an effort to force the Werneckes to submit Katie to conventional cancer treatments, the modern-day "governmental Gestapo" (Child Protective Services) took Katie away from her parents in 2005, after receiving a tip that Katie and her mother were hiding out at a family ranch in order to avoid the radiation that doctors claimed she needed to survive. Authorities promptly took Katie into custody and arrested her mother on charges of interfering with child custody. That's right, the Texas government kidnapped a child from her family in order to poison her, and then they arrested her mother for attempting to keep her child from being poisoned.

Her mother had to pay $50,000 bail to get out of jail. Imagine that...$50,000 for protecting your own child! This is ludicrous! I have heard of murderers who were out on less than $50,000 bail! In addition to kidnapping her daughter, CPS placed her three sons in a foster home. Attorneys for the Texas Department of Family and Protective Services have stated in court that the Werneckes are "medically neglectful" for refusing radiation. Apparently, these attorneys are blissfully unaware of the irony of that statement. In late 2005, a Texas judge ruled that the Werneckes would be "allowed" to take Katie out of state to consult with alternative cancer doctors, but not before she underwent five more days of chemo-poison. Eventually, Katie was released and reunited with her family. Fortunately, the chemotherapy did not kill Katie, and she survived despite this horrible cancer treatment. This story is a prime example of how the Medical Mafia is out of control.

If you think that we live in a "free" society, think again. Right now, under the direct supervision of ill-advised cancer specialists, a judge can order CPS to kidnap your own kids from your own home, haul them into hospitals, and drip chemical toxins into their veins!

According to Mike Adams: *"This is not a system of health care at all, folks. It's a system of control. How do you control a population? Drug them, from cradle to grave. Keep 'em in a mental haze. Bewilder them with television images. Bankrupt them with medical bills. And if they don't comply, arrest them at gunpoint and terrorize their family to set an example. I call it state-sponsored medical terrorism. In this case, the state is Texas. Personally, I think that in a just society, the Texas CPS personnel would be arrested and charged with kidnap-ping, and the oncologists who took part in this cancer conspiracy would be tried in an international court for crimes against humanity. Is it not a crime to inject a child with deadly chemicals against her will and against her parents' will? If I loaded a syringe with the exact same chemicals used on this girl, and injected them into your arm without your permission, I would be (rightly) charged with attempted murder."* www.naturalnews.com/016387.html

THOMAS NAVARRO'S STORY

In the sobering and eye-opening documentary, *"Cut Poison Burn,"* producers Louis Cimino and Wayne Chesler bring to light the sinister nature of the multi-billion dollar Cancer Industry, the insidious nature of the Medical Mafia, the suppression of natural cancer treatments, and the "forced medication" of individuals who wish to choose their own personalized, natural forms of treatment.

At the core, the heartbreaking true story of Jim and Donna Navarro as they encountered road-blocks and a lack of freedom in choosing treatment options for their son Thomas, who (*at 4 years old*) was diagnosed with medulloblastoma, a malignant brain tumor. The conventional treatment methods, which included toxic chemotherapy drugs and radiation, offered virtually no hope. Even if their son survived the treatment, side effects could include hearing loss, brain damage, cumulative reduction in IQ and other cancers, just to name a few.

Rather than undergo conventional chemotherapy and radiation, the Navarros instead wanted to pursue an alternative route (*Dr. Stanislaw Burzynski's non-toxic antineoplaston treatment*) which has been shown to be particularly effective (50% to 60%) at treating brain cancers, but the FDA blocked them from getting this "unapproved" treatment. You see, if a child is under a certain age, then the Medical Mafia **requires** that he/she undergo the prescribed treatment regimen (i.e. toxic chemo and radiation) even though these forms of treatment are virtually useless at treating medulloblastoma. To add insult to injury, the state threatened Donna and Jim that if they did not subject him to these barbaric poisons, they would remove Thomas from their custody.

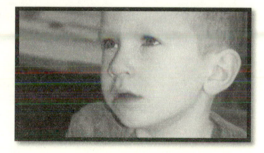

Like so many others, they realized that they were **not** free to seek whatever treatment they saw fit for their child. Yes indeed, the freedoms for which many of America's forefathers sacrificed their lives seem to have gradually eroded to this sad state of affairs. In the film, Jim Navarro makes a statement that really highlights the sheer ludicrousness of the current model of cancer care. Although the doctor admitted that chemotherapy "**would not work**" for their son's particular cancer, and the package insert stated that the drug "**has not been proven safe or effective for pediatric use**," he **still** insisted that chemotherapy had to be used, and if the Navarro's refused to submit their son to this "standard care," they could go to jail and their son could be legally taken from them. This is a dementedly inhuman game, where a child's quality of life and entire future is tossed aside in order to maintain a highly profitable status quo in the Cancer Industry.

After an 18 month legal battle with the Federal Death Administration and tens of thousands of dollars in legal expenses, the Navarros were finally "allowed" to take their son to Dr. Burzynski. However, by then he had already had his second brain surgery, and had already been forced to undergo chemotherapy, and had already suffered recurring tumors which were induced by the toxicity of the chemotherapy. Thomas died at the tender age of six. His death certificate states the cause of death as: *"Respiratory failure and pneumonia due to **chronic toxicity of chemotherapy**."* In the end, it was the chemo that killed Thomas ... **not** his brain cancer ...

How can we allow these murderers to get away with this? How can the death certificate state (unequivocally) that Thomas died from *"chronic toxicity of chemotherapy,"* but the doctors who administered the chemotherapy are **not** in jail? I am speechless.

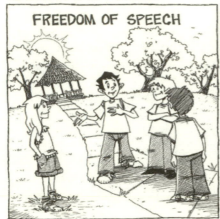
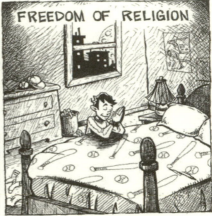
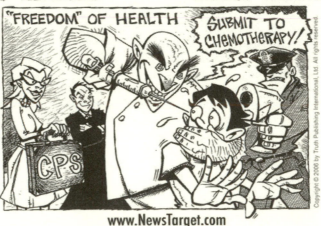

Thanks to Mike Adams and *www.NaturalNews.com* for the cartoon above.

PART 2

BIOLOGY BASICS

NON-TOXIC TREATMENTS

COMMON CANCERS

&

"CACHEXIA"

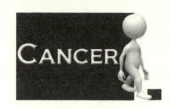

CHAPTER 5
BIOLOGY 101 & CANCER

> "CANCER DOES NOT CAUSE CELLS TO TURN ANA-
> EROBIC, BUT RATHER IT IS STABILIZED ANAEROBIC
> RESPIRATION THAT IS THE SINGLE CAUSE (*OR
> ESSENTIAL REQUIREMENT*) THAT TURNS THE NORMAL
> CELLS THAT DEPEND ON AEROBIC RESPIRATION INTO
> CANCER CELLS."   -DR. DAVID GREGG

Before we get into the causes of cancer, it is important that we obtain a grasp of the basics of biology as well as define the terms which will be used throughout the remainder of this book. So, let's get started, shall we?

CELL BIOLOGY

God has made our bodies in a miraculous way. Our heart pumps blood through our veins, arteries, and capillaries to every cell in our body. Imagine that your body is a country and the cells are its citizens. In order for the country to be strong, its citizens must have various jobs, proper tools to perform those jobs, proper nutrition to stay healthy, a transportation system, a communication system, a waste disposal system, a safe place to rest, and protection from toxins who wish to do them harm. Our goal is to provide our cells with all of these requirements.

Just like people, our cells come in all shapes and sizes, and they all have different abilities and jobs. But they are all essential to the health of your body. The "trash collector" cells are just as important as the "food server" cells and the "communication" cells. All of our cells are highly structured. At the center of a cell is its nucleus, which is basically the equivalent of a "brain." The nucleus is covered by a plasma membrane. Interestingly, other than red blood cells, all of the cells in our bodies have a nucleus.

Extending from the nucleus to the cell membrane (the "skin" of the cell) are cell fibers, which are basically the cell's scaffolding. These cell fibers also serve as the "muscles" of the cells, allowing the cell to contract and expand into different shapes. This ability to change shapes is called pleomorphism. In these cell fibers are embedded organelles, which are like "little organs," since each of them has a specific function. As I mentioned, the cell "skin" is called a membrane which is made of protein molecules. Some of these proteins act like a "name tag" to identify the type of cell, while other proteins act as a "door" to the cell.

Healthy cells are aerobic, meaning that they function properly in the presence of sufficient oxygen. Healthy cells metabolize (burn) oxygen and glucose (blood sugar) to produce adenosine triphosphate (ATP), which is the energy "currency" of the cells. This process is referred to as aerobic respiration (or aerobic metabolism). This cycle of creating energy, called the Krebs cycle, takes place in the mitochondria, which are organelles composed of an outer membrane and an inner membrane. The enzymes used to produce energy lie on top of the inner membrane.

ATP is composed of three phosphates. The breaking of the bond between the second and third phosphates releases the energy to power virtually all cellular processes. Amazingly, we all generate enough metabolic energy to produce our own body weight in ATP every day just to function! Every second, each of our approximately 60 trillion cells consumes and regenerates 12 million molecules of ATP, the production of which is the essential core function of every human cell. Without it, basic activities such as cellular repair, and protein, enzyme, hormone, and neurotransmitter synthesis would not occur. DNA repair and cell reproduction would cease. Many factors such as aging, poor diet, improper nutrition, and external toxins can impede this critical energy generation. Negatively charged electrons from hydrogen are the source of the energy needed to generate this staggering amount of ATP.

Once the ATP is produced, it is stored in the Golgi bodies of the mitochondria until it is needed by the cells for their activities. The byproduct of this energy making process is carbon dioxide. Carbon dioxide, in turn, is responsible for releasing oxygen from hemoglobin (the protein pigment in red blood cells). The oxygen then is burned to produce more ATP with more carbon dioxide byproduct, which is then used to extract the oxygen from hemoglobin. It's a miraculous state of continual perpetuity.

The immune system is a collection of cells, chemical messengers, and proteins that work together to protect the body from potentially harmful, infectious microbes such as bacteria, viruses, and fungi; thus, the immune system plays a role in the control of cancer and other diseases. Our remarkable immune system is composed of leukocytes (white blood cells), antibodies (proteins in the blood), the thymus, spleen, and liver. It even has its own network of vessels (the lymphatic system) which drains waste products from tissues and transports it from lymph node to lymph node where macrophages filter out debris.

Leukocytes are the body's "first line of defense." When foreign "invaders" enter the body, our immune system comes to the rescue in two ways:

1. Leukocytes directly attack the invader.
2. Antibodies either damage the invaders directly, or alert leukocytes to mount an attack.

There are two main subgroups of leukocytes. The first subgroup is called polymorphonuclear leukocytes (aka granulocytes). These leukocytes are filled with granules of toxic chemicals that enable them to digest microbes by a process called phagocytosis (literally "cell-eating"). Three types of granulocytes are neutrophils (which kill bacteria), eosinophils (which kill parasites), and basophils.

The second subgroup of leukocytes is called mononuclear leukocytes, which include both monocytes and lymphocytes. Monocytes ingest dead or damaged cells (through phagocytosis) and provide immunological defenses against many infectious organisms. Monocytes migrate into tissues and develop into macrophages. Macrophages contain granules or packets of chemicals and enzymes which serve the purpose of ingesting and destroying microbes, antigens, and other foreign substances.

Lymphocytes, found in the lymph system, are mononuclear leukocytes which identify foreign substances and germs (bacteria or viruses) in the body and produce antibodies and cells that specifically target them. It takes from several days to weeks for lymphocytes to recognize and attack a new foreign substance. The main lymphocyte subtypes are B-Cells, T-Cells, and NK ("natural killer") Cells.

AEROBIC VS. ANAEROBIC RESPIRATION

The cycle of creating energy is called the Krebs cycle and takes place in the mitochondria. Cells typically create energy via a process known as aerobic (*i.e.,* "with oxygen") respiration. However, if something happens which either inhibits the bloods ability to transport oxygen, lowers the amount of oxygen in the blood, decreases our carbon dioxide, prohibits the cells from absorbing the oxygen in the blood, or damages the mitochondria's ability to produce ATP, then the Krebs cycle has been disrupted, the cells have no energy, and we have a serious problem.

Since there is not enough oxygen for the cell to breathe, it changes to anaerobic (*i.e.,* "without oxygen") respiration to survive. According to Dr. David Gregg, *"Cancer does not cause cells to turn anaerobic, but rather it is stabilized anaerobic respiration that is the single cause (or essential requirement) that turns the normal cells that depend on aerobic respiration into cancer cells."* www.krysalis.net

The cell stops breathing oxygen and starts fermenting glucose (blood sugar) to make energy. The waste byproduct of the fermentation process is a sea of lactic acid, which further inhibits the cell from receiving oxygen. Calcium and oxygen are used up trying to buffer this acid. This is what enables a cancer cell to stabilize.

Anaerobic respiration is extremely inefficient and a severe drain on the body, since anaerobic cells must work much harder than aerobic cells to produce ATP from the glucose they metabolize. As a matter of fact, aerobic respiration creates as many as 36 ATP molecules from each glucose molecule, while **an**aerobic respiration creates only two ATP molecules. Thus, anaerobic respiration releases only 1/18 of the available energy. So, when we do the math, we calculate that in order for a cancer cell to obtain the same energy as a normal cell it must metabolize at least 18 times more glucose. Now do you see why we hear the phrase "cancer loves sugar?"

To be honest, the cancer cell has no possibility of actually utilizing 18 times more sugar to come up to the energy level of a good cell. Therefore, the cancer cell is chronically weak. This weakness prevents it from making the protective antioxidant enzymes [*superoxide dismutase (SOD), glutathione peroxidase (GPx), glutathione reductase (GR), and catalase*], thus leaving the cell wide open to oxidative attack by ozone.

As I've already mentioned, healthy cells metabolize oxygen and glucose to produce ATP while releasing carbon dioxide. Carbon dioxide, in turn, is responsible for releasing oxygen from hemoglobin, which are the red blood cells that transport oxygen from the lungs to cells. However, cancer cells cannot extract the oxygen from hemoglobin since their anaerobic respiration does not produce carbon dioxide which is required to get the oxygen out of the hemoglobin.

Now, different cells have different life spans. God created our neurons (nerve cells) to last our entire life, but He made our leukocytes to last only a couple of days. When cells are damaged, they can die prematurely; these dead cells are constantly being replaced to insure proper tissue function. This sort of cell replacement occurs constantly through a process known as mitosis, which is basically cell division where one cell divides into two smaller "daughter" cells. The new cells are structurally and functionally similar to each other. I say similar because the two daughter cells receive about half rather than exactly half of their parent cell's organelles. Much more important, however, is that each daughter cell inherits an exact replica of the DNA (heredity information) of the parent cell.

However, even though there is always a considerable amount of mitosis occurring, there is no real change in the total number of cells in our bodies. How does this happen? Well, in accounting lingo, your body has to *"balance its books."* Simply put, in order for the body to stay balanced, for every new cell that is generated via mitosis, another cell must die. Programmed cell death is a process referred to as apoptosis. Amazingly, every year the average human loses half of his/her body weight in cells via apoptosis!

Deregulation of apoptosis is associated with several diseases and syndromes, including cancer and AIDS. In the case of cancer, inhibition of the normal process of apoptosis can lead to the development of tumors, since cells that would normally have died live indefinitely. However, cancer is not necessarily a result of a problem with the p53 gene (which regulates apoptosis). The centers of solid cancer tumors are dead cells – no shortage of apoptosis in these tumors. It is the edges of growing tumors that are alive, where they can get a good supply of sugar, and not drown in their own lactic acid.

A cancer cell is described as being undifferentiated. What this means is that a cancer cell has no useful function. As a result, a cancer cell cannot become part of the tumor tissue itself, since tumor tissue must be composed entirely of healthy cells. The cancer cells just sit inside the tumor tissue, doing nothing except multiplying and refusing to die. However, what kills cancer patients is the **spreading of their cancer cells**. This is exactly why biopsies are so dangerous! Cutting the tissue can release the cancer cells into the bloodstream, thus enabling them to travel throughout the body! When the cancer spreads throughout the body, eventually there are enough cancer cells to kill a person.

Of course, cancer cells spread even without biopsy. There is a colonizing effort made with the spreading of "daughter" cells from the "mother" tumor. The daughter cells are mostly held in check by statins released by the mother, until the mother tumor is removed by surgery, or destroyed by radiation, whereupon the daughter cells have nothing to suppress them, and therefore start to grow.

Tumors have been shown to become self sustaining by creating their own blood supply. Angiogenesis is the process by which new blood vessels are formed and is a normal, essential process for biological development. However, angiogenesis is also required for cancerous tumors to grow. The primary initiating event for angiogenesis is a **lack of oxygen** (hypoxia). The growth of blood vessels is an external event, so that more sugar can be brought into the edges of the tumor, where the cells are alive. Many things can be done to inhibit angiogenesis, including taking large amounts of pancreatic enzymes. (*"Cells deprived of oxygen emit angiogenic signals." The Townsend Letter*, June, 2002, pg. 97)

According to Dr. David Gregg, *"The complex process of new blood vessel formation follows from there. In a way this makes sense in that one would expect a normal cell to respond in such a manner, not just tumor cells. In fact, that might be happening. Normal cells in the oxygen deficient environment of the anaerobic tumor cells may be creating the new blood vessels, not the cancer cells. **I have always wondered why all cancers are anaerobic in metabolism.** It is almost like it is a requirement. I think I now understand the answer. It is well-known that in order for tumors to grow they must form new blood vessels to supply the increased tumor size. If they can't do this they can't grow. This is a fundamental requirement for all cancers. If the angiogenesis theory...is correct, they have to create an oxygen deficient environment to stimulate the growth of new blood vessels. The anaerobic metabolism accomplishes this. Thus, anaerobic metabolism is not just a secondary consequence of cancer; it is a requirement for cancer to grow. Cells that are not anaerobic have no means of stimulating the formation of new blood vessels and thus cannot support tumor growth. Lacking this ability they would eventually die off."*

One scientist who contributed much to cancer research was P.G. Seeger, who published almost 300 scientific works and was twice nominated for the Nobel Prize. In the 1930s, he showed that cancer starts in the cytoplasm of the cell, not in the nucleus. The cytoplasm is the gel-like fluid inside the cell, and it provides a platform upon which other organelles can operate within the cell. All of the functions for cell expansion, growth, and replication are carried out in the cytoplasm of a cell. The cytoplasm contains the mitochondria, which are sometimes described as "cellular power plants," because they produce ATP through a series of steps which he called the "respiratory chain."

Seeger showed that in cancer cells, the respiratory chain was blocked by the destruction of important enzymes; thus, the cell can only produce energy **an**aerobically by converting glucose into lactic acid. In 1957, Seeger successfully changed normal cells into cancer cells within a few days by introducing chemicals that blocked the respiratory chain. Perhaps his most important discovery: certain nutrients have the ability to restore cellular respiration in cancer cells, thus transforming them back into normal cells. In other words, Seeger believed that cancer is reversible. One of these nutrients is the B vitamin inositol, which has been used (in conjunction with IP6) by University of Maryland Professor of Pathology, Dr. AbulKalam M. Shamsuddin, PhD to successfully revert cancer cells into normal cells.

German born Dr. Otto Warburg, a cancer biochemist and the 1931 Nobel Laureate in Medicine, first discovered that cancer cells have a fundamentally different energy respiration than healthy cells. He discovered that cancer cells are anaerobic; thus, whatever causes this anaerobic respiration to occur is the cause of all cancers. He believed that cancer occurs whenever any cell is denied 60% of its oxygen requirements, and showed that cancer cells exhibit anaerobic respiration. His thesis was that cancer is a fermentative disease caused by cells which have mutated from aerobic respiration to anaerobic respiration, resulting in glucose fermentation and uncontrolled cellular growth. He theorized that tumors are nothing more than walled-off toxic waste dumps inside the body sustained by fermenting sugar. According to Warburg, most, if not all degenerative diseases, are a result of lack of oxygen at the cellular level.

Some researchers claimed that Warburg's theory was not valid after they had measured a particularly slow growing cancer, and found no fermentation at all. Dean Burn and Mark Woods, two researchers at the National Cancer Institute, checked those results. Using more sophisticated equipment, they determined that the equipment these researchers used to measure fermentation levels was not accurate enough to detect fermentation at low levels. Using newer and more accurate equipment, Burn and Woods showed that even in those very slow growing cancer cells, fermentation was still taking place, albeit at very low levels.

THE pH BALANCE

"Indeed, the entire metabolic process depends on a balanced pH." (Dr. Robert Young, Sick & Tired, page 59)

After years and years of research, I have learned that, in addition to modulating the immune system, most successful non-toxic alternative cancer treatments have two other common denominators:

1. maintaining the acid/alkaline balance of our body
2. increasing the amount of oxygen at the cellular level

So let's take a quick look at these two concepts. Back in high school chemistry, we learned about our acid/alkaline balance, also referred to as the body's **pH** ("potential Hydrogen" or "powers of Hydrogen"). Our pH is measured on a scale from 0 to 14, with around 7.35 being neutral (normal). The pH numbers below 7.35 are acidic (with 0 being the most acidic) and the numbers above 7.35 are alkaline (with 14 being the most alkaline).

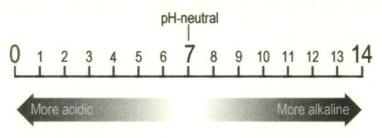

Hydrogen is both a proton and an electron. If the electron is stripped off, then the resulting positive ion is a proton. Without going into all the details about protons ("+" charge) and electrons ("-" charge), it's important to note that alkaline substances (also called "bases") are proton "acceptors" while acids are proton "donors." What does that mean to someone who isn't a doctor? Let me simplify it for you. Since bases have a higher pH, they have a greater potential to absorb hydrogen ions and vice versa for acids.

Why is hydrogen so important? Our universe is composed of millions of compounds, all derived from just 106 atoms. Of these elements, hydrogen is the first and most fundamental. Hydrogen is also the most abundant element, comprising 90% of all atoms in the cosmos. In our sun and stars, hydrogen nuclei fuse to produce helium, the second element. This generates the enormous energy that powers life on earth. And just as hydrogen fuels the sun, so, in the human body, it is the crucial factor in the electrochemical process that produces ATP, as we just discussed.

In chemistry, we know that water (H_2O) decomposes into hydrogen ions (H+) and hydroxyl ions (OH-). When a solution contains more hydrogen ions than hydroxyl ions, then it is said to be acid. When it contains more hydroxyl ions than hydrogen ions, then it is said to be alkaline. As you may have guessed, a pH of 7.35 is neutral because it contains equal amounts of hydrogen ions and hydroxyl ions.

Over 70% of our bodies are water. When cells create energy via aerobic respiration, they burn oxygen and glucose. I don't want to get overly scientific here, but the fact is that in order to create energy, the body also requires massive amounts of hydrogen. As a matter of fact, each day your body uses about ½ pound of pure hydrogen. Even our DNA is held together by hydrogen bonds. And since the pH of bases is higher, they have a greater potential to absorb hydrogen, which results in more oxygen delivered to the cells.

The hydrogen ion concentration varies over 14 powers of 10, thus a change of one pH unit changes the hydrogen ion concentration by a factor of 10. The pH scale is a common logarithmic scale. For those of you who never liked math, what this means is that a substance which has a pH of 5.2 is 10 times more acidic than a substance with a pH of 6.2, while it is 100 (10^2) times more acidic than a substance with a pH of 7.2, and it is 1,000 (10^3) times more acidic than a substance with a pH of 8.2, etc...

Our blood must always maintain a pH of approximately 7.35 so that it can continue to transport oxygen. Thus, God has made our bodies resilient with the ability to self-correct in the event of an imbalanced pH level through a mechanism called the buffer system. In chemistry, a buffer is a substance which neutralizes acids, thus keeping the pH of a solution relatively constant despite the addition of considerable amounts of acids or bases. However, due to our poor diet of junk foods, fast foods, processed foods, and sodas, most of us are putting our bodies through the ringer in order to maintain the proper pH in our blood. Although our bodies typically maintain alkaline reserves which are utilized to buffer acids in these types of situations, it is safe to say that many of us have depleted our reserves.

When our buffering system reaches overload and we are depleted of reserves, the excess acids are dumped into the tissues. As more and more acid is accumulated, our tissues begin to deteriorate. The acid wastes begin to oxidize ("rust") the veins and arteries and begin to destroy cell walls and even entire organs. According to Dr. Robert Young, "*A chronically over-acidic body pH corrodes body tissue, slowly eating into the 60,000 miles of our veins and arteries like acid eating into marble. If left unchecked, it will interrupt all cellular activities and functions, from the beating of your heart to the neural firing of your brain. Over-acidification interferes with life itself, leading to all sickness and disease.*" (Sick & Tired, page 59)

As we learned earlier, normal cells create energy via aerobic (with oxygen) respiration. Alkaline cells are able to absorb sufficient quantities of oxygen to support aerobic respiration. However, when cells become more acidic, less oxygen is absorbed, and the cells begin to ferment glucose in order to survive. This concept is essential to understand, because cancer cells thrive in an acidic, anaerobic environment and don't do very well in an aerobic, alkaline environment. Having an acidic pH is like driving your car with the "check engine" light on. It's a sign that something is wrong with the engine; and if we don't get it fixed, then eventually the car will break down.

According to Keiichi Morishita in his book, <u>Hidden Truth of Cancer</u>, as blood starts to become acidic, the body deposits acidic substances into cells to get them out of the blood. This allows the blood to remain slightly alkaline. However, it causes the cells to become acidic and toxic. Over time, he theorizes, many of these cells increase in acidity and some die. However, some of these acidified cells may adapt in that environment. In other words, instead of dying (as normal cells do in an acidic environment) some cells survive by becoming abnormal cells. These abnormal cells are called malignant cells, and they do not correspond with brain function or with our own DNA memory code. Therefore, malignant cells grow indefinitely and without order. **This is cancer.**

Putting too much acid in your body is like putting poison in your fish tank. Several years ago, we purchased a fish tank and a couple of goldfish for our children. After killing both goldfish, we quickly learned that the key factor in keeping fish alive is the condition of the water. If their water isn't just right, then they quickly die. We also learned that you can kill a fish rather quickly if you feed it the wrong foods! Now, compare this to the condition of our internal "fish tank." Many of us are filling our fish tanks with chemicals, toxins, and the wrong foods which lower our pH balance, and an acidic pH results in oxygen deprivation at the cellular level. As I have already mentioned, this is the beginning of degenerative disease.

Since we are beginning to understand what internal conditions make cancer cells thrive (an acidic pH and hypoxia), then it stands to reason that the opposite conditions (an alkaline pH and oxygen) should make cancer cells revert to being inert, or harmless. So, one way to make our pH more alkaline is to stop consuming things that make our bodies more acidic. A soda pop has a pH around 2, thus it is 100,000 (10^5) times more acidic than water with a pH of around 7. People that consume huge amounts of sodas (as well as coffee and alcohol) are typically very acidic and are "cancer magnets." One can of soda pop also reduces the immune response by 50% for a period of six hours!

So, what other things can we do to keep our tissue pH in the proper range? The easiest thing is to eat mostly alkaline foods. One of our favorite cookbooks is called <u>Back to the House of Health</u> by Shelly and Robert Young. The general rule of thumb is to eat 20% acid foods and 80% alkaline foods. Fresh fruit juice also supplies your body with a plethora of alkaline substances. You can also take supplements, such as potassium, cesium, magnesium, calcium, and rubidium, which are all highly alkaline.

Some excellent **alkaline-forming** foods are as follows: most raw vegetables and fruits, figs, lima beans, olive oil, honey, molasses, apple cider vinegar, miso, tempeh, raw milk, raw cheese, stevia, green tea, most herbs, sprouted grains, sprouts, wheatgrass, and barley grass. Foods such as yogurt, kefir, and butter are basically neutral. Several **acid-forming** foods are as follows: sodas, coffee, alcohol, chocolate, tobacco, aspartame, meats, oysters, fish, eggs, chicken, pasteurized milk, processed grains, sugar, peanut butter, beans, and pastas.

SOME STATISTICS

One American dies of cancer every minute! That's over 1,400 people per day – enough to fill four fully loaded jet planes. That's over half a million Americans each year. In his book, <u>Don't Waste Your Life</u>, John Piper quotes Ralph Winter on pages 115-116. *"Satan has, horrifyingly, employed his rebellious freedom in the development of destructive germs and viruses at the microbial level, which today account for 1/3 of all deaths on the planet...(however all of the) funded projects of the federal National Cancer Institute are focused on chemo and radiation treatment, not prevention. It's like getting caught up in 150 Vietnam wars at the same time – as far as battle deaths are concerned. And yet we act as though no war exists!* **How can the consciousness of America be aroused to the fact that 1/3 of all women and 1/2 of all men will contract cancer before they die?"**

Have you lost a loved one to cancer? It seems like everyone I know has cancer or has a loved one with cancer. Finding out that you or a loved one has cancer can be absolutely terrifying. When my father died in 1996, it inspired me to get to the bottom of what causes cancer and what treatments actually work to stop this terrible disease.

Consider these facts:

- ➤ Each year, we spray over a billion pounds of pesticides on our crops.
- ➤ We feed millions of pounds of antibiotics to our farm animals.
- ➤ We inject our cattle with cycle after cycle of growth hormone.
- ➤ We eat grains contaminated with mycotoxins (*fungal toxins*).
- ➤ We dump billions of tons of toxic waste into our waste sites and rivers.
- ➤ We unknowingly poison our children with vaccinations.
- ➤ We drink water that has been poisoned by chlorine and fluoride and other chemicals.
- ➤ We drink diet sodas contaminated with aspartame.

➢ We have mouths full of mercury fillings and root canals.
➢ We breathe air that has been polluted with "chemtrails."
➢ We let doctors destroy our bodies with x-rays.
➢ We smoke cigarettes and drink lots of alcohol.
➢ We eat mainly junk food, fast food, and processed food.

Is it any wonder we are sick all the time?

WHAT CAUSES CANCER?

God has miraculously made our bodies with trillions of living cells. Each cell is unique, has its own identity, and performs a specific task. In the body, these trillions of cells have to discover how to interact and work together in order to maintain health and vigor. Cancer cells are constantly being created in the body, but God has miraculously created our immune systems with the ability to seek out and destroy these cells. However, tumors begin when more cancerous cells are being created than an overworked, depleted immune system can destroy. Cutting out the tumor does not usually fix the problem. Remember, a tumor is just an uncontrolled growth of cells, and is just a **symptom** of cancer, not the cause.

However, tumors **do** have the ability to migrate to different parts of the body and grow out of control there as well, so I am not saying that tumors are irrelevant. They may compress surrounding structures, and their waste products may be toxic to the rest of the body. This being so, they oftentimes interfere with the function of organs such as the brain, liver, kidney, and lungs, thus resulting in death. Overcoming cancer is a process of reversing the conditions that allowed the cancer to develop. It is critical to note that cancer is a systemic imbalance. In other words, it is a problem with the entire system of the interrelated parts of the body. This being so, appropriate treatment must be for the total environment of the body.

There are many different theories on what actually causes cancer:

1. **The External Toxin Theory** – this theory holds that the proliferation of cancer cells is caused by external toxins, such as chemicals and other materials created largely from industry and carelessness. These chemicals have saturated our water, food, and the very air we breathe. You can't see, feel, or smell many toxins – at least, not right away. We don't realize their affects until we come down with a chronic disease (like cancer) after years of exposure. Over four billion pounds of toxic chemicals are released by industry into the nation's environment each year, including 72

million pounds of recognized carcinogens. The link between external toxins and cancer cells is irrefutable.

2. **The Microbe Theory** – this theory holds that cancer is caused by pleomorphic ("shape changing") microbes, such as fungi, yeasts, bacteria, and parasites. It is irrefutable that these pathogenic microbes are related to cancer. It is well-known and well documented that some fungal infections were actually misdiagnosed as leukemia. Many prominent researchers over the last century have observed cellular "pleomorphism" with the aid of dark field microscopes. Pleomorphism is based on the belief that fungi, molds, yeasts, and bacteria are all merely different stages in the life cycle of microbes.

3. **The Immune System Theory** – this theory maintains that cancer is fundamentally a disease of the immune system, and it takes root when your exposure to contaminants gets too high and/or the strength of your immune system drops too low. Quite simply, in your body, as part of the normal metabolic process, you produce anywhere from a few hundred to as many as 10,000 cancerous cells each and every day of your life. If your immune system is functioning properly, it has the ability to recognize each and every one of those aberrant cells and remove them from your body. The reason that everybody doesn't get cancer is because their immune systems are designed to prevent it. According to Jon Barron, *"That's just what a healthy immune system does."*

4. **The Hypoxia Theory** – this theory, based largely upon the research of Dr. Otto Warburg, holds that cancer is caused by a poor diet and lifestyle which results in toxic buildup, thus overloading the body's self-cleansing mechanism. Cancer is believed to be a manifestation of long-term nutritional and environmental irritation as well as a deficiency in the immune system, resulting in cellular oxygen starvation (hypoxia), leading to uncontrolled cell replication. Since oxygen is our main life force, it is understandable to think that a lack of it would cause damage to our bodies and organs. This fact is, of course, true.

5. **The Internal Rebel Theory** – this is the predominant theory of Big Medicine. This theory holds that the wild overgrowth of cancer cells is a kind of genetic rebellion within the body, where one's own cells rebel and destroy the body which produced them. Logically, if this theory is correct, then it only makes sense to do whatever it takes to squelch the rebel. This is why doctors try to cut and burn the cancer out of the body, or poison the cancer with toxic medicines, or send radiation throughout the body to kill these internal rebels. With orthodox medicine's adherence to the "internal rebel theory," the standard treatment protocols are **slash, poison, and burn**.

My research over the past decade has resulted in a theory, which is a synthesis of what causes cancer and also of what we can do to stop cancer. Summarized in a few words, I believe that the prime causes of cancer are a compromised immune system (created by an overload of toxicity) coupled with the replacement of the respiration of oxygen in normal body cells by a fermentation of sugar. In other words, **hypoxia** (lack of oxygen) at the tissue level and **immune failure** (oftentimes resulting from **toxicity**) and are the prime causes of cancer.

Of course, microbes are definitely associated with cancer. However, I used to believe that cancer was caused by microbes or fungi, but I now believe that microbes and fungi follow as the "cleanup crew." In other words, they are the resultants of hypoxia and immune system failure due to toxic overload. According to Dr. Saul Pressman, *"The cause of cancer is clear: poor diet, lifestyle and poor mental attitude result in toxic buildup which overloads the self-cleansing mechanism. Cancer is manifestation of long term nutritional and environmental irritation, resulting in cellular oxygen starvation, leading to uncontrolled cell replication."*

Under normal conditions, the cells of the human body function by burning sugar in oxygen to provide energy. The waste products are carbon dioxide and water. However, if there is insufficient oxygen at the cellular level, the burn will be incomplete, and anaerobic respiration will begin, forming carbon monoxide and lactic acid, which lower the intracellular pH of the cell. The body cannot easily rid itself of carbon monoxide since it prevents the hemoglobin from picking up fresh oxygen at the lungs, and the body temperature is lowered. The lactic acid can build up in the system, clogging nerve signal pathways, eventually crystallizing and causing degeneration.

Once anaerobic respiration has begun, it perpetuates and reinforces itself, due to the fact that the process doesn't produce carbon dioxide, which is responsible for extracting oxygen out of hemoglobin. Without oxygen, there is no carbon dioxide...thus there is no oxygen...thus there is no carbon dioxide...and the cycle continues. In this state of hypoxia, the oxygen-starved cancer cell rapidly duplicates and grows out of control. Many researchers believe that cell replication occurs as a result of damage to the p53 gene. This may be one of the reasons that cancer cells replicate, but it's definitely not the only reason. According to Dr. Stephen Ayre, *"...cancer cells get their energy by secreting their own insulin, and they stimulate themselves to grow by secreting their own insulin-like growth factor (IGF). These are their mechanisms of malignancy."*

Recent research by Dr. Gregg L. Semenza at Johns Hopkins University in Baltimore has shown that the reason why the cells replicate is not necessarily because there is damage to the p53 gene, but rather because the exposure of cancer cells to IGF causes them to self-stimulate and also induces the expression of hypoxia-inducible factor 1 (HIF-1) transcription factor, which controls oxygen delivery (via angiogenesis) and also metabolic adaptation to hypoxia (via fermentation). Some causes of hypoxia include a buildup of toxins within and around cells, which blocks and then damages the cellular oxygen respiration mechanism. Clumping up of red blood cells slows down the bloodstream and restricts flow into capillaries, which also causes hypoxia. Even lack of the proper building blocks for cell walls (essential fats) restricts oxygen exchange and leads to hypoxia.

UK Researchers from the Gray Laboratory Cancer Research Trust concluded, *"Cells undergo a variety of biological responses when placed in hypoxic conditions, including activation of signalling pathways that regulate proliferation, angiogenesis and death. Cancer cells have adapted these pathways, allowing tumours to survive and even grow under hypoxic conditions..."* (*Int'l Journal of Radiation, Oncololgy, Biology, Physics*, August 1986, p. 1279-1282). When the solid tumor is large enough and the disease progresses, cancer starts to invade other tissues. This process is called metastasis. Does poor oxygenation influence it? According to M. Kunz and S.M. Ibrahim, *"Tissue hypoxia has been regarded as a central factor for tumor aggressiveness and metastasis."* (Molecular Cancer 2003, p. 23-31)

WHY SOME GET CANCER AND NOT OTHERS

Let me ask you this question: **Why don't we have a forest fire each time that someone throws a burning cigarette out a car window**? There are many reasons why a burning cigarette may not start a forest fire.

1. Perhaps the cigarette falls on the pavement rather than the grass.
2. Perhaps there was a recent rain and the grass is wet and won't ignite.
3. Perhaps the grass is dry, but the cigarette is snuffed before it can start a fire.
4. Perhaps it starts a fire but the grass is surrounded by water and cannot spread into the forest.
5. Or perhaps a fire begins, but then the wind blows so hard that it blows the fire out.

In the burning cigarette example above (used with permission from Tanya Harter Pierce in her book <u>Outsmart Your Cancer</u>), the cigarette represents one of the many potential causes of cancer, like toxins, while the forest fire represents cancer. The pavement and the wet grass and the wind all represent the internal control mechanisms that prevent cancer, such as a healthy immune system, a balanced pH, and oxygenated cells.

Given the same exposure to the same toxins over the same period of time, someone with a healthy immune system may have no adverse effects while someone with a compromised immune system may develop hypoxia and eventually cancer. Do you follow my drift? We see the evidence of this truth constantly around us. One person in an office gets a very bad cold. The one sitting next to him doesn't get a sniffle. Certainly both were exposed to the same microorganisms. But what is the difference? One of them has a healthy immune system while the other does not.

Some people are better able to resist cellular mutations and damage by outside toxins and carcinogens. Perhaps their acid buffering systems are better suited to maintaining homeostasis within the body's pH system. So, despite years of exposure to external toxins, chemicals, tobacco, and eating a poor diet, they will not develop cancer, while others exposed to the same toxins will develop cancer. Human cancer is primarily attributable to chemical pollutants, horrible eating habits, and unhealthy lifestyles, not genetics, according to recent research by Paul Lichtenstein of the Karolinska Institute of Stockholm, Sweden, who led a giant study of 89,576 twins and reported results in the 2000 *New England Journal of Medicine*. The researchers found that even an identical twin has only a 10% chance of being diagnosed with the same cancer as his or her cancer-afflicted twin.

So, no matter what your genetic predisposition, there are a multitude of steps you can take to minimize your cancer risk if you don't have cancer, and there are scores of successful treatment protocols you can use if you do have cancer. Or, you can choose to bury your head in the sand, allow your irrational trust in Big Medicine to blind you from the truth, and think happy thoughts (like many of our friends have done).

HISTORY 101

In order to better understand the scientific basis behind my cancer theory, let's travel back in time to the 1850s and learn about the scientific "duel" of two Frenchmen – Louis Pasteur and Antoine Beauchamp. Both men had bacteriological theories of disease, but they disagreed about the origin and character of the bacteria. Little did they know that the winner of their duel would influence the course of medicine forever. Pasteur promoted what is referred to as the "germ theory" of disease. He hypothesized that disease arises from microbes outside the body (germs). He believed that each microbe has a constant shape and color (*i.e.,* monomorphic). He also believed that each disease and illness was caused by a unique microbe which entered the body, and that disease can only be caused by microbes or bacteria that invade the body from the outside. Therefore, the only way to cure diseases is to kill the invader.

Beauchamp promoted what is referred to as the "cellular theory" of disease. He hypothesized that disease arises from microbes within the cells of the body. He hypothesized that microbes can go through diverse stages of growth and they can mutate into various growth forms within their life cycle. In other words, he believed that the microbes were pleomorphic, which means "many forms." His theory was that when the host organism (*i.e.,* person) became unbalanced and unable to maintain homeostasis, then these microbes would mutate and become pathogenic. In other words, it is the condition of the host organism is the primary cause of disease. Beauchamp called these organisms "microzymas," meaning "small ferments." Beauchamp believed that the bacteria, microbes, viruses, and fungi that were being blamed as the **cause** of disease, were actually part of God's "clean-up crew," breaking down sick tissue and ultimately decomposing a no-longer-occupied body.

Claude Bernard, another French scientist, entered into the debate with the theory that it was actually the environment that is the determining factor in disease. He agreed with Beauchamp in his belief that microbes do mutate, but Bernard asserted that these mutations are all a result of the environment to which they are exposed. Therefore, Bernard's theory was that disease in the body is dependent upon the state of the internal biological terrain. Pasteur went to great lengths to disprove Beauchamp and Bernard's theory. Due largely to his wealth and political connections, he was able to convince the scientific community that his theory was correct, despite the fact that he had never been educated in science! However, on his deathbed, Pasteur admitted that his germ theory had flaws and that Bernard was correct. He said, "*Bernard was correct ...The terrain is everything.*" I think his pride prohibited him from admitting that Beauchamp was also correct, as he had been Pasteur's nemesis for so long. However, it was too little, too late. The mainstream scientists had already embraced his monomorphic germ theory.

In the 150 years since the birth of Pasteur's erroneous germ theory, it has become so widely accepted that it is seldom even discussed in conventional medical circles today. His theory was the genesis of modern allopathic (conventional) medicine, which claims that germs from an external source invade the body and are the first cause of infectious disease. The germ theory also gave birth to the technique of

vaccination in 1796 by Edward Jenner, who took pus from the running sores of sick cows and injected it into the blood of his patients. Thus, the vile practice of vaccination / immunization was born.

Unfortunately, conventional cancer treatments do not address the underlying conditions of cancer, such as our pH balance, immune system failure, and hypoxia (lack of oxygen) at the cellular level. Rather, conventional cancer treatment protocols focus on treating the **symptoms** of cancer, such as tumors. If you decide to pursue conventional treatments for cancer or even for the flu, you are doing nothing more than **gambling** with your health. Personally, I would prefer to utilize a natural cancer treatment, the most proven of which are outlined in the next few chapters.

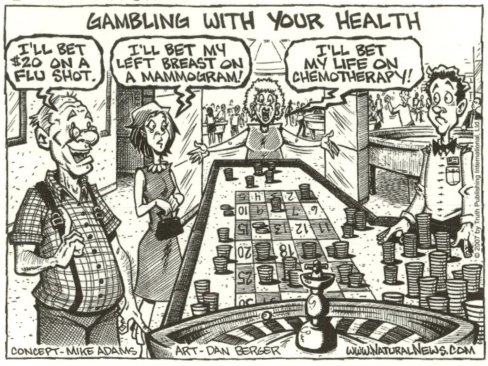

Thanks to Mike Adams and *www.NaturalNews.com* for the cartoon above.

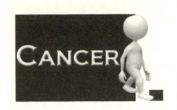

CHAPTER 6

NON-TOXIC TREATMENTS

> "ALL OF MY KNOWLEDGE IS LEARNED BY STANDING ON THE SHOULDERS OF GENIUSES."
> -DR. ALBERT SCHWEITZER

The reason I begin this chapter with this quote is that I want to make it crystal clear that these treatments are not "my" treatments, per se. They have been formulated and tested by medical mavericks and have been shown to be effective at treating cancer. I have merely summarized them for you in order to make all this information readily available and understandable, since it is next to impossible to successfully navigate the millions of websites on cancer, wade through the lies propagated by the Medical Mafia, and get to the truth on alternative cancer treatments.

This entire chapter is devoted to the non-toxic alternative cancer treatments which have been shown to be the most effective at treating **advanced cancer** (*i.e.*, Stages III and IV). The title of this chapter highlights the chief difference between conventional cancer treatments and alternative cancer treatments. Without exception, conventional cancer treatments are all toxic, while all successful alternative cancer treatments are **non**-toxic.

Back in 2006, the controlled mainstream press seemed downright giddy when Coretta Scott King (widow of Reverend Martin Luther King, Jr.) died of cancer after exploring an alternative cancer treatment clinic in Mexico. What the press didn't report is that conventional medicine had already given up on her and left her to die. It's no surprise she would want to check out alternatives. Sadly, she was too late.

The truth is that many patients only seek alternative care after they been "slashed, poisoned, and burned" by the "Big 3." Blaming an alternative cancer clinic for the death of a patient who was considered terminal when they walked in the door is like blaming an auto body shop worker for damaging the car you towed in after it was totaled in a high-speed collision. But unfortunately, this is the point at which most cancer patients finally decide to try alternative cancer treatments.

If you have cancer, the good news is that there is hope with alternative cancer treatments. **Real hope**. Not the false, dishonest, deceitful hope that doctors give you when they try to convince you that the "Big 3" treatments are the answer. Remember, that's what they have been taught in medical school, so that's all they know. But, you also need to remember to **follow the money trail**. When your doctor is skeptical about a new natural treatment, you can bet that he is only regurgitating the lies that he has read in the latest medical journal, sponsored by Big Pharma.

It is painfully obvious that the Medical Mafia has absolutely no interest in saving lives or in the truth. According to Walter Last, *"There is widespread suppression of natural cancer therapies, and persecution of successful therapists. The undisputed leader in this field is the USA, and other governments and medical authorities happily follow the US example. The rationale for this suppression is the claim that natural cancer therapies have not been scientifically proven to be effective, and such treatment, even if harmless, would delay the more effective conventional cancer treatment. This argument would be laughable if it were not so tragic for millions of sufferers."*

Why is there "no *official* scientific evidence" for alternative treatments? This is vital to understand. According to Webster Kehr, *"the reason there is no **official** 'scientific evidence' for alternative cancer treatments is that they are not highly profitable to Big Pharma. It is impossible, by law, for a substance to be considered to have 'scientific evidence' unless Big Pharma submits it to the FDA, and they will only submit things that are very, very profitable to them. Thus, the many thousands of studies of natural substances that have cured or treated cancer are not 'scientific evidence' and they are ignored by our government, because they were not done under the control of Big Pharma."*

However, despite the Medical Mafia's efforts to completely suppress and squelch the truth about alternative cancer treatments, sometimes the word still gets out about an effective treatment, thanks largely to the internet. But the Mafia is prepared for just such an occasion and has a standard operating procedure for these "leaks."

They typically handle them in one of the following ways:

➢ The testimonials are explained as "unreliable" or "anecdotal"
➢ The alternative cancer treatments are ignored and suppressed
➢ The patients are said to have undergone "spontaneous remission" unrelated to the alternative cancer treatment
➢ The patients are said to have actually been cured from the delayed effects of conventional cancer therapy which was administered before the alternative cancer treatment.
➢ The physicians who administer the alternative cancer treatment are persecuted

Do **not** believe the **lies** of the Medical Mafia! There are several non-toxic alternative cancer treatments that work with advanced cancer patients. However, due to the fact that Big Pharma pumps billions of dollars into the advertising each year, you are probably **only** familiar with the "Big 3" cancer treatments. And since most alternative cancer treatments are very inexpensive and non-patentable, they do not provide the Cancer Industry with a single penny of revenue; thus, they are relatively obscure.

Remember, the successful alternative treatments **target cancer cells** and **do not harm healthy cells**. This is a key difference between alternative cancer treatment protocols and conventional cancer protocols, which are not selectively toxic (*i.e.*, they kill all cells, including healthy cells). Big difference, isn't it? Alternative cancer treatments focus on cleansing the body and stimulating the natural immune system with special diets, supplementation, detoxification, and oxygenation.

Alternative doctors regard cancer as a systemic disease (one that involves the whole body); they focus on correcting the underlying **root** of the disease, not the tumor, which is merely a **symptom**. So why doesn't every doctor get on the bandwagon and begin to treat cancer with treatments that really work? Well, we live in the real world, don't we?

There are well over 300 non-toxic alternative cancer treatments that I have studied. This chapter focuses on the most effective of these 300 treatments. If you have advanced cancer, then you are considered to be "terminal." You do **not** have time to waste monkeying around with unproven cancer treatments. The clock is ticking! After careful consideration and voluminous research, I have detailed the most effective non-toxic cancer treatments in this chapter. Some of them are "stand alone" treatments while others can be combined.

If you had a six inch gash on your abdomen, you wouldn't treat it with a band aid. Neither should you treat advanced cancer with a less potent cancer treatment. If you have cancer and have been given up on by orthodox medicine, then please pay close attention to these treatments. Perhaps one of them will save your life.

The treatments in this chapter are listed in alphabetical order, not according to their success record. Honestly, these are the treatments that I would consider if I had advanced cancer. Guaranteed to work? **Sorry. No guarantees**. But if you have advanced cancer, you have likely already been given a guaranteed "death sentence" from your doctor and you have basically a **0%** chance of survival with conventional cancer medicine.

Unless otherwise specified, these advanced non-toxic cancer treatments **should never be combined**, except in a clinical setting. This is because the dosages for these treatments are established based on the ability of the body to rid itself of dead cancer cells. By combining these treatments at home, the number of dead cancer cells could be far too high and toxicity could occur.

If you decide to do one (or more) of these treatments at home, it is **vital** that you get a formal test (before, during, and after) to insure that the cancer is completely gone before stopping the treatment. I recommend the AMAS test. Unlike tests such as CEA and PSA, the AMAS test measures a well-defined antibody. Learn more at www.oncolabinc.com.

ALOE ARBORESCENS

In 1988, while presiding in the shantytown of Rio Grande dol Sul, Brazil, Father Romano Zago (a Franciscan friar and scholar) learned from local natives about a potent all-natural recipe derived from the Aloe arborescens plant which they used to promote supreme immune health. He began to recommend it to his friends and church, and this was where he first observed the positive results from Aloe arborescens.

Zago was sent to Jerusalem and Italy, where he continued to see great success in the improvement of the immune system of people who used the recipe made with the whole leaf of the Aloe arborescens plant which grows naturally in those regions. This inspired him to devote his life to research and education on the Aloe arborescens botanical and the Brazilian recipe for the benefit of mankind worldwide. Eventually, Zago published two books on the Brazilian Aloe arborescens recipe, which is as follows:

1. Half a kilo (1.1 pounds) of pure honey (*i.e.*, **not** synthetic or refined honey).
2. 350 grams (.77 lbs) of Aloe arborescens leaves (approximately 3 or 4 leaves, depending on their size),
3. 40 to 50 ml (6-8 teaspoons) of distillate (whisky, cognac, or other pure alcohol) to preserve the product and open the path for the main treatment to get all over the body by dilating the blood vessels. The distillate is only 1% of the formula, but it is very important.

The doses are measured in tablespoons, meaning one tablespoon is a single dose. The person takes one dose, three times a day (*i.e.*, three tablespoons a day). The doses are taken 10 to 20 minutes before a meal on an empty stomach. Shake the bottle very well just before pouring into a tablespoon. And remember that the product should **never** come into direct contact with sunlight. In fact, when taking the product try to avoid any type of light as much as possible. For example, after you pour the product into the tablespoon drink it immediately.

Generally, It should be stored in a cool, dark place. This treatment will clean your body (*i.e.*, detox). As with any protocol which releases toxins, there may be some uncomfortable experiences. A wide range of detox symptoms may be experienced. It is important that the patient does not stop the protocol until the cancer is completely in remission. Otherwise, the cancer will likely come back.

When made from scratch, this combination is mixed together in a blender, and because it is a pure plant product (with honey and a distillate), it can be added to any other non-toxic treatment. In fact, this is an excellent "supplemental" treatment to be used in conjunction with other protocols. Even though I hate to even mention the "c" word, this protocol can be combined with chemotherapy and may considerably reduce the side effects. This treatment has also been shown to alleviate radiation burns.

While the formula appears quite simple, if you actually want to make it at home there are many important rules about when to cut the leaves, how to process the leaves, etc. If you decide to make this formula at home, then you really need to read Zago's book entitled <u>Cancer Can Be Cured!</u> The book also features an encyclopedic bibliography of current information on the scientific studies and writings validating the healing and curative properties of Aloe arborescens. Zago cites numerous scientific articles which demonstrate Aloe's therapeutic and anti-tumor potential.

There has been much publicized scientific research and literature on the synergistic benefits of the 300 phytotherapeutic biochemical and nutrient constituents of Aloe vera to aid the body's defenses to enhance the immune system and protect against diseases. However, this is the first book to reveal the little known potency to be found in the constituents of its "cousin plant" species of Aloe arborescens, which contains 200% more medicinal substances than Aloe vera and almost 100% more anti-cancer properties.

Zago also wrote another book (for ailments other than cancer) entitled Aloe Isn't Medicine, and Yet...It Cures. If you don't want to make the product at home but would rather purchase Aloe arborescens, please contact Tom Waid at 800-665-3318 or visit the following website: www.aloeproductscenter.com.

BIO-OXIDATIVE THERAPIES

The body can survive weeks without food, days without water, but only minutes without oxygen. Our bodies are composed mostly of water, which is over 90% oxygen. Each cell of the body requires an incessant supply of oxygen to feed the chemical reactions that generate energy, detoxify waste products, and sustain production of the structural cell components. Remember Otto Warburg's Nobel Prize? It was based on his research of cytochromes in cellular respiration. He firmly believed that all degenerative diseases are a result of **lack of oxygen** at the cellular level. He is often quoted as saying, *"Cancer has only one prime cause. The prime cause of cancer is the replacement of normal oxygen respiration of body cells by an anaerobic cell respiration."*

Dr. Warburg pointed out that any substance that deprived a cell of oxygen was a carcinogen. In 1966, he stated that it was useless to look for new carcinogens, because the end result of each one was the same, cellular deprivation of oxygen. He further stated that the incessant search for new carcinogens was counter-productive because it obscured the prime cause, lack of oxygen, and therefore prevented appropriate treatment. Once the level of oxygen available to a cell drops below 40% of normal, the cell is forced to switch to an inferior method of energy production, called fermentation. The cell then loses its governor on replication because it is self-stimulating with growth factors (such as IGF) in response to **hypoxia**.

Simply defined, "oxidation" is the interaction between oxygen and any substance it contacts. Breathing oxygen is an "oxidative" process. There can be no life if oxidation does not occur. The body uses oxidation as the first line of defense against bacteria, viruses, yeast, and parasites. When we use the principals of oxidation to bring about improvements in the body, it is called "oxidative therapy."

Most biochemical reactions in the body are "balanced" through "redox" mechanisms. "Redox" means **red**uction **ox**idation. Anytime a substance is "reduced" (*i.e.*, gains electrons), something else must be "oxidized" (*i.e.*, loses electrons) for the reactions to stay "in balance." As an example, oxidation is the process that causes rust on metals (slow oxidation) or fire (rapid oxidation).

There are two simple natural substances whose clinical use has been documented in medical literature since the 1920s and which have been proven effective in treating some of our most common serious diseases, including heart disease, cancer, and AIDS. They are **hydrogen peroxide** (H_2O_2) and **ozone** (O_3), used in a therapeutic approach known collectively as "bio-oxidative therapies." The foremost researcher of bio-oxidative therapies, Dr. Charles H. Farr, was nominated for the Nobel Prize in Medicine in 1993 for his work.

The philosophy behind bio-oxidative therapies is a simple one. If the oxygen system of the body is weak or deficient (due to lack of exercise, poor diet, environmental pollution, smoking, or improper breathing), then the body is unable to adequately eliminate toxins. Bio-oxidative therapies are used to provide the body with active forms of oxygen (orally, intravenously, or through the skin) in order to eliminate toxins and fight disease.

Once in the body, the hydrogen peroxide or ozone breaks down into various oxygen subspecies, which contact **an**aerobic viruses and microbes (*i.e.*, viruses and microbes which have the ability to live without air), as well as diseased or deficient tissue cells. It oxidizes these cells while leaving the healthy cells intact. When the body becomes saturated with these special forms of oxygen, it reaches a state of purity wherein disease microorganisms are killed, while the underlying toxicity is oxidized and eliminated. The result is a stronger immune system and improved overall immune response.

Ozone was discovered by Fridereich Schonbein in 1840. It is oxygen in a "ménage á trios," an activated form of oxygen with three atoms. (Oxygen is O_2 whereas ozone is O_3.) Ozone was originally used to disinfect wounds during World War I. Ozone therapy accelerates the metabolism of oxygen and stimulates the release of oxygen atoms from the bloodstream. Over a period of twenty to thirty minutes, ozone breaks down into two atoms of regular oxygen by giving up one atom of singlet oxygen leaving a single, reactive oxygen atom. It is this oxygen singlet that does most of the work for a cancer patient.

153

It has been shown that ozone can "blast" holes through the membranes of viruses (HIV), fungi, yeasts, bacteria, and abnormal tissue cells (cancer cells) before killing them, without harming normal tissues. Ozone was the focus of considerable research during the 1930s in Germany, where it was successfully used to treat patients suffering from inflammatory bowel disorders, ulcerative colitis, Crone's disease, and chronic bacterial diarrhea.

Medical ozone is made from pure oxygen mixed with electrical energy (using an ozone generator) to form ozone. Ozone (O_3) has one extra molecule of oxygen (oxygen singlet) that doesn't want to be there, so it breaks off and tries to join other elements like carbon monoxide (which is deadly) and changes it into carbon dioxide (which the body knows what to do with). Our bodies love oxygen, so that extra oxygen singlet is gobbled up by everything that is good in the body and destroys all that is bad, because pathogens like bacteria, viruses, molds, fungi, parasites, and cancer hate ozone. After the extra singlet is gone, oxygen (O_2) is left.

So, how do you get the ozone into the body? One excellent method is via ozone IV (injecting a fluid saturated with ozone into the blood). Another effective method is autohemotherapy (via infusion bottle) where 10-15 mL of blood is removed from the body, saturated with ozone, and then put back into the body. Perhaps the most effective ozone therapy of all is the ozone sauna, with the dual application of ozone and hyperthermia. Direct injection is powerful, but not nearly as readily available as the ozone sauna, which virtually any person can apply at home to themselves and their family with excellent success.

Remember, it is the **energy** of ozone that does the work. That is why ozone has always been considered an electrotherapy. As Tesla said, oxygen is just the carrier to get electricity into the body. Ozone stimulates the production of cytokines. Cytokines are "messenger cells" such as interferons and interleukins, which set off a cascade reaction of positive changes throughout the immune system. The increased availability of oxygen in turn supports the metabolic and detoxification functions of all organs of the body.

As I have already mentioned, unlike the majority of bacteria, fungi, and viruses, God has miraculously designed our bodies to protect themselves against single reactive oxygen. The protection is provided through the cellular production of defensive enzymes [*superoxide dismutase (SOD), glutathione peroxidase (GPx), glutathione reductase (GR), and catalase*]. These enzymes require a good deal of energy to make, but the weak cancer cell doesn't have the energy to make them. Therein lays its vulnerability to singlet oxygen.

Thus ozone does not harm healthy cells, but has *"highly pronounced bactericidal, fungicidal and virostatic properties and is thus widely used in disinfecting wounds, as well as bacterially and virally produced diseases."* (R. Viebahn Haensler, <u>The Use of Ozone in Medicine - 3rd English Edition</u>, page 132) Ozone is selectively toxic, thus the end result is that ozone therapy kills harmful bacteria, viruses, fungi, and yeasts but leaves the healthy cells alone.

In the August 22, 1980, edition of *Science*, there was a report written by several medical doctors (Sweet, Kao, Hagar, and Lee) entitled: *"Ozone Selectively Inhibits Growth of Human Cancer Cells."* It stated, *"The growth of human cancer cells from lung, breast and uterine cancers was selectively inhibited in a dose-dependent manner by ozone at 0.3 to 0.8 parts per million of ozone in ambient air during eight days of culture. Human lung diploid fibro-blasts served as non-cancerous control cells. The presence of ozone at 0.3 to 0.5 parts per million inhibited cancer cell growth at 40 and 60% respectively. The non-cancerous lung cells were unaffected at these levels. Exposure to ozone at 0.8 parts per million inhibited cancer cell growth more than 90% and control cell growth less than 50%. Evidently the mechanisms for defense against ozone damage are impaired in human cancer cells."* The evidence from these doctors' research is irrefutable.

Both the EPA and the FDA acknowledge ozone's ability to oxidize over 99.99% of all waterborne pathogens. Ozone has been used for human health since 1860, and is presently employed in over 16 countries. Its widest use is in Germany, where over 7,000 doctors have treated more than 12,000,000 people since World War II. However, as you might expect, the FDA has not allowed testing of ozone, and has actively persecuted physicians who use it.

According to Dr. Hans Nieper, who used ozone in Hanover, Germany, *"You wouldn't believe how many FDA officials or relatives or acquaintances of FDA officials come to see me as patients in Hanover. You wouldn't believe this, or directors of the AMA, or ACA, or the presidents of orthodox cancer institutes. That's the fact."* Also, many well-known folks traveled to Germany to be treated by Dr. Nieper, including President Ronald Reagan, Sir Anthony Quinn, William Holden, John Wayne, Yul Brynner, and Princess Caroline of Monaco.

Hydrogen peroxide is involved in all of life's vital processes and must be present for the immune system to function properly. Colostrum (found in mother's milk) contains tremendously high concentrations of H_2O_2. The cells in the body that fight infection produce H_2O_2 naturally as a first line of defense against invading organisms (*i.e.,* parasites, viruses, bacteria, and yeast). Dr. Charles Farr has shown that H_2O_2 stimulates oxidative enzyme systems throughout the body, which triggers an increase in the metabolic rate, causes small arteries to dilate and increase blood flow, clears out toxins, raises body temperature, and enhances the body's distribution and consumption of oxygen. (*Proceedings of the International Conference on Bio-Oxidative Medicine*, 1989-1991) H_2O_2 also stimulates the production of white blood cells, which are necessary to fight infection.

In the 1950s, Dr. Reginald Holman conducted experiments involving the use of H_2O_2 added to the drinking water of rats that had cancerous tumors. The tumors completely disappeared within fifteen to sixty days. In the 1960s, European physicians began prescribing H_2O_2 to their patients. Before long, the use of H_2O_2 became an accepted part of the medical mainstream in Germany and Russia, as well as Cuba. In an article for a publication called *Alternatives*, Dr. Kurt Donsbach wrote: *"One ounce of 35% hydrogen peroxide (per gallon of water) in a vaporizer every night in an emphysemic's bedroom, and they will breathe freer than they have breathed in years! I do this for my lung cancer patients."*

Have you ever wondered why H_2O_2 foams when you put it on a wound? The reason why it foams is because blood and cells contain an enzyme called "catalase." Since a cut or scrape contains both blood and damaged cells, there is lots of catalase floating around. When the catalase comes in contact with hydrogen peroxide, it turns the hydrogen peroxide (H_2O_2) into water (H_2O) and oxygen gas (O_2). Catalase does this extremely efficiently -- up to 200,000 reactions per second! The bubbles you see in the foam are pure oxygen bubbles being created by the catalase.

One excellent method to administer H_2O_2 is as follows: weak, very pure H_2O_2 (0.0375% or lower concentration) is added to a sugar or salt-water solution, the same as used for intravenous feeding in hospitals. This is injected in doses from 50 to 500 mL into a large vein usually in the arm, slowly over a period of one to three hours depending on the amount given and the condition of the patient. It is painless, excluding the very small needle stick. Treatments are usually given about once a week in chronic illness, but can be given daily in patients with illnesses such as HIV and cancer. Your physician will determine the total number of treatments necessary to treat your specific condition. Over the past half century, tens of thousands of patients have received H_2O_2 treatment without serious side effects.

I want to emphasize very strongly that, for internal purposes, you should not use any type of hydrogen peroxide unless it is "35% food grade." The hydrogen peroxide you buy at the grocery store is only 3% and contains toxic chemicals. It is for **external use only**. Cancer patients should stay away from this form of H_2O_2. Also, cancer patients who use H_2O_2 internally should also use a quality proteolytic enzyme (such as Vitälzym) which will cut through the protein coating on the cancer cells and will enable the H_2O_2 to penetrate the cell wall. If you are on the Budwig Diet, you should avoid ingesting food grade H_2O_2 since the interaction of the fats with the H_2O_2 may cause stomach damage.

Oxycyclene ™ is a liquid composed of natural substances that works like an engine that forces the production of H_2O_2 within the white blood cells, resulting in the destruction of both the disease organism and the harboring white cell. Oxycyclene ™ utilizes the body's own natural defenses to recognize and annihilate the sick, diseased cells. Unlike vaccines and immunization, it is essentially free of side effects, and initial results have been extremely promising.

Almost 200 years ago, during the reign of Queen Victoria, people in India (a British colony then) found that H_2O_2 added in small amounts to drinking water cured a variety of sickness, including colds, flu, cholera, and malaria. This knowledge threatened the "British Big Pharma" drug sales, so Britain sent an "undercover" agent who masqueraded as a doctor and claimed that taking H_2O_2 causes viral brain damage. He even made up a story about a (nonexistent) child who supposedly died of brain damage after taking H_2O_2. Coming from a "doctor," the fabricated story was accepted as "truth," and the Indian people began purchasing the British drugs.

Sounds familiar, doesn't it? The same technique is still being utilized today by the Medical Mafia. Despite the voluminous amount of scientific data which validates the amazing chemical and biological effects of ozone and hydrogen peroxide, a large portion of the medical community continues to overlook or purposely ignore these incredibly simple and inexpensive treatments.

One clinic that uses bio-oxidative therapies is Dr. Frank Shallenberger's Nevada Center for Alternative and Anti-Aging Medicine, located in Carson City, Nevada. According to Dr. Shallenberger, both ozone and hydrogen peroxide actually increase the efficiency of the antioxidant enzyme system, which scavenges excess free radicals in the body. This then also enhances cellular immunity further. Their website is www.antiagingmedicine.com. Another excellent clinic is Caring Medical & Rehabilitation, run by Dr. Ross Hauser, located in Illinois. Their website is www.CaringMedical.com.

Lastly, if you decide to use ozone therapy, you must contact Dr. Saul Pressman, whom I call *"the Ozone Guru."* He moderates the following email group: *ozonetherapy@yahoogroups.com.* Just join the group and email Dr. Pressman with any questions. He is incredibly responsive and always willing to help. He also assisted me with the information in this section of the book.

BOB BECK PROTOCOL

The Bob Beck Protocol started out as an electromedicine treatment for AIDS; however, it has incredible potential for being a superb advanced cancer treatment.

Back in 1990, two medical doctors, Dr. William D. Lyman and Dr. Steven Kaali, discovered that a small electric current could disable microbes from being able to multiply, thus rendering them inert or harmless. This was one of the greatest discoveries in the history of medicine because virtually all diseases are caused by, or enhanced by, a microbe. The discovery was a cure for almost every disease known to mankind.

However, even though their technology is very well documented, orthodox medicine is not interested in their discovery. Orthodox medicine is interested in "treatments" **not** "cures" because "treating" a person is much more profitable than "curing" them.

Dr. Beck, who died in 2002, held a PhD in physics and had 30 years of electromedicine research behind him. He learned of Lyman and Kaali's discovery and found a non-invasive way to use it.

According to Dr. Beck, *"I read an article in Science News that was published March 30, 1991. On page 207, it described the "shocking" treatment proposed for AIDS by Albert Einstein College of Medicine in New York City, which had accidentally discovered a way to cure all AIDS. So I looked into this, and I found that a paper on an AIDS cure had been presented to a Joint Congress on Combination Therapies in Washington, D.C., on March 14, 1991, at the First International Symposium on Combination Therapy.*

*When I attempted to find a copy of this paper to see what it said, I found that they had all **vanished** or were cut out of the proceedings. We hired a private investigator who got a personal abstract copy from one of the conference attendees. I also did a computer search and found that the only other mention of this technology was in "Outer Limits" in Longevity Magazine which appeared in the December 1992, issue. It stated that Steven Kaali, M.D., from Albert Einstein College of Medicine, had found a way of inhibiting AIDS in blood, but that* *years of testing would be required before the virus-electrocuting device was ready for use. In other words, they discovered it and then tried to cover it up immediately.*

But a very funny thing happened. Two years later, a patent popped up. The U.S. Government Patent Office described the entire process. You can obtain Patent #5188738 in which the same Dr. Kaali describes a process, which will attenuate any bacteria or virus (including AIDS/HIV), parasites and all fungi contained in the blood, rendering them ineffective from infecting a normally healthy human cell. This is in a government document! This was in 1990! Why haven't they told the public about it? I decided if there was a sure-fire cure for AIDS, I had to find out about it.

When I looked into Dr. Kaali's work, I decided to go ahead and fund it. We found that it worked all of the time. For two and a half years, we gave full credit for this invention to Dr. Kaali, whose name is on the patent. Then I discovered that there was a long history of this technology. We followed a trail of these patents back 107 years! We found a patent, #4665898, that cured all cancer, dated May 19, 1987.

Why has this been suppressed? Why hasn't your doctor told you about an absolutely proven, established cure for cancer? The answer is that doctors get $375,000 per patient for surgery, chemotherapy, x-ray, hospital stays, doctors and anesthesiologists. This is the official statistic from the U.S. Department of Commerce. Unfortunately, the medical patient cured is a customer lost."

Dr. Beck's early research had to be done outside of the USA. His first electromedicine machine is called the Blood Purifier or Blood Electrifier. The Blood Electrifier creates a very small alternating electric current which destroys a key enzyme on the surface of a microbe and prevents the microbe from multiplying. The body safely excretes the disabled microbes.

However, Dr. Beck found out that in some cases, viruses were hiding in the body and were dormant, and thus were not circulating with the blood. He then developed his second electromedicine machine (the Magnetic Pulser) to disable those microbes which were not circulating in the blood. Dr. Beck's protocol also included colloidal silver and ozonated water. Since this protocol could potentially destroy the "friendly" bacteria in the digestive tract, you should consider adding some potent probiotics to your diet to help replenish them.

At least one person has been thrown in jail for selling Bob Beck Protocol equipment and two others have mysteriously died. Bob Beck believed that his treatment, which clearly removes every type of microbe from the body of a person, is a potent way to restore the immune system of that person. He felt that that was a large reason his treatment had been so successful on cancer patients.

IMPORTANT: No other alternative cancer treatment or orthodox cancer treatment can be used with the Bob Beck Protocol. All other cancer treatments must be stopped at least two days prior to starting the Bob Beck protocol. The Bob Beck Protocol must be used by itself. No prescription drugs, no herbs, etc. If you decide to use the Bob Beck protocol, please visit www.cancertutor.com/Cancer02/BobBeck.html. Be sure to study the list of "forbidden substances" as well as read the entire article.

BRANDT/KEHR GRAPE CURE

In the 1920s, Johanna Brandt of South Africa said she cured her stomach cancer with what she called The Grape Cure. A few years later, she wrote a fascinating book that revealed the specifics of how she rid herself of cancer. Basically, Brandt ate grapes ... lots of grapes ... including their skins and seeds. As it turns out, grapes have been show to contain a substance called **resveratrol.**

According to a well-known researcher, Dr. John Pezzuto of the University of Illinois at Chicago, this naturally occurring phenol "*has multiple modes of action, inhibiting cancer growth at a lot of different stages, which is unusual.*" It is also believed that resveratrol activates the p53 gene which induces apoptosis (normal cell death). In addition to resveratrol, grapes (especially purple Concord grapes) contain several other nutrients that are known to kill cancer cells, such as ellagic acid, lycopene, OPCs, selenium, catechin, quercetin, gallic acid, and vitamin B_{17}. **What an amazing cancer fighting arsenal!**

Since many things have changed since Brandt published her Grape Cure diet in the 1920s, I have adapted this diet based upon recommendations from Webster Kehr; thus, I have called it "the Brandt/Kehr Grape Cure." For example, the trace minerals in the soil have largely been depleted over the past half century, and chlorine and fluoride are now added to water supplies, just to name a few. I mention these items because all grape juice, including organic, may have been mixed with chlorine water. Also, all grape juice has been pasteurized, by law, thus destroying the enzymes which are critical to the digestion of grape juice. This being so, the Brandt/Kehr Grape Cure requires a certain amount of whole grapes.

A typical day on the Brandt/Kehr diet involves twelve hours of fasting followed by twelve hours of grape consumption. During the consumption period, you are supposed to consume absolutely nothing except for grapes, grape mush, and fresh squeezed grape juice, which should be consumed slowly over the twelve hour period, not just at meal times. During this period, you should consume between ½ gallon and one gallon of pure "grape mush" made from putting the grapes into a food processor. To avoid nausea and maximize the effectiveness of the grape mush, divide it into eight equal portions to be eaten slowly every 1½ hours of the twelve hour consumption period.

Be sure to drink at least a gallon per day of pure spring water or artesian well water, spread out over both twelve hour periods, and taken with the grape mush during the consumption period. Make sure your water is **not** treated with chlorine or fluoride. The grape juice mush should include crushed seeds and the skins, and the grapes should be purple Concord grapes. Don't buy seedless grapes or green grapes, as they don't have all the "goodies" that purple Concord grapes do. And purchase **organic** grapes if possible, since grapes are heavily sprayed with pesticides. If you are unable to obtain organic grapes, be sure to wash your grapes in warm spring water for at least fifteen minutes and rinse.

During the water fast, the cancer cells get very hungry. Then, when they finally do get food, what they get is grapes, which they gobble up since grapes contain high concentrations of natural sugar. And cancer cells love sugar! However, those same grapes also contain several major cancer killing nutrients listed above. So, in essence, we "fool" the cancer cells into ingesting an entire myriad of cancer-fighting nutrients. It's like putting poison in candy and then giving it to a starving child. And since cancer cells are extremely inefficient at producing energy, they require much more sugar than regular healthy cells, so they gobble up even more grapes! And as we learned previously, cancer cells consume eighteen times more sugar (and eighteen times more of the cancer-fighting nutrients found in grapes) than normal healthy cells. Thus, the Brandt/Kehr Grape Cure diet is one of the ultimate ways to **kill cancer cells**!

What supplements should be taken with the Brandt/Kehr Grape Cure?

1. Grape seed extract – check the ingredients to get the most OPCs.

2. Grape skin extract – check ingredients to get the most resveratrol.
3. Quercetin – available as an over the counter supplement.
4. Vitamin C – 12 to 15 grams spread out during the day (build up to this amount over two weeks, do **not** start out at 12-15 grams).
5. Cayenne pepper – as hot and as close to raw as possible.
6. Niacin – one gram per day.

Both cayenne pepper and niacin increase blood flow, which helps get the grape juice to the cancer cells. Cancer cells frequently thrive in areas where circulation is poor. What treatments can you use along with the Grape Cure? **Do not** use cesium chloride, since cesium blocks glucose from getting into the cancer cells, and the Brandt/Kehr Grape Cure uses the glucose as a transport agent for the cancer-fighting nutrients.

There is a six week cycle on this treatment. The first five weeks are the pure Brandt/Kehr Grape Cure treatment. Do not eat or drink anything other than grapes. **Period**. During the sixth week, eat only *raw* fruits and vegetables. The sixth week will allow certain other foods to be eaten. Repeat the six week cycle as many times as necessary to cure your cancer.

BUDWIG DIET

A remarkable alternative cancer treatment was devised by a German biochemist, Dr. Johanna Budwig, also a seven time Nobel nominee. Her most important medical contributions involved her research into the roles of essential fatty acids (EFAs). In order to mass produce and distribute foods high in oils, food manufacturers deliberately alter the chemical composition of the oils, which gives them longer shelf lives. In the 1950s, she proved that these chemically-altered, hydrogenated fats (which she called "pseudo" fats) are rigid fats which stick to the cell membranes, thus causing them to malfunction.

Dr. Budwig believed that these hydrogenated, processed fats and oils shut down the electrical field of the cells and make us susceptible to chronic and terminal diseases, since the beneficial oxidase ferments are destroyed by heating or boiling. She also demonstrated that the absence of essential unsaturated fats is responsible for the production of oxidase, which induces cancer growth and causes many other chronic disorders. She came to believe that cancer was not the result of too much cell growth, but defective cell growth (*i.e.*, cell division), caused by the combination of too much "pseudo" fats and too few healthy fats in the cell membrane.

But exactly what happens to fats when they are processed? In healthy fats there is a vital electron cloud which enables the fat to bind with oxygen. Healthy, oxygenated fats are capable of binding with protein and in the process become water-soluble. This water solubility is vital to all growth processes, cell damage restoration, cell renewal, brain and nerve functions, sensory nerve functions, and energy development. In fact, the entire basis of our energy production is based on lipid metabolism. Hydrogenation destroys the vital electron cloud and as a result, these "pseudo" fats can no longer bind with oxygen or with protein. These fats end up blocking circulation, damaging the heart, inhibiting cell renewal, and impeding the free flow of blood and lymph. It would be wise to remember this fact the next time you want to buy some margarine or fried foods, since both typically contain these harmful fats.

Dr. Budwig began to study fats in the 1950s, and she quickly discovered much more about the metabolism of fats than had previously been known. She began her research by analyzing the blood samples of thousands of seriously ill patients, and then she compared these samples to the blood of healthy people. She soon found that the blood of seriously ill cancer patients was deficient in certain important essential ingredients, including phosphatides and lipoproteins, whereas the blood of a healthy person always contained sufficient quantities of these ingredients. She hypothesized that the lack of these ingredients resulted in the proliferation of cancer cells. When she analyzed the blood of cancer patients, instead of finding healthy, red, oxygen-rich hemoglobin, she discovered a greenish-yellow substance. She found that when these natural ingredients were replaced, that the cancerous tumors began to shrink. The strange greenish elements in the blood were replaced with healthy red blood cells as the lipoproteins and phosphatides amazingly reappeared. She then discovered that eating a combination of two foods would replace the lipoproteins and phosphatides and turn the blood healthy again.

The two EFAs are linoleic acid (LA), an omega-6 fat, and alpha-linolenic acid (ALA), an omega-3 fat. Good health requires the proper ratio of omega-6 and omega-3 fats; the ideal ratio is around 2:1. Vegetables and nuts (corn, safflower, cottonseed, peanuts, and soybeans) are the highest in omega-6 fats. LA is the primary omega-6 fat, which a healthy human will convert into gamma linolenic acid (GLA). Other omega-6 fats include conjugated linoleic acid (CLA), dihomo-gamma-linolenic acid (DGLA), and arachidonic acid (AA). Ocean fish (such as salmon, tuna, and mackerel) and certain nuts/seeds (such as flax/linseed, and walnuts) are the highest in omega-3 fats. ALA is the principal omega-3 fat, which a healthy human will convert into eicosapentaenoic acid (EPA) and later into docosahexaenoic acid (DHA) and docosapentaenoic acid (DPA).

Budwig believed that chronic disease is a result of a body lacking EFAs, which are full of electrons and bind to oxygen and proteins. When they are absorbed into the cell wall, they pull oxygen into the cell. And when bound to sulfur-based proteins, they become water-soluble. **This is the theory behind the Budwig Diet: The use of oxygen in the organism can be stimulated by lipoproteins (sulfur-rich proteins and linoleic acid).**

On page 85 of his book, Oxygen Therapies, Ed McCabe discusses his point of view on EFAs: *"The red blood cells in the lungs give up carbon dioxide and take on oxygen. They are then transported to the cell site via the blood vessels, where, they release their oxygen into the plasma. This released oxygen is 'attracted' to the cells by the 'resonance' of the ... fatty acids. Otherwise, oxygen cannot work its way into the cell. 'Electron rich fatty acids' play the decisive role in respiratory enzymes, which are the basis of cell oxidation."* EFAs combined with sulfur-rich proteins (such as those found in cottage cheese) increase oxygenation of the body, since the electrons are naturally protected until the body requires the energy.

Of course, as you would expect, Dr. Budwig was persecuted for her work. Just think of the money generated each year from the fat and oil industry. The hydrogenation process is central to both of these industries, and Dr. Budwig's theory was based upon the foundation that hydrogenated fats contribute to the formation of cancer cells! Eventually, she was prevented from doing further research and prevented from publishing her findings. In her own words, *"I have the answer to cancer, but American doctors won't listen. They come here and observe my methods and are impressed. Then they want to make a special deal so they can take it home and make a lot of money. I won't do it, so I'm blackballed in every country."*

Several excellent sources of sulfur-rich proteins are nuts, onions, chives, garlic, and especially cottage cheese and yogurt. The flaxseed oil should optimally be virgin, cold-pressed, organic, liquid, refrigerated, and unrefined. One of the best brands is Barlean's Flaxseed Oil. The blend of flaxseed oil and cottage cheese should be a part of every cancer patient's diet. You simply mix one cup of organic cottage cheese with two to three tablespoons of flaxseed oil. Be sure to blend them together and let them sit for several minutes. This will convert the oil-soluble omega-3 into water-soluble omega-3. It is also a good idea to grind fresh flax seeds and add to the mixture. It is important to note that neither foods rich in EFAs nor sulfur-rich proteins **alone** will accomplish these tasks. This is because the oils must first bind to the proteins before oxygen can be bound and before the body can assimilate the combination.

Thanks to the tireless work of Dr. Budwig we now know that electron-rich fats interact with sulfur-rich proteins to bind oxygen and promote aerobic metabolism which restores health. According to oncologist and former cardiologist, Dr. Dan C. Roehm, *"What she (Dr. Budwig) has demonstrated to my initial disbelief but lately, to my complete satisfaction in my practice is:* **CANCER IS EASILY CURABLE,** *the treatment is dietary/lifestyle, the response is immediate; the cancer cell is weak and vulnerable. The precise biochemical breakdown point was identified by her in 1951 and is specifically correctable, in vitro (test-tube) as well as in vivo (real)... This diet is far and away the most successful anti-cancer diet in the world."* (*Townsend Letter for Doctors*, July 1990)

Bill Henderson has worked with over a thousand "terminal" cancer patients. The keystone to his treatment protocol is the Budwig Diet. His book, Beating Cancer Gently, is excellent as is his new book, Cancer-Free. Bill is a wonderful man and will "coach" you over the phone. His protocol includes some very advanced attributes that make it one of the most potent cancer treatments available. He really focuses on a strict cancer diet, which is one of the reasons that so many people have been cured using his treatment. And as the name says, it is also one of the most "gentle" treatments. Anyone who chooses the Budwig protocol should use Bill Henderson's protocol. His book may be purchased at www.beating-cancer-gently.com.

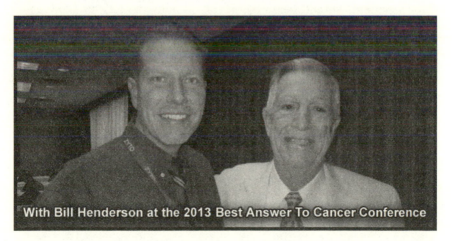

With Bill Henderson at the 2013 Best Answer To Cancer Conference

Please be aware that if you are on the Budwig Diet, you should **not** take Protocel™, since it works in the opposite manner. Also, do **not** take any product with Paw Paw or Graviola since these plants lower ATP and may offset the Budwig Diet.

CELLECT-BUDWIG

This section of the book focuses on **five cancer treatments** (to be used together) which comprise the Cellect-Budwig protocol. This is one of the most potent, non-toxic, and highly effective alternative cancer treatments.

The heart and soul of this treatment is Cellect, a multi-mineral, multi-amino acid, multi-vitamin supplement, with some anti-cancer products added. Cellect was designed by a biochemist named Fred Eichhorn who had "terminal" pancreatic cancer in 1976. He is still alive today and is the president of the National Cancer Research Foundation (www.ncrf.org).

By itself, Cellect has shown excellent results treating advanced cancer. Mike Vrentas, board member of the Independent Cancer Research Foundation, Inc. has added the Budwig Diet, Vitamin B_{17} (apricot seeds), and juicing to the Cellect, making it a very potent treatment.

#1 – Cellect Powder

As I mentioned, the key product in this protocol is a powder called Cellect, which has shown excellent results with all forms of cancer. Cancer patients should begin by quickly building up to four scoops per day. Children, of course, should take smaller doses. Advanced patients should build up to between six and eight servings per day. Cellect occasionally causes constipation, so be sure to take three of the Cod Liver Oil capsules (included with the Cellect) with each serving. Psyllium husk and fresh vegetable juice also helps to alleviate constipation.

Cellect can be purchased at www.cellect.org. Click on "products" then choose a "maxi-blend" powder. I recommend that you mix it with purple grape juice. They also sell the product as capsules.

#2 – The Budwig Diet

The previous section of the book detailed the Budwig Diet, so I won't spend much time here to reiterate. However, I will state emphatically that you should **not** take the Cellect and the Budwig Diet within 1.5

hours of each other. Also, be sure to take the cod liver oil with the Cellect and the flax oil with the Budwig Diet.

#3 – Vitamin B₁₇

I will spend several pages later in this chapter describing vitamin B_{17} so I won't spend much time here. The fact is that this vitamin is selectively toxic to cancer cells, so it fits perfectly with this protocol. It is recommended that you eat the apricot seeds rather than taking the pill form of the vitamin. According to Dr. Krebs, cancer patients should start with a few apricot seeds a day and build up to around thirty apricot seeds per day, preferably eaten on an empty stomach and spread throughout the day between meals, taking around ten seeds between breakfast and lunch, then ten more between lunch and dinner, then ten more at bedtime.

#4 – Organic Vegetable Juicing

As with the Budwig diet and vitamin B_{17}, I explain fresh juicing in another section of the book, so I won't go into too much detail here. Just remember that organic vegetable juicing is critical for two major reasons. First of all, vegetables are typically very high in cancer-fighting nutrients and phytochemicals. Also, by filling up on fresh, organic vegetable juice, you won't have as much room left for the toxic junk food that most folks love to eat, such as sodas, donuts, and chips. It is **not** necessary to do a juice fast, but cancer patients should drink (daily) about one ounce of fresh vegetable juice for every four pounds of body weight. So, a 200 pound person should have 50 ounces per day, a 160 pound person should have 40 ounces, etc. It is recommended that you drink the juice in several smaller amounts spread over the entire day, not drinking the entire juice at one sitting.

#5 – Sunshine (Vitamin D)

See the following chapters for more information on vitamin D. It is recommended that you get thirty minutes of sunshine each day, if possible. Do **not** use sunscreen, as it filters out helpful light and also **causes cancer.**

Liver Cleansing

I can say with 99% certainty that an advanced cancer patient on the Cellect-Budwig protocol will need to stimulate their liver to clean out toxins captured from other parts of the body. So, following the Gerson Therapy and Dr. Kelley's treatment, coffee enemas are recommended, since the coffee will open up the bile ducts and stimulate the production of bile in the liver. How many enemas per day? Well, some folks need a few and some need only one per day. It all depends on what kind of shape your liver is in. Most of us have livers that are overloaded with toxins, so it's quite likely that you'll need three or more enemas per day.

My friend, Mike Vrentas, is the alternative cancer researcher who developed this protocol. His website is www.CellectBudwig.com. If you decide on this treatment, you **must** visit Mike's website and listen to **all** of his CDs explaining this treatment. He is also available for telephone consultations.

DMSO/MSM/CESIUM CHLORIDE ("DMCC")

Dimethyl sulfoxide ("DMSO") is a highly non-toxic, 100% natural product that comes from the wood industry. Methyl sulfonyl methane ("MSM") is basically DMSO with an additional oxygen atom attached to the sulfur atom, forming a molecule with a total of two attached oxygen atoms. MSM occurs in fresh fruit and vegetables, raw milk, wheat grass juice, and aloe vera.

Both DMSO and MSM have the property of being quite soluble in both oil and water based liquids. In this book, I use the term "DMSO" to refer to both substances, since according to biochemist Dr. David Gregg, *"DMSO and MSM, which form each other in the body, should be essentially indistinguishable in their biochemical effects."*

DMSO, as a healing agent, was introduced in the 1960s by a research team headed by Stanley W. Jacob, M.D., at the University of Oregon Medical School. A study was conducted in which DMSO was mixed with a haematoxylon (a purple dye) and injected into patients with cancer. The purpose of the study was to determine which cells would attract the DMSO.

They learned that DMSO has an affinity for cancer cells. As a matter of fact, some of the cancer patients were cured during this study, even though DMSO was only being combined with a dye! ("Haematoxylon Dissolved in Dimethylsulfoxide [DMSO] Used in Recurrent Neoplasms" by E. J. Tucker, M.D., and A. Carrizo, M.D., June 1968) The study also showed that DMSO could not only dissolve substances, but it could also penetrate human skin and carry the dissolved substances along with it!

How does it work?   According to Dr. David Gregg, *"In the body DMSO forms equilibrium with MSM (the oxidized form of DMSO), and the combination becomes an oxygen transport system, enhancing aerobic metabolism. This operates at only one point, the respiratory chain (at the inner membrane of the mitochondria)."* www.krysalis.net

Over the past four decades, more than 10,000 articles on the biologic implications of DMSO have appeared in the scientific literature, and 30,000 articles on the chemistry of DMSO have also been published. The results of these studies strongly support the view that DMSO is a remarkable new therapeutic principle.   In his book, Cancer & Natural Medicine, John Boik cites a number of publications where DMSO solutions have caused numerous forms of cancer in vitro (outside the living organism) to differentiate, thus reverting into normal cells through reestablishing aerobic metabolism.

Once aerobic metabolism is reestablished, the previously cancerous cells will eventually be eliminated via apoptosis. Remember, apoptosis is programmed cell death that happens to most normal cells in a matter of a couple of weeks. Reestablishing aerobic metabolism with DMSO will not correct genetic damage, but holding the cancer cells in a normal state long enough gives the natural process associated with healthy cells (*i.e.*, apoptosis) time to kill the cancer cells. This is a bit of a paradox, but one way that DMSO kills cancer cells is through making them healthy.

Of course, with an effective alternative treatment, you can expect the Cancer Industry's cronies to go to work. According to Webster Kehr, *"The FDA took note of the effectiveness of DMSO at treating pain and made it illegal for medical uses in order to protect the profits of the aspirin companies (In those days aspirin was used to treat arthritis). Thus, it must be sold today as a 'solvent.' Few people can grasp the concept that government agencies are started for the sole purpose of being the 'police force' of large, corrupt corporations. Buying the souls of politicians is as easy as giving candy to a baby."* www.cancertutor.com/Cancer/DMSO.html

While DMSO has been called *"the most controversial therapeutic advance of modern times,"* the controversy seems to be based on politics and money rather than science. Honestly, I wish we lived in a world where physicians would treat cancer patients with the ***proper*** treatment rather than have patients treat themselves at home. Unfortunately, due to the influence of Big Pharma, physicians are using treatments that have been chosen solely on the basis of their profitability rather than their effectiveness. When you consider the fact that DMSO is not a patentable drug, is cheap, safe and effective, and knowing what you should know about the Cancer Industry, is it any wonder that there is a smear campaign against DMSO?

One of the most important attributes of DMSO and MSM is that they both work in synergy with other treatments, such as **cesium chloride**, which is the most alkaline mineral. It's a fact that many parts of the world that have high levels of strong alkaline minerals in their water have a very low incidence of cancer. The Hunzakuts of Northern Pakistan have water high in cesium and **never** develop cancer unless they move away from their homeland. The Hunzakuts also eat apricot kernels (which contain vitamin B_{17}) on a regular basis. I will discuss B_{17} therapy later in the book.

When cesium is transported into the cell, it is able to radically increase the intracellular pH of the cell. Once inside the cell, the cesium begins to pull potassium from the blood; thus, it eventually blocks the cell's intake of glucose, stops the fermentation process, and starves the cell. The cesium also neutralizes the lactic acid which is produced with anaerobic respiration, thus stopping the cell from proliferating and stopping the "cachexia cycle" at the cellular level.

Perhaps the most well-known physician to use cesium to treat cancer is Dr. H. E. Sartori. He began his cesium cancer therapy program in April 1981 at Life Sciences Universal Medical Clinics in Rockville, Maryland, where 50 patients with "terminal" cancer were treated. In other words, their cancer had metastasized to other organs, and they were sent home to die. The Cancer Industry labeled their conditions as "hopeless" and "terminal." Of the 50 patients, 3 were comatose, and 47 had already completed maximum dosages of the "Big 3" before cesium was tried.

Cesium chloride was given to patients, along with vitamin A, vitamin C, vitamin B_{17}, zinc, and selenium. The diet consisted primarily of whole grains, vegetables, and foods rich in omega-6 fats. To increase efficiency of the treatment and improve the circulation and oxygenation, the patients received the chelating agent EDTA and DMSO. The study included ten patients with breast cancer, nine with colon cancer, six with prostate cancer, four had pancreatic cancer, six had lung cancer, three had liver cancer, three had lymphoma, one had pelvic cancer, and eight had cancer from an unknown site of origin.

The results were astounding. Approximately 50% of patients with breast, colon, prostate, pancreatic, and lung cancer survived for at least three years, despite the fact that conventional doctors gave them only a few weeks to live! Thirteen (13) patients died in the first two weeks of therapy. Autopsy results in each of these thirteen disclosed reduced tumor size from the cesium therapy. Amazingly, pain disappeared in all the patients within one to three days after initiation of cesium therapy. The write up of these studies can be found in Dr. Sartori's book, <u>Cancer – Orwellian or Utopian?</u>

Considering the fact that cesium chloride is typically only used on advanced cancer patients, Dr. Sartori's fifty percent cure rate is astonishing. **Here's why**: All of the patients had already been given their "death sentence" by conventional doctors. They were labeled as "terminal" and sent home to die. They likely had damage to their major organs from the toxic chemo treatments and/or radiation. Yet, still half of them were saved! This is truly remarkable. Remember, the cure rate for similar advanced cancer patients by orthodox medicine is close to **zero percent**.

Dr. Keith Brewer (a physicist) became very interested in cancer in the 1930s. He discovered that **cancer cells have an affinity for cesium**. This fact is the reason that a radioactive isotope of cesium is commonly used as a "marker" to trace the movement of conventional chemotherapy drugs into a tumor. Introducing substantial amounts of cesium into the body, he reasoned, might cause a cancer cell to absorb enough to change its pH and disrupt anaerobic metabolism and the fermentation process it needed to stay alive.

After extensive testing, Brewer determined that cesium or rubidium could raise the pH of cancer cells. Ultimately he focused on cesium because it was the more alkaline of the two. The question, however, was how to get enough cesium into the cancer cell to change its pH. Brewer determined that there were a number of vitamins and minerals (including vitamin B_{17}) that greatly enhanced the absorption of these elements by the cancerous cells. By administering these substances in conjunction with the cesium, the level of the cesium absorbed was sufficient to kill the cancer cells.

Here's how: The cesium proceeded to alkalize the cancer cells, thus causing them to reestablish aerobic metabolism and causing cell replication to cease. It also caused normal apoptosis to occur within a few days. In 1981, tests were performed on 30 patients with cancer, and in all 30 patients, the cancerous tumors disappeared and the pain ceased within a couple of days. This protocol became the basis for what is now commonly referred to as "High pH Therapy." <u>www.mwt.net/~drbrewer/highpH.htm</u>

Remember the story of Neal Deoul? He had financed research on cesium and aloe vera to battle cancer and AIDS. He was sued and his name was dragged through the mud in a lengthy court battle initiated by the Cancer Industry. During the court battle, Deoul was diagnosed with cancer, and turned to a form of high pH therapy, which eventually cured him of cancer. **Great** news for alternative cancer treatments; **horrible** news for the Cancer Industry. Since their court battle began in the late 1990s, Neal and his entire family have been horribly persecuted by the Cancer Industry. Read more about their story here: www.cancer-coverup.com.

DMSO binds with cesium chloride to get inside of cancer cells. However, what DMSO is really used for is to get the cesium chloride through the skin into the blood stream. The DMCC protocol is especially effective with brain cancer patients because of how quickly it gets past the blood-brain barrier, but it can be used productively with any type of cancer.

In a case study, one brain cancer patient had a tumor in his brain pressing against one of his optic nerves. When he mixed DMSO with the cesium chloride, he could literally feel the cesium flooding into the tumor's cancer cells within just a few minutes, since the tumor was pressing against his optic nerve.

According to Dr. Robert R. Barefoot in his book, <u>The Calcium Factor: The Scientific Secret of Health and Youth</u>, *"Cesium chloride is a natural salt, and where it is found, cancer does not exist. This is because cesium is the most caustic mineral that exists, and when it enters the body, it seeks out all of the acidic cancer hotspots, dousing the fire of cancer, thereby terminating the cancer within days. Also, when dimethyl sulfoxide (DMSO) is rubbed near a painful cancer, the pain is removed, and the DMSO causes the cesium to penetrate the cancer tumor much faster, thereby terminating the cancer much faster."* However, since this can also cause excessive swelling, in some cases it is better not to rub the cesium directly above the tumor.

There are multiple theories on why and how the DMCC protocol stops cancer in its tracks. The most logical explanation is that the DMCC protocol transports enough oxygen to the cells that the condition of hypoxia is reversed and the cells reestablish aerobic metabolism.

According to Dr. David Gregg, the cesium "cancer-kill mechanism" is one (or a combination of) the following:

1. It changes the osmotic pressure in the cancer cells relative to the surrounding media, causing them to swell and burst. This is why the tumor swells, which can be dangerous in some cases.
2. It results in an opposing cesium & potassium concentration gradient that arrests the continued operation of the sodium-potassium

pump, arresting the sodium-glucose co-transport system feeding glucose into the cancer cell, thus starving the cancer cell.

3. It results in an accumulation of negative ions inside the cancer cell, canceling the potential gradient across the cell membrane, which is required to energize the sodium-glucose co-transport system, thus starving the cell.

4. It results in a breakdown of the cancer's disguise which "deceives" the immune system, thus the cancer cell is made visible and is attacked/destroyed by the immune system.

I suppose that it's possible that all four mechanisms described by Dr. Gregg play a role in killing the cancer cells. In any event, regardless of the exact cancer-kill mechanism, the fact of the matter is that the DMCC protocol kills cancer cells (either directly or indirectly), stops cancer from metastasizing (spreading), shrinks tumors within weeks, and alleviates pain within a few days, depending upon what is causing the pain. However, please understand that any level of swelling, inflammation, and/or congestion can be very dangerous; thus, the DMCC protocol is not recommended for everyone.

ENZYME/METABOLIC THERAPY

The primary basis of the enzyme/metabolic therapy for cancer emanates from the recognition that cancer cells are virtually indistinguishable from placental cells found in pregnancy. This theory, called the "trophoblast" theory, was proposed by Scottish embryologist Dr. John Beard around 1900. First he observed that the invading placental (trophoblast) cells were astonishingly similar to cancer cells, and other observations led him to believe there was an intimate correlation between these trophoblasts and cancer cells.

In early fetal development, the placental trophoblasts produce a protective environment (placenta) and a source of nutrition (umbilical cord), much in the same manner as cancer cells form a protective environment (tumor) and a source of nutrition (new blood supply). Another observation was that the placental trophoblasts seem to take a downturn in activity around the 8th week of pregnancy. It became clear to Beard that this downturn coincided with the completion of the digestive system in the fetus and the activation of the fetal pancreas.

Modern medical research has also shown that these trophoblast cells secrete a hormone called human chorionic gonadotropin (hCG), and the quantities of this hormone rise until around the 8th week and then begin to taper off. It is this very hormone that coats the trophoblast cells and cancer cells and makes them impervious to our immune system. It has been proven that hCG is found in all types of cancers.

Other than the trophoblast cell and the cancer, no other human cells produce hCG. So, if you take an hCG urine test and get a positive result, then you are either a pregnant woman or you have cancer. The Navarro Urine Test is the most accurate hcG test, according to my research.

Trophoblasts are also surrounded by a coating of glycoprotein including a molecule that gives them a negative charge. This same type of negative-charged coating is found around the cancer cell; and in fact, this is one of the chief reasons for classifying all cancer cells as trophoblastic. Also, the leukocytes (white blood cells) of the immune system are negatively charged; and as we all know, like charges repel, while opposites attract. This being so, both trophoblasts and cancer cells are impermeable to the immune system's natural defense mechanism.

Remember that the placental trophoblasts produce hCG until the eighth week of pregnancy, when they taper off. **This is a direct result of the fact that the fetal pancreas begins to produce enzymes!** And when certain enzymes, namely trypsin and chymotrypsin and amylase, encounter a trophoblast cell, they are able to break down its negatively charged protein coating. This is why "morning sickness" typically begins around the 8th week of pregnancy – the fetal pancreas is not yet fully developed and does not yet produce amylase, which is responsible for digesting glycogen (the "glyco" part of the glycoprotein coating). As a result, the glycoproteins are not broken down into their smallest units, and the mother's kidneys and pancreas are both forced to compensate and become overloaded. The result is nausea, pain in the lower back, and low energy. Thus, the pregnant mother can supplement her diet with amylase to minimize morning sickness.

Interestingly, one of the rarest cancers is cancer of the duodenum, which is the area of the intestines that is highest in pancreatic enzymes. The reason that we **do** find cases of pancreatic cancer is that the enzymes have not yet been "activated" in the small intestine. This is also the reason that pancreatic cancer has such a high mortality rate – the pancreas loses its ability to produce enzymes, thus there is no control mechanism for the cancer!

In 1911, Dr. Beard published a paper entitled <u>The Enzyme Therapy of Cancer</u>, which summarized his therapy and the supporting evidence. After his death in 1923, the enzyme therapy was largely forgotten, especially with the advent of Marie Curie and her radiation work. The pioneer in the development of Enzyme/Metabolic therapy was Dr. William Donald Kelley (a Texas orthodontist). Around 1960, at the age of 35, his health began to deteriorate. In 1964, a series of x-rays showed the signs of advancing pancreatic cancer, including lesions in his lungs, hip and liver. The surgeon said Kelley was too sick to operate on and told Mrs. Kelley (his wife and the mother of his four children) that he had four to eight weeks to live. Kelley was ready to give up, but his mother was not! She threw out the junk food and meat and instructed him to eat only fresh and raw fruits, vegetables, nuts, grains, and seeds. After several months, Kelley began to feel better, and he was even able to return to work.

However, after 6 or 7 months, he stopped improving and developed severe digestive problems, probably from the advancing cancer. He therefore began taking pancreatic enzymes to aid his digestion, and eventually increased the dose to 50 enzyme capsules per day. It was at this point that he discovered the work of Dr. John Beard concerning the relationship of pancreatic enzymes to cancer. He also encountered the writings of Dr. Edward Howell, an early advocate of the raw plant food diet. In time, Kelley fully recovered from his cancer. Considering the fact that the Cancer Industry still considers pancreatic cancer incurable, this was very impressive!

Kelley theorized that the formation of cancer was attributable to excess female hormones which were responsible for changing a stem cell into a trophoblast cell. Simply put, this means that cancer is the growth of normal tissue, but at the wrong place at the wrong time. He believed that cancer progresses due to a lack of pancreatic enzymes that digest the cancer cells. Eventually, Kelley went on to treat over 33,000 patients who had cancer. Dr. Kelly had a cure rate of **93%** in patients that lived at least 18 months after starting his treatment. In other words, those that weren't "on their last leg" had tremendous success with his treatment protocol, since this is not necessarily a fast-acting treatment.

Of course, the building blocks of his treatment protocol were pancreatic enzymes. He also instructed patients to eliminate pasteurized milk, peanuts, white flour and sugar, chlorinated water, and all processed foods. Dr. Kelley developed a line of over 50 nutritional formulations for different types of cancers, and he always individualized plans for patients according to their own metabolic type. The typical Kelley diet restricts protein, is 70% to 80% raw, and emphasizes whole grains, fruits, vegetables, raw juices, sprouts, and pancreatic enzymes. Coffee enemas are taken to help the body detoxify and to eliminate toxins secreted by tumors as they dissolve.

The Medical Mafia, in their pompous ignorance and diabolical greed, didn't like Dr. Kelley curing cancer with inexpensive enzymes! So, they sent a young medical intern, Dr. Nicholas Gonzalez, to investigate Kelly's claims and debunk him. Dr. Gonzalez traveled to Dallas in 1981 to interview and to investigate Dr. Kelley. He was astonished to find case after case of appropriately diagnosed, advanced cancer patients who were healthy and active 10 to 15 years after their diagnosis. Kelley made all his records available (over 10,000 patients) and encouraged Gonzales to contact any and all of them. Eventually, the study sample was narrowed down to 50 cases which represented 25 different types of cancer. All 50 patients were initially diagnosed as terminal. The median survival of this group was 10 years!

As incredible as these results seemed, Dr. Gonzalez decided to go a step further. He wanted to focus on pancreatic cancer, since the five year survival rate with orthodox treatments is virtually **zero percent**. He searched and found 22 pancreatic cancer patients who had been treated by Dr. Kelley between 1974 and 1982.

The twenty-two patients fell into three categories:

1. Ten patients consulted with Kelley only once and never went on the protocol – All died.
2. Seven patients followed the protocol only partially and sporadically (as determined by interviews with family members, doctors, and records) – All died.
3. However, five patients followed the protocol completely – All achieved long-term remission (although one died of Alzheimer's disease after 11.5 years of survival). The median survival rate of these five pancreatic cancer patients was nine years!

Of course, as with other medical mavericks, Dr. Kelley had his share of persecution from the Medical Mafia and its leg breakers. He was issued a restraining order which prohibited him from treating anything but dental disease. When he violated this order, he was thrown in jail. A Texas court also made it illegal for him to distribute his self-published booklet, entitled One Answer To Cancer. This makes Dr. Kelley the first *(and only)* doctor ever to be prohibited by court decree from publishing!

Although he appealed the decision to the United States Supreme Court, arguing that his First Amendment rights were being flagrantly violated, the ruling was upheld. He eventually had to move his clinic to Mexico. Not surprisingly, his enzyme/metabolic therapy protocol was put on the American Cancer Society's "Unproven Methods" blacklist in 1971 where it remains today. However, One Answer To Cancer can be found at this website: www.drkelley.com/CANLIVER55.html. Dr. Kelley died in 2005, but before he died, he wrote a book entitled Cancer: Curing the Incurable Without Surgery, Chemotherapy or Radiation. This book is even better than his first book and is available on Amazon.com. His work is currently being continued by Dr. Nicholas Gonzalez, who runs a clinic in New York City. His website is www.dr-gonzalez.com. I know Dr. Gonzalez personally and highly recommend his clinic.

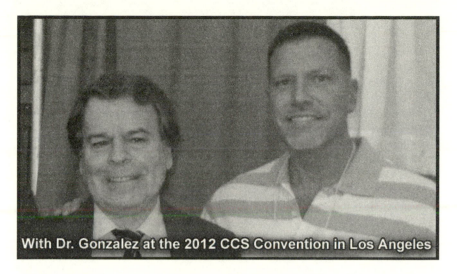

With Dr. Gonzalez at the 2012 CCS Convention in Los Angeles

Essiac Tea

My grandmother, Helen Cade, "Mama Helen" as we all affectionately called her, was the church visitor for Castle Hills First Baptist Church in San Antonio for over 40 years. She and my mom had been two of the 18 charter members of the church way back in 1952. (The church now has over 10,000 members.) As the church visitor, Mama Helen's job was to travel to hospitals and visit sick people ... dying people ... injured people. I remember traveling with her; and everywhere she went, to everyone she met, she would say, *"Honey, do you know Jesus?"* And then she would proceed to give them one of her "pet rocks" on which was painted "Jesus Loves You;" then she would tell them about Jesus' death and resurrection. What a woman she was! I can only guess that there are literally thousands of souls in heaven as a direct result of Mama Helen's witness for Jesus.

Mama Helen was diagnosed with terminal cancer in 1988. I'm not sure where she learned of it, but almost immediately she began to brew her own Essiac Tea. I remember going to her house in San Antonio and helping her make the tea, fill those amber bottles, and stick them in the fridge. She drank it faithfully, almost as faithfully as she shared the gospel with everyone she met. I say **almost** as faithfully, because I honestly don't know of anything that she did more faithfully than share the gospel. Anyway, Mama Helen lived another 10 years with her terminal cancer, largely as a result of taking Essiac Tea, in my opinion. I'm not sure why, but she had stopped drinking the tea about two years before she died.

Back in 1922, a Canadian nurse named Rene Caisse noticed some scar tissue on the breast of an elderly woman. The woman told her that doctors had diagnosed her with breast cancer years before. However, the woman didn't want to risk surgery, nor did she have the money for it. Providentially, she had met an old Indian medicine man who told her that he could cure her cancer with an herbal tea. The woman proceeded to tell Caisse about the ingredients in the tea. About a year later, Caisse was walking beside a retired doctor who pointed to a common weed and stated, *"Nurse Caisse, if people would use this weed there would be little or no cancer in the world."* This "weed" (sheep sorrel) was one of the herbs in the medicine man's formula. The doctor had watched his horse cure itself of cancer by repeatedly grazing in a particular part of the pasture where sheep sorrel grew.

In 1924, Caisse wanted to test the tea on her aunt who had been diagnosed with terminal stomach cancer and was given less than six months to live. Caisse asked the physician, Dr. R. O. Fisher, for permission to try the tea on her aunt, and he consented. Her aunt drank the herbal tea daily for two months and recovered. Amazingly, she lived for 20 more years! Caisse also tested the tea on her mother who had been diagnosed with terminal liver cancer and had been given less than two months to live. Remarkably, her mother lived another 18 years!

Dr. Fisher and nurse Caisse immediately began treating cancer patients with the magic tea, which she eventually named *"Essiac,"* which is *"Caisse"* spelled backwards. She healed thousands of terminal cancer victims with Essiac in her clinic between the mid 1920s and the late 1930s. **At the height of her involvement, Caisse saw up to 600 patients a week**. The majority of those whom she treated came on referral with letters from their physicians certifying they had incurable or terminal forms of cancer and that they had been given up by the medical profession as untreatable. It was typical for Nurse Caisse to give her patients the Essiac treatment at no cost.

After word of her impressive results spread to the United States, a leading diagnostician in Chicago introduced Caisse to Dr. John Wolfer, director of the tumor clinic at Northwestern University Medical School. In 1937, Wolfer arranged for Caisse to treat 30 terminal cancer patients under the direction of five doctors. She commuted from Canada across the border to Chicago, carrying her bottles of freshly prepared herbal brew. After supervising 18 months of Essiac therapy, the Chicago doctors concluded that the herbal mixture *"prolonged life, shrank tumors, and relieved pain."* So effective were her free treatments that in 1938 her supporters gathered 55,000 signatures for a petition to present to the Ontario legislature to make Essiac Tea an official cancer treatment. She fell three votes short.

Caisse was not aware of the vast influence of Big Pharma and Big Medicine, which were (and still are) more interested in making money than in helping people. Essiac was cheap and non-toxic. It could cut into the huge lucrative profits generated from the "Big 3." Caisse constantly played cat and mouse with Canadian federal health officials. They demanded clinical tests, but she stubbornly refused to divulge her formula unless she got official assurance that Essiac would not be lost to the people who needed it, since her primary loyalty was to the people who had come to depend on her. The authorities couldn't give her the assurance she needed; thus, she never divulged the formula.

Even the world's largest cancer research center, Memorial Sloan-Kettering Cancer Center in New York, could not convince Caisse to divulge her formula. A steady stream of doctors visited her in Canada, observing case files and talking to patients, pressuring her to sell them the formula. She was offered huge sums of money to commercialize Essiac but refused all but minimal amounts of payment for her services. Not surprisingly, Caisse was heavily persecuted and continually threatened with arrest. Finally, fearing prosecution, she closed the clinic in 1942 and went into seclusion.

Rene Caisse died in 1978, at the age of ninety. Before she died, she signed over the rights to the Essiac formula to two parties: Resperin Corporation of Toronto, to test, manufacture and distribute it, and to a long-trusted friend, Dr. Charles Brusch of Cambridge, Massachusetts, Director of the prestigious Brusch Clinic and personal physician to former President John F. Kennedy. Dr. Brusch himself had cancer of the lower bowel, which completely disappeared after Essiac treatments. Brusch once stated "*I know Essiac has curing potential. It can lessen the condition of the individual, control it, and it can cure it.*"

Rene Caisse never published her formula. The only person she trusted to help her make Essiac was her best friend, Mary McPherson, who knew the formula by heart. Anyone with internet access can verify the correct Essiac formula that Caisse entrusted to Mary McPherson. Simply visit *"The Rene M. Caisse Memorial Room"* at www.octagonalhouse.com and click on the "Essiac" hotlink.

There you will see this formula:

> ➢ 6 1/2 cups cut up Burdock Root (cut into pea-sized pieces)
>> o For centuries, burdock root has been regarded as an effective blood purifier that neutralizes and eliminates poisons from the body. Studies have shown anti-tumor activity in burdock. Japanese scientists have isolated an anti-mutation property in burdock, which they call

179

the "B factor." A memo from the WHO revealed that burdock is effective against HIV.

> 1 pound powdered Sheep Sorrel (including the roots)
> - o Caisse isolated sheep sorrel leaves as the main essiac herb that dissolves cancerous tumors. Sheep sorrel contains aloe emodin, a natural substance that shows significant anti-leukemic activity. Sheep sorrel contains antioxidants, is diuretic and has been used to check hemorrhages. Be sure to include the roots of Sheep Sorrel as well, as they are essential.

> 1/4 cup powdered Slippery Elm Bark
> - o Slippery elm is well-known for its soothing properties. It reduces inflammations such as sore throat, diarrhea, and urinary problems. It contains beta-sitosterol, which has shown anti-cancer activity.

> 1 ounce powdered Turkish Rhubarb Root
> - o "Turkey Rhubarb" has been shown to have anti-tumor activity. It is diuretic, anti-inflammatory, and antibacterial.

The preparation of Essiac Tea is as important as the formula itself. Essiac is a decoction, not an infusion. An infusion is what people do when they put a tea bag in a cup of hot water. Generally speaking, an infusion tends to extract vitamins and volatile oils. A decoction is used to extract minerals, etc. from roots, bark or seeds by boiling for several minutes and then allowing the herbs to steep for several hours. Entrepreneurs often sell Essiac imitations in tincture form (herbs in alcohol) or in gelatin capsules; neither form is Essiac because Essiac is a decoction.

1. Using a stainless steel pot and lid, boil ½ cup of herb mix in one gallon of pure, unchlorinated water for 10 minutes.
2. Turn off heat and allow herbs to steep for 12 hours.
3. Heat up tea to steaming, but not boiling. Allow herbs to settle a couple minutes.
4. Strain off hot liquid into sterilized canning jars. The remaining pulp can be used for healing poultices.
5. Refrigerate tea. For long-term storage use the boiling water bath canning method and store in a cool, dark, dry place.

For preventive purposes, people take one to two ounces per day diluted with about ½ cup of hot water. Be sure to drink plenty of water (at least half a gallon) each day to help flush the toxins out of your system. If you have cancer, you should take Essiac three times a day. Do not eat or drink anything (except water) one hour before to one hour after taking Essiac. Essiac tea is compatible with other alternative cancer treatments, except for Cancell. Do not take Protocel™ with Essiac tea, since they tend to neutralize each other.

Some of the best information on the internet concerning Essiac tea can be found at www.healthfreedom.info/Cancer_Essiac.htm. I highly recommend that you visit their frequently asked questions page. Perhaps the best book written on this topic is called The Essiac Book and can be found at www.ReneCaisseTea.com. If you are going to use this treatment, you really should purchase the book.

FREQUENCY GENERATORS

Much of this section is excerpted (with permission) from Webster Kehr's www.cancertutor.com; thus, much of the verbiage and hypotheses are related to the microbial theory of cancer. The term "electromedicine" has a very specific meaning in the alternative cancer world. It means very low amperage electrical currents or electro-magnetic waves which travel through the body. There are many kinds of "electromedicine" devices. "Frequency generators" are electromedicine devices which can generate a vast number of different electrical currents in the body and are able to revert cancer cells into normal cells. Let me discuss the theory behind how frequency generators can cure cancer.

Cancer is caused by an imbalance between the immune system and the number of cancer cells which form. We all have cancer cells, but when the immune system is weakened, the cancer cells can overwhelm the immune system and a person is said to "have cancer." However, while the balance between the immune system and the number of cancer cells which form may cause cancer, this imbalance is not typically what causes a normal cell to become cancerous! Many researchers believe that a normal cell becomes cancerous when a highly pleomorphic "cell-wall-deficient" bacterium is able to get inside the cell.

Once inside the cell this bacterium blocks the formation of ATP molecules. The cell then reverts to fermentation to create ATP molecules, and the cell is then defined to be "cancerous." Note that DNA damage does **not** cause a cell to become cancerous, rather DNA damage is the result of the DNA of the bacteria interacting with the DNA of the cell. What this means is that if you can kill the microbe inside the cancer cell, the cell will be able to restore its normal metabolism and revert into a normal cell. In fact, this is the ideal way to cure cancer because there are no dead cancer cells and in fact no cancer cells at all (because the cancer cells have reverted into normal cells).

Dr. Royal Raymond Rife, a microbiologist who did much of his research in the 1930s, fully understood all of these things. With this understanding he designed a frequency generator (aka "Rife Machine") to vibrate the microbes (inside the cancer cells) to death. While frequency generators have been around since the 1930s, a new breed of frequency generator has been developed which has matched and surpassed the original work of Dr. Rife.

Treating cancer is a race. It is a race between your cancer cells destroying your non-cancerous cells versus getting rid of your cancer cells quickly in order to protect your non-cancerous cells. The faster you get rid of your cancer cells the better your chance of survival. To understand the importance of electromedicine, suppose you are on a battlefield and are in a gun battle (firefight) with the enemy. While your main weapons are guns, machine guns, tanks, etc., I can assure you that you would be greatly pleased to hear the roar of friendly jets overhead. In exactly a similar way, when frequency generators are used as the secondary cancer treatment, your primary cancer treatment can be likened to your guns and tanks. The roar of the jet engines is the quiet workings of frequency generators.

Unfortunately, you will not find any frequency generator manufacturer or vendor which advertises that their product treats diseases (including cancer), nor will they likely use the term "electromedicine" in their literature, nor will they answer your questions about using their device for the treatment of any health condition! This is due to the potential persecution from the FDA and the Medical Mafia.

This section contains the information you will **not** get from your vendor because of possible (probable) persecution. The fact that manufacturers and vendors are not allowed to make medical claims about their equipment (even if accurate and fully documented) is proof that the FDA and FTC have achieved their goal of separating truthful information from products. In other words, honest information about a product and the product itself are not allowed to be combined on the same website or in marketing literature or even in sales pitches! This is totally absurd, in my opinion. But this is why you will never see any information like this displayed on a manufacturer's website or a vendor's website.

Frequency generators when properly used are extremely effective in the treatment of cancer.

While every cancer patient can benefit from frequency generators, there are seven situations for which frequency generators are critical:

1. The patient cannot digest foods (usually due to stomach or colon surgery),
2. The patient cannot extract nutrients from foods (usually due to chemotherapy),
3. The patient has a very fast growing cancer,
4. The cancer has spread throughout the body,
5. They have cancer in their bones or bone marrow,
6. Their type of cancer involves massive infections,
7. They have significant cachexia (*i.e.*, lactic acid problems).

These are situations where diet and supplements may not be enough to deal with the cancer. What electromedicine provides patients in these situations is an outside source of safely getting rid of cancer cells without causing any swelling or inflammation. Frequency devices are also helpful for newly diagnosed patients and may be the only treatment needed for newly diagnosed cancer patients.

Please note that because electromedicine protocols **only** focus on quickly getting rid of cancer cells and not on rebuilding the immune system with nutrition, the cancer patient should always use an electromedicine protocol in conjunction with a nutrition-based protocol. For patients who have had a lot of chemotherapy, not only should they use an electromedicine protocol, they should also use several highly potent liquid supplements/foods which are more easily digested than solid foods and solid supplements (such as Aloe arborescens).

There is one cardinal rule when combining electromedicine with other alternative cancer treatments or prescription drugs. That rule is to not use the electromedicine device and the other cancer treatment or prescription drug at the same time. To be more specific, starting 120 minutes **before** using the electromedicine device until 60 minutes **after** the patient is finished with the electromedicine device (the "120/60 rule"), the patient should **not** take any portion of any other cancer treatment or any prescription drugs.

The reason for this rule is "electroporation," which is a phenomenon in which an electrical current will "open" cells which are exposed to it, such that just about anything in the bloodstream can get inside that cell. Electroporation essentially opens the door of the cell to anything passing by. Electroporation can be good or bad, depending on what substances are in your blood.

For example, because electroporation "opens" all cells in an area of the body (not just the cancer cells) the frequency generator should not be used within four days of chemotherapy, since many non-cancerous cells would be killed. Here is why: It takes 35 hours for the chemotherapy to work out of the system (1½ days), and another day for it to do the cellular damage it inflicts on the body. It then takes two weeks for the body to recover from the damage to the cellular structure and the immune system (actually the body never fully recovers from chemotherapy). It is not necessary to wait the two weeks, but it is best to allow four days after intravenous chemo before beginning a frequency generator program. If the patient is taking oral chemo weekly, allow one or two days off, and then hit it hard with the frequency machine. In addition, because chemotherapy literally destroys a person's immune system, opportunistic infections are highly likely to exist. Careful monitoring of the patient is critically important to watch for early signs of opportunistic infections.

Just like electroporation can be bad, it can also be good. An example would be that electromedicine has the potential to help advanced cancer patients who have cachexia. Because cancer cells "steal" nutrients and glucose from non-cancerous cells (and the lactic acid created by cancer cells can also block nutrients from getting to non-cancerous cells), non-cancerous cells are frequently very, very weak. Electromedicine has the potential to create reversible electroporation which can open up all cells (not just cancer cells) in an area of the body.

If the body is then flooded with super-nutrients (such as the Brandt/Kehr Grape Cure with Cellect and colloidal silver mixed in), the healthy cells would be able to get an extra shot of super-nutrients which normally would be "stolen" by the cancer cells. At the same time the cancer cells would get an extra shot of Cellect, resveratrol, ellagic acid, lycopene, selenium, catechin, quercetin, gallic acid, vitamin B_{17}, and colloidal silver, all of which will kill the microbes inside of the cells.

Because of this, during the electromedicine treatment the patient is allowed to take very pure colloidal silver (like MesoSilver®) and/or pure grape juice. The patient should mix the colloidal silver and grape juice together. The reason that colloidal silver and grape juice are allowed is that they are healthy for non-cancerous cells and deadly for the microbes that are inside the cancer cells.

If you need support for using a frequency generator protocol, I recommend that you visit the website of the Independent Cancer Research Foundation (www.new-cancer-treatments.org). The ICRF board members are experienced at frequency machines and will be a big asset if you pursue this line of treatment. They endorse the GB-4000 frequency machine for two reasons. First, it was designed specifically to meet or exceed the specifications of an original Rife Machine. Secondly, an exact button-by-button protocol has been made public for using the GB-4000 to treat cancer. For more information on the GB-4000 machine and protocol, please visit the following website: http://cancertutor.com/Cancer03/Spec01_GB4000.pdf.

GERSON THERAPY

Gerson Therapy is a metabolic therapy which uses a special diet, along with supplements, and coffee enemas. The first two editions of this book did not contain details on this cancer treatment, but due to additional research over the past couple of years, I now believe that the Gerson Therapy is one of the best cancer treatments available. It is undoubtedly the most basic, the best recognized, the most complete, and the longest existing effective cancer treatment available today. It is also very rigorous and requires that patients adhere to a very strict protocol in order to succeed.

Dr. Max Gerson was a German refugee physician who came to New York and preached a gospel of pure organic food and farming. Prior to immigrating to the USA, while he was a resident physician in Germany, Gerson was able to cure his own migraine headaches through changing his diet. The foods that Gerson was sensitive to included many of the staples of young German medical students (creamy fish dishes, spicy sausages, alcohol, salt, and fatty meats). Later, when he entered private practice, he began prescribing his migraine diet to his own patients and reported great success.

One migraine patient reported that his lupus vulgaris (skin tuberculosis) had also cleared up on Gerson's migraine diet. Gerson began to use his dietary approach to cure other lupus sufferers. He even began to have success with treating tuberculosis. A prominent pulmonary surgeon, Dr. Ferdinand Sauerbruch, heard about Gerson's successes and invited him to conduct a clinical trial of his therapy at Sauerbruch's Munich tuberculosis ward.

Gerson's dietary regime was applied to 450 tuberculosis patients. At that time, tuberculosis was considered to be "incurable." After the trial, it was reported that 446 patients completely recovered. For those of you who like percentages, that's a 99.1% cure rate on terminal patients!

Gerson's dietary therapy quickly became well-known in Europe, and it was adopted by many as standard treatment for immune system disorders of all kinds, including tuberculosis. Advocates of the therapy claim many Swiss mountain tuberculosis sanatoria were put out of business by Gerson's discoveries and are now ski resorts, including Davos, Gstaad and others.

In 1928, Gerson received a call from a woman who was told she had incurable bile-duct cancer. According to Gerson, she begged him to treat her with his migraine and tuberculosis therapy, accepting that he knew nothing about cancer and could not predict the outcome of his treatment. Gerson claimed she totally recovered on his therapy, as did two friends of hers who had cancer. Of course, with any successful cancer treatment, there will be "hit men" from the Medical Mafia that attempt to slander and criticize the provider, and Gerson was no exception.

He embarked on a clinical trial of his therapy that would attempt to silence his critics once and for all. He decided to treat only patients who had been declared "terminal" in writing by at least two specialists, so there was no doubt as to the disease or its prognosis. On April 1, 1933, just six weeks before he was to present the results of his study, Adolf Hitler began arresting Jews and sending them to concentration camps. Gerson literally escaped arrest by accident, and left Germany for good, leaving behind the results of his study.

As a German Jew, Gerson was forced to flee Germany with his family in 1933, first to Vienna and then to Ville d'Avray (near Paris) and London. He settled in New York City in 1936. Once in the USA, Gerson began applying his dietary therapy to advanced cancer patients. In 1946, along with five of his cured cancer patients, he testified in court that he had discovered a cure for cancer. On the evening of July 3, 1946, it was announced publicly on radio that Gerson had discovered a cure for cancer. Not surprisingly, this public declaration was condemned by his "holier-than-thou" colleagues in the New York State Medical Society.

After several more years of successful medical practice, but under increased scrutiny, Dr. Max Gerson died suddenly on March 8, 1959, under mysterious circumstances. Charlotte Gerson, his youngest daughter and founder of the Gerson Institute, stated: *"My father, aged 78, was in perfectly good health when, from one day to the next, he felt awful. They tested his blood and found a high level of arsenic."* When asked if she had called the police, she replied: *"No, we had our suspicions but knew from experience that justice would not be done."*

According to Dr. Gerson, cancer is the result of two things: **deficiency** and **toxicity**. Our body simply doesn't get enough nutrition on the modern diet and is exposed to too many chemicals and toxins and as a result develops cancer. Gerson believed that cancer could be reversed if the patient would cleanse the body from these toxins and restore the immune system with proper nutrition.

As a result of this belief, the underlying foundation of Gerson Therapy is detoxification and rejuvenation of the body, based upon the principle of flooding the body with micronutrients from salt-free, fat-free, organic, vegetarian food, including 13 fresh-pressed fruit and vegetable juices daily. This treatment utilizes a "whole body" approach, unlike toxic conventional treatments, since Gerson did not believe that treating only the localized area of concentrated cancer cells was a good idea.

Pancreatic enzymes are vitally important to the Gerson Therapy. Here's why: Before the body can deteriorate into cancer, all the body's defense systems have to be depressed and out of balance. If your pancreas is working properly and if you have adequate pancreatic enzymes, you cannot develop cancer. As I mentioned in the chapter on nutrition, pancreatic enzymes (specifically trypsin and chymotrypsin) dissolve the protective protein coating which covers malignant tissue and makes it impossible for the body's natural immune system to recognize the cancer cells as foreign. So, in a body with cancer, pancreatic enzymes must be supplemented.

Correlated to its adherence to pancreatic enzymes, Gerson Therapy also holds tightly to the axiom that excess protein in the diet is carcinogenic. As a former competitive bodybuilder, I used to follow the advice of doctors and nutritionists and consume massive amounts of animal protein on a daily basis. For instance, I would typically have eight small meals of at least thirty grams of protein, comprised primarily of chicken, fish, and eggs. I mistakenly believed that meat, fish, eggs, and milk products had complete proteins (containing the eight essential amino acids not produced in the body), while all vegetable proteins were incomplete proteins.

However, research at the Karolinska Institute in Sweden and the Max Plank Institute in Germany has shown that most vegetables, fruits, seeds, nuts, and grains are excellent sources of complete proteins. In fact, their proteins are easier to assimilate than those of meat, and they are non-toxic. Whereas the Karolinska researchers also discovered that when meat was heated to 212° (regardless of whether it was boiled, broiled, fried, or baked) the protein in the meat changed into toxic, cancer-causing amides. Research done at the University of California at Irvine showed that children who eat as few as three hotdogs a week were 10 to 12 times as likely to develop leukemia and brain tumors. In a vast study conducted in China by T. Colin Campbell, PhD., it was found that the groups of people who ate the most animal protein had, by far, the most heart disease and cancer.

One of the reasons to avoid excess protein is that the body stores very little protein. Our kidneys and liver are responsible for getting rid of the protein; so the more protein we eat, the harder the kidneys and liver must work to excrete it. Gerson was also very interested in treating the liver, since he believed that the liver was actually the most important organ in the body due to the fact that it is the filtration system for detoxification. As a matter of fact, he saw a parallel between the deterioration of the liver and the growth and progression of the cancer!

Due to his concern for liver problems, he was opposed to fasting and instead, his regimen called for fresh pressed juice every waking hour of the day. By drinking the juice, patients receive an enormous flooding of nutrients, minerals, enzymes, and vitamins which start to flush out the kidneys. The nutrients go into the tissues, into the cells and force out the poisons, and all those poisons are released into the blood stream. The liver filters them out. You have to help the liver get rid of them, and there is only one way to do this – by opening the bile ducts. Gerson accomplished this task with his much maligned and ridiculed coffee enemas. Even today, half a century after his death, he remains a favorite "whipping boy" of the Cancer Industry.

Until recently, I was unaware of the fact that sodium stimulates tumor growth. Also, it's a fact that all processed foods contain reduced potassium and increased sodium. So, with the Gerson Therapy's focus on high potassium and low sodium (in the same ratio which can be found in fresh live foods), it's no wonder that all processed foods are forbidden. With the Gerson Therapy, most fats are strictly prohibited since they stimulate tumor growth. However, Gerson was aware that cancer patients do need a certain amount of essential fatty acids. He became aware of the work of Dr. Johanna Budwig in Germany who showed that flaxseed oil, which helps to stimulate the immune system, is well tolerated by cancer patients. As a general rule, with the exception of coconut oil, you should never cook with oils, since their chemical nature changes (deteriorates), acrylamides are formed, and they cause health problems. So the flaxseed oil must only be used raw and cold.

The Gerson Institute was established in 1977 in San Diego by Charlotte Gerson, solely for the purpose of educating the public and cancer patients about the Gerson Therapy. Is it any surprise that the corrupt United States government does not support the Gerson Therapy? As a matter of fact, it is illegal in the USA to treat and cure patients with the Gerson Therapy. In response, Charlotte opened a hospital in Tijuana, Mexico. You can visit the Gerson Institute's website (www.Gerson.org) for more information on Gerson Therapy.

An excellent book on the Gerson Therapy was written by Max Gerson himself and is entitled <u>A Cancer Therapy: Results of Fifty Cases and the Cure of Advanced Cancer</u>. It's available on Amazon.

HEMP

A 1938 article from *Popular Mechanics* stated that there are more than 25,000 uses for hemp ... from food, paint and fuel to clothing and construction materials. There are even hemp fibers in your Lipton® tea bags. And several cars made today contain hemp. One acre of hemp can produce as much raw fiber as 10 acres of trees. Pulping hemp for paper would produce a stronger paper that lasts incredibly long and doesn't yellow with age. Hemp oil (derived from hemp seeds) has long been recognized as one of the most versatile and beneficial substances known to man.

Back in the early days of America's founding, hemp was a commonly grown and used resource. America's hemp heritage includes the following facts:

> ➢ Early laws in some American colonies actually required farmers to grow hemp, and they could go to jail for refusing to grow it!
> ➢ According to their diaries, many of our early presidents, including George Washington and Thomas Jefferson, grew hemp.
> ➢ The Declaration of Independence and the Constitution of the USA were both drafted on hemp paper.
> ➢ Abraham Lincoln used hemp seed oil to fuel the lamps in his home.
> ➢ Henry Ford built an experimental car body out of hemp fiber, which is 10 times stronger than steel. The first Model-T was actually built to run on hemp gasoline. (*Popular Mechanics*, 1941)

Hemp is considered to be a superfood (like spirulina and chlorella) due to its high essential fatty acid content and the unique ratio of omega-3 to omega-6, specifically gamma linolenic acid (GLA). Hemp oil contains up to 5% of pure GLA, a much higher concentration than any other plant. For millenia, hemp has been used in medicinal teas and tonics because of its healing properties. Hemp not only relieves pain and helps with the appetites of cancer patients; it also has been shown to have curative properties.

The chemicals in hemp which are responsible for many of the medical benefits are called "cannabinoids." The most notable cannabinoid is "Delta-9-tetrahydrocannabinol" but most folks call it "THC." Before I go any further, let me explain the difference between the terms "hemp" and "marijuana" and "cannabis." The word "hemp" is English for a number of varieties of the cannabis plant, particularly the varieties like "industrial hemp" that were bred over time for industrial uses such as fuel, fiber, paper, seed, food, oil, etc. The term "marijuana" is of Spanish derivation, and was primarily used to describe varieties of cannabis that were more commonly bred over time for medicinal and recreational purposes (like *cannabis indica* and *cannabis sativa*).

Two cannabinoids are preeminent in cannabis – 1) THC, the psychoactive ingredient, and 2) CBD, which is an anti-psychoactive ingredient. "Marijuana" (which is actually a slang term to make it sound more "sinister") is high in the psychoactive cannabinoid, THC, and low in the anti-psychoactive cannabinoid, CBD. The reverse is true for industrial hemp, which has minimal THC and a much higher percentage of CBD. I prefer to use the terms "hemp" or "cannabis" for all varietals of the cannabis plant. Using the term "marijuana" is actually acquiescing to the pejorative intentions of the Medical Mafia that wants to ban this miracle plant ... not miracle "drug" ... miracle **plant**. You see, "marijuana" was one of the battle line words that marked the difference between "straights" and "stoners" ... between "Feds" and "heads."

As late as the 1930s in the USA, medicinal hemp tinctures with THC were available in most pharmacies. About that same time (the late 1930s), William Randolph Hearst and the Hearst Paper Manufacturing Division of Kimberly Clark owned millions of acres of timberland. The Hearst Company, which supplied most of the paper products in the USA and also owned most of the newspapers, stood to lose billions because of the hemp industry. In 1937, Dupont patented the processes to make plastics from oil and coal. Dupont's Annual Report urged stockholders to invest in its new petrochemical division. Synthetics such as plastics, nylon, and rayon could now be made from oil. Natural hemp industrialization would have ruined over 80% of Dupont's business.

Andrew Mellon became President Hoover's Secretary of the Treasury and Dupont's primary investor. He appointed his future nephew-in-law (Harry J. Anslinger) to head the Federal Bureau of Narcotics and Dangerous Drugs. Secret meetings were held by these financial tycoons. Hemp was declared "dangerous" and a threat to their billion dollar enterprises. For their dynasties to remain intact, hemp had to go. They took an obscure Mexican slang word ("marijuana") and pushed it into the consciousness of America. A media blitz of "yellow journalism" raged in the 1920s and 1930s; Hearst's newspapers ran stories emphasizing the horrors of "marijuana." Readers were led to believe that it was responsible for car accidents, loose morality, and countless acts of violence, incurable insanity, and vicious murders. Films like "Reefer Madness" and "Marihuana: The Devil's Weed" were propaganda designed by these industrialists to create an enemy. Their purpose was to gain public support so that anti-marijuana laws could be passed. http://www.tpuc.org/content/marijuana-conspiracy

In the 1930s, people were very naïve, even to the point of ignorance. The masses were "sheeple" waiting to be led by the few in power. They did not challenge authority. Much like the sheeple today, if the news was in print or on the radio, they believed it had to be true. So, despite the fact that the brainwashing campaign was based on total lies, hemp was outlawed in the late 1930s. Hemp was too much of a threat to the paper industry and the oil industry. Plus, Big Pharma didn't like the non-toxic and inexpensive medicinal applications! Hemp was plentiful and economical, and to make matters worse for the Medical Mafia, it didn't cause any additional medical conditions that required prescriptions for more of their toxic poisons.

The medical evidence for the effectiveness of THC at treating cancer and also reducing pain is overwhelming. We have known this since 1974 when the first experiment documenting marijuana's anti-tumor effects took place at the Medical College of Virginia at the behest of the U.S. government and the National Institute of Health (NIH). The purpose of the study was to show that marijuana damages the immune system and causes cancer. However, the study found instead that THC slowed the growth of three kinds of cancer in mice (*lung and breast cancer, and a virus-induced leukemia*). **OOPS!** We can't have that information made public, can we? So, the DEA quickly shut down the Virginia study and all further research on the anti-cancer effects of hemp, even though research proved that **THC cures cancer**!!

In 2000, researchers in Madrid learned that the THC in hemp inhibits the spread of brain cancer through selectively inducing programmed cell death (*apoptosis*) in brain tumor cells without negatively impacting surrounding healthy cells. They were able to destroy **incurable** brain tumors in rats by injecting them with THC. But sadly, most Americans don't know anything about the Madrid discovery, since virtually no major US newspapers carried the story.

A 2007 Harvard Medical School study showed that the THC in hemp decreases lung cancer tumors by 50% and significantly reduces the ability of the cancer to metastasize (spread). "*The beauty of this study is that we are showing that a substance of abuse, if used prudently, may offer a new road to therapy against lung cancer,*" said Anju Preet, Ph.D., a researcher at the Division of Experimental Medicine. http://www.sciencedaily.com/releases/2007/04/070417193338.htm

Other researchers have also shown that THC is an effective treatment for Hodgkin's disease and Kaposi's Sarcoma. A recent study out of

191

Thailand demonstrated that THC can also fight bile duct cancer, which is rare and deadly. As a matter of fact, the International Medical Verities Association includes hemp oil on its cancer protocol. Studies have also shown that cannabinoids (and endocannabinoids) inhibit the proliferation of other various cancers, including:

> Breast cancer http://cancerres.aacrjournals.org/content/66/13/6615.abstract
> Colorectal cancer http://gut.bmj.com/content/54/12/1741.abstract
> Prostate cancer http://cancerres.aacrjournals.org/content/65/5/1635.abstract
> Stomach cancer http://ar.iiarjournals.org/content/33/6/2541.full.pdf
> Skin cancer http://www.jci.org/articles/view/16116
> Leukemia http://www.ncbi.nlm.nih.gov/pubmed/16908594
> Lymphoma http://onlinelibrary.wiley.com/doi/10.1002/ijc.23584/abstract
> Lung cancer http://www.nature.com/onc/journal/v27/n3/abs/1210641a.html
> Uterine cancer http://americanmarijuana.org/Guzman-Cancer.pdf
> Thyroid cancer http://www.ncbi.nlm.nih.gov/pubmed/19047095
> Pancreatic cancer http://cancerres.aacrjournals.org/content/66/13/6748.abstract
> Cervical cancer http://jnci.oxfordjournals.org/content/100/1/59.abstract
> Mouth cancer http://www.ncbi.nlm.nih.gov/pubmed/20516734
> Glioma Brain Cancer http://www.ncbi.nlm.nih.gov/pubmed/16899063
> Billary tract cancer http://www.ncbi.nlm.nih.gov/pubmed/19916793

Rick Simpson successfully treated his terminal cancer with hemp oil, and since then has been leading the way to promote hemp oil as a viable cancer treatment. Ironically, on November 25th, 2009, one day before he was crowned the "Freedom Fighter of the Year 2009" at the Cannabis Cup in Amsterdam, Simpson received word that he had been raided again by the RCMP in Canada. Simpson has been heavily persecuted for his stance on medicinal marijuana and for his efforts to help folks cure their cancer with hemp oil.

Folks, I definitely believe that we are living in the matrix! Almost every natural substance that God created (such as hemp, apricot seeds, and sunlight) is considered to be "dangerous" while toxic drugs being pushed by Big Pharma are considered to be safe! It is legal for doctors to attack people with their poisons but you can go to jail for trying to save yourself or a loved one from cancer with the oil of a simple garden weed or the seed of a simple fruit.

Two drugs which are legal in this country (alcohol and tobacco) are known killers. Every year in the USA, tobacco causes 435,000 deaths and alcohol causes 85,000 deaths. (www.drugwarfacts.org/cms/node/30) The same study showed **no deaths** attributed to use of marijuana. Nevertheless, the US government continues its phony "war on drugs," which is just as much of a failure as the fraudulent "war on cancer" and the fake "war on terror." It has been proven that anytime the corrupt government declares a "war" on anything, the problem only gets much worse. Who's kidding who?

> "Marijuana,in the its natural form, is one of the safest therapeutically active substances known ... It would be unreasonable, arbitrary, and capricious for the DEA to continue to stand between those sufferers and the benefits of this substance."
> ~ *Francis L. Young, DEA Chief Administrative Law Judge, 1988*

On March 29, 2001, the *San Antonio Current* printed a story by Raymond Cushing titled, *"Pot Shrinks Tumors – Government Knew in '74"* which detailed government and media suppression of news about marijuana cancer benefits. Cushing noted in his article that it was hard to believe that the knowledge that cannabis can be used to fight cancer has been suppressed for almost thirty years and aptly concluded his article by saying: *"Millions of people have died horrible deaths and in many cases, families exhausted their savings on dangerous, toxic and expensive drugs. Now we are just beginning to realize that while marijuana has never killed anyone, marijuana prohibition has killed millions."*

The science for the medicinal use of hemp is overwhelming. It should be produced and distributed to each and every cancer patient that needs it. But the reality is that we live in a corrupt world run by the Medical Mafia who would rather make money while cancer patients die cruel deaths than give them access to a non-toxic, effective, natural treatment like hemp. If you want to obtain the highest quality hemp oil, I recommend that you visit http://hempmedspx.com/ and check out the Real Scientific Hemp Oil (RSHO) ™.

Some of the information in this section was taken, with permission, from an article entitled "The Marijuana Conspiracy" written by Doug Yurchey published in the March-April 2009 issue of *The Dot Connector* Magazine and can be found at www.thedotconnector.org/mag/.

HYPERTHERMIA

Hyperthermia is an artificially induced fever. Hippocrates noted that *"illness not cured by heat is incurable."* In 1893, Dr. William B. Coley observed the regression of cancer in 10 patients into whom he injected bacterial toxins (aka Coley's toxins) directly into the tumor and created a high fever. The modern name for Coley's toxins is Mixed Bacterial Vaccine (MBV). In a German study, advanced non-Hodgkin's lymphoma patients receiving MBV had a 93% remission rate, compared to 29% for controls receiving chemotherapy. (Dr. Ralph W. Moss, The Cancer Industry, page 160) In 1927, Julius Wagner-Jauregg received the Nobel Prize in medicine for work involving the therapeutic application of hyperthermia.

Fever has long been a misunderstood and mistreated symptom. Most orthodox doctors try to combat and suppress fever, hence the need for Advil and Tylenol. However, the fact is that fever is a constructive, health-promoting symptom, initiated and created by the body in its own effort to fight infections and other conditions of disease and to restore health. You see, fever speeds up metabolism, inhibits the growth of invading virus or bacteria, and accelerates the healing processes.

Hyperthermia is a therapeutic procedure used to raise the temperature of cancerous tumor to at least 108°F for one hour. It is based on a simple and easily verifiable scientific fact that a temperature of 108°F **kills cancer cells** but not normal human tissue cells. In normal tissues, blood vessels open up (dilate) when heat is applied, dissipating the heat and cooling down the cell environment. Unlike healthy cells, a tumor is a tightly packed group of cells, and circulation is restricted and sluggish. When heat is applied to the tumor, vital nutrients and oxygen are cut off from the tumor cells. This results in a collapse of the tumor's vascular system and destruction of the cancer cells.

All we need is some way to raise the body's temperature, and we create a selectively negative environment for the renegade cancer cells, which can be mopped up by the immune system. Microwave energy is very effective in heating cancerous tumors, because tumors typically have high-water content. In 1990, Dr. Alan J. Fenn (an electrical engineer at Massachusetts Institute of Technology) developed a concept for heating deep tumors by means of adaptive microwaves. These adjust to the properties of a patient's tissue to concentrate the microwave energy at the tumor.

There are several other methods used to induce hyperthermia, such as full-body submersion in hot water, ultrasound, and saunas, to name a few. Personally, I prefer saunas, since the skin is our largest eliminative organ and is sometimes called the "third kidney." As a general rule, the skin should eliminate 30% of the body's toxic wastes by way of perspiration. However, due to lack of physical work and an overly sedentary life, the skin of most people today has degenerated as an eliminative organ (since most people never sweat). If health is to be restored, it is of vital importance that the eliminative activity of the skin is revitalized. Taking sauna or steam baths regularly will help to restore and revitalize the cleansing activity of the skin. Hyperthermia combined with low dose radiation is a very effective treatment for many forms of cancer. There are few side effects and the body has the ability to recover from the low dose radiation in most cases.

Dr. A. Lwoff, a famous French bacteriologist, has demonstrated in repeated scientific experiments that fever is indeed a "great medicine," and that it can help to cure many "incurable" diseases. Renowned oncologist, Dr. Josef Issels, stated: *"Artificially induced fever has the greatest potential in the treatment of many diseases, **including cancer.**"* Keep in mind that this remark was made by one of the leading cancer specialists in the world!

Hyperthermia gives cancer a "triple whammy" by:

1. removing accumulations of toxic chemicals that cause cancer
2. improving circulation so that tissues are both nourished with oxygen and flushed of acidic wastes
3. weakening or even killing cancer cells that have a lower tolerance for heat than healthy cells.

In May 2009, the BSD Medical Corporation (based in Salt Lake City) attained a Humanitarian Use Device (HUD) designation for the company's BSD-2000 Hyperthermia System for use in conjunction with radiation therapy for the treatment of some cervical carcinoma patients. But if you try to get hyperthermia treatment in an American hospital, you will mostly experience frustration. If you want to have a reasonable chance of adding hyperthermia to your own cancer treatment program you will still have to go to Germany, China or some other country that welcomes innovation.

Please note that because hyperthermia **only** focuses on destroying cancer cells in tumors and not on rebuilding the immune system with nutrition, the cancer patient should always use hyperthermia in conjunction with a nutrition-based protocol. Over 2,000 years ago, the famous Greek physician, Parmenides, stated *"Give me a chance to create fever, and I will cure any disease."* This traditional wisdom has certainly stood the test of time.

INTRAVENOUS VITAMIN C

Vitamin C is essential to the formation of collagen, the protein "cement" that holds our cells together. Think of cells like bricks in a wall. The strength of a brick wall is not really in the bricks but it is in the cement between the bricks. Collagen is this cement that holds your cells together. If collagen is abundant and strong, your cells hold together well. If cells stick together, tumors have a tough time spreading through them. Strong collagen can thereby arrest the spread of cancer.

Cancer cells secrete an enzyme called "hyaluronidase," which helps them eat away at collagen and break out into the rest of the body. This is described in great detail in the book Hyaluronidase and Cancer by Dr. Ewan Cameron. In order to prevent the hyaluronidase enzymes from dissolving collagen, Dr. Matthias Rath advocates increased consumption of the amino acids L-Lysine and L-Proline and EGCG (a polyphenol catechin found in Green Tea) as companion nutrients with vitamin C. Laboratory trials have demonstrated the effectiveness of the combination of these four substances at blocking the hyaluronidase enzymes.

Vitamin C is required for our immune systems to generate and mobilize the leukocytes that fight cancer. Maximum immune function is vital if we want the body to fend off cancer. As I have mentioned, orthodox treatments like chemo and radiation destroy the immune system. In a 1995 publication, several physicians presented evidence that ascorbic acid is **preferentially toxic** to cancerous cells. In other words, vitamin C kills cancer cells while leaving normal cells alone. So, it appears that vitamin C not only strengthens the immune system, but it also preferentially kills cancer cells. This is fascinating. Preferential toxicity occurred in vitro in multiple tumor cell types. They also presented data suggesting that plasma concentrations of ascorbate required for killing tumor cells is achievable in humans. (Riordan, Meng, Li, Jackson, "Intravenous ascorbate as a tumor cytotoxic chemotherapeutic agent," *Medical Hypotheses*, 1995)

And if that's not enough reason to take vitamin C, then check this out: vitamin C assists with oxygen transport and is a powerful antioxidant. According to Dr. David Gregg, *"Basically, the vitamin C is transported to the lungs in the blood where it is oxidized. It then is transported to the cells where it diffuses to the mitochondria and delivers its oxidation potential, powering the respiratory chain, and cycle repeats."*

Dr. Gregg theorizes that the primary effect of the large doses of vitamin C is to serve as an oxygen transport molecule in the blood, substituting for hemoglobin, which cannot provide oxygen to cancer cells. He recommends a combination of vitamin C and vitamin E, since vitamin C transports oxygen in the cytoplasm and vitamin E carries oxygen through the cell walls.

Dr. K.N. Prasad's theory is that normal cells require only a minute, precisely controlled amount of antioxidants in order to function. They reject any excess. But among other defects, malignant cells have lost the capacity to regulate their uptake of antioxidants such as vitamin C and E. Antioxidants can therefore accumulate in cancer tissue in levels that can lead to the breakdown and death of malignant cells. (Prasad KN. "Antioxidants in cancer care: when and how to use them as an adjunct standard and experimental therapies" *Expert Rev Anticancer Therapy,* 12/2003, 903-15)

Doctors A. Goth and I. Littmann in a paper entitled "Ascorbic Acid Content in Human Cancer Tissue" (*Cancer Research,* Vol. 8, 1948) described how cancer most frequently originates in organs with ascorbic acid (vitamin C) levels below 4.5 mg% and rarely grows in organs with higher levels. Do you see the connection? Remember how hydrogen peroxide is poured on wounds to kill germs? Research published in September of 2005 by Dr. Mark Levine has shown that high-dose intravenous vitamin C can increase hydrogen peroxide (H_2O_2) levels within cancer cells and eradicate the cancer cells. www.pnas.org/cgi/content/abstract/102/38/13604

The awareness that vitamin C is useful in the treatment of cancer is chiefly attributable to the pioneering work of Dr. Linus Pauling. In 1976, he and a Scottish surgeon, Dr. Ewan Cameron, reported that patients treated with high doses of vitamin C had survived three to four times longer than similar patients who did not receive vitamin C supplements. The study was conducted during the early 1970s at the Vale of Leven Hospital in Loch Lomonside, Scotland. Dr Cameron treated 100 advanced cancer patients with 10,000 milligrams of vitamin C per day.

The progress of these patients was then compared with that of 1,000 patients (*of other doctors*) who had **not** received vitamin C. The findings were published in 1976, with Pauling as co-author, in the *Proceedings of the National Academy of Sciences.* The 1976 report emphasized that all of the patients had previously received conventional treatment (*i.e.,* the "Big 3"). The vitamin C patients were reported to have a mean survival time of 300 days longer than the other patients, with an improved quality of life. Their experiments proved conclusively that vitamin C is a superior treatment for terminal patients versus chemotherapy.

The Cancer Industry was furious with Pauling and Cameron. There was no way that these two "quacks" and their vitamin therapy were going to cut into the chemotherapy **cash cow**! There was too much at stake for the Cancer Industry. Shareholders needed huge profits! The Boards of Directors needed 7-figure salaries and golden parachutes! Children needed Ivy League educations! So, following standard operating procedure, there was a "smear" campaign to discredit Dr. Pauling. The truth about what Cameron and Pauling had discovered had to be crushed. But they had a big problem: The results of these tests had already been published in Cameron and Pauling's book, Cancer and Vitamin C.

So, the Cancer Industry and their cronies quickly went to work. They conducted three bogus studies with "predetermined" outcomes, all of which contradicted the findings of Cameron and Pauling. Here's their dirty little secret: in all three studies, they failed to follow the selection protocol, failed to follow the treatment protocol, and performed some fancy linguistic and statistical tricks.

Is it any wonder that, in the end, the Cancer Industry proudly proclaimed that Cameron and Pauling were quacks and that their research was not to be trusted? However, four totally independent studies used the same treatment protocol and got the same results as Pauling and Cameron. The three bogus studies did **not** use the same treatment protocol and did **not** get the same results.

According to Webster Kehr, *"The Mayo Clinic studies were done specifically to discredit the work of two-time Nobel Prize winner Linus Pauling. Linus Pauling was getting people to believe there was "scientific evidence" for Vitamin C, and he had to be stopped. It is totally unacceptable (from the viewpoint of Big Pharma) for our corrupt government to allow **any** scientific evidence for alternative treatments of cancer. Because there **was** scientific evidence for Vitamin C, and because they could not shut-up a two-time Nobel Prize winner, there had to be bogus studies designed to divert people's attention from the valid studies. Once the bogus studies were finished, the media could then take over the suppression of truth and immediately start blacklisting the valid studies."* www.cancertutor.com

Dr. Abram Hoffer is commonly credited with being the principal founder of the alternative health movement using nutritional (orthomolecular) treatment methods. During his practice, extending more than 40 years, he treated thousands of patients primarily for cancer and schizophrenia, authoring many journal articles and books. As part of this effort, he collaborated with Dr. Linus Pauling in his focus on utilizing vitamin C (along with other nutrients) for the treatment of cancer.

How much vitamin C should you take? Studies have shown that in order to pump adequate levels of vitamin C into the cancerous cells, intravenous vitamin C (IVC) is the best protocol. Of course, you will need to be under the supervision of a doctor – you don't want to try to give yourself an IV of vitamin C! The key is to be consistent with large quantities of vitamin C. It needs to be taken several times every day.

The Riordan Clinic, a large research clinic, in Wichita, Kansas, offers IVC therapy. Their website is http://riordanclinic.org. For a good video on IVC therapy, visit www.internetwks.com/cathcart/Cathcart2low.rm. Dr. Cameron's entire protocol is available at the following website: www.doctoryourself.com/cameron.html.

I.P.T. (INSULIN POTENTIATION THERAPY)

Although I am opposed to traditional "high dose" chemotherapy, the IPT protocol does involve chemotherapy, albeit in **extremely low doses**. Over time, traditional chemotherapy dosages compromise the patient's blood counts, immune system, and organ function to such an extent that they preclude further treatment and oftentimes cause organ damage resulting in the patient's death. However, IPT eliminates the decision between the "lesser of two evils" that cancer patients face when they are diagnosed.

By targeting a low dose of chemotherapy (less than 1/10 of the typical chemo dosage) to the cancer cells, IPT enhances toxicity to the cancer while reducing toxicity to the patient. It is an extremely safe, effective, and relatively inexpensive cancer therapy used successfully for over 60 years.

Readers will recognize insulin as being the hormone used to treat diabetes. Secreted by the pancreas in healthy people, insulin is a powerful hormone with many actions in the human body, a principal one being to manage the delivery of glucose across cell membranes into cells. Insulin communicates its messages to cells by joining up with specific insulin receptors scattered on the outer surface of the cell membranes. Every cell in the human body has between 100 and 100,000 insulin receptors. Insulin actually opens the cell membrane or "door" to the cell, thereby allowing sugar and other substances to be transported inside. That's why diabetics, who are unable to produce insulin properly, cannot admit sugar into their cells; thus, they develop hyperglycemia (high blood sugar).

What does this have to do with cancer? It is a well-known scientific fact that cancer cells have an insatiable appetite for glucose. Remember, **cancer loves sugar!** Also, remember that cancer cells are **an**aerobic. So, they produce energy via fermenting glucose, an extremely inefficient way to produce energy, and also one of the reasons that cancer patients lose so much weight. Their cancer cells require so much glucose that they literally steal it away from the body's normal cells, thus starving the cancer patient.

With IPT, insulin acts as a "potentiator," tricking the cancer cells into believing they are going to be fed sugar (which they thrive on) when, in fact, they are going to be destroyed by chemotherapy. Since insulin acts as a potentiator and increases the effectiveness of the chemo, far less chemo is needed than with traditional chemo. This means far less side-effects as well as a much more effective treatment.

The interesting connection between cancer cells and insulin is that recent findings published in the scientific medical literature report that cancer cells actually manufacture and secrete their own insulin.

According to Dr. Stephen Ayre, one of the experts in IPT, "*Cancer cells get their energy by secreting their own insulin, and they stimulate themselves to grow by secreting their own insulin-like growth factor (IGF). These are their mechanisms of malignancy. Insulin and IGF work by attaching to special cell membrane receptors, and these receptors are* **sixteen times** *more concentrated on cancer cell membranes than on normal cells. These receptors are the key to IPT. Using insulin in IPT, the end result is that the low dose chemotherapy gets channeled specifically inside the cancer cells, killing them more effectively, and with no chemotherapy side-effects. IPT is ingenious; it kills cancer cells by using the very same mechanisms that cancer cells use to kill people.*" www.contemporarymedicine.net/ipt_main.htm

The above quote is very important in understanding the mechanism of IPT therapy. IPT kills the cancer cells ... and **only** the cancer cells. Just as cancer cells have their own independent secretion of insulin, they also have their own independent secretion of IGF to provide them with an unlimited stimulus for growth. And cancer cells have 16 times more receptors for insulin and IGF on their cell membranes. Not only can insulin join up with its own specific receptors on cell membranes, but insulin is also able to join up with the receptors for IGF and to communicate messages about growth to the cell. While it may seem highly undesirable for a cancer therapy to actually promote cancer cell growth, this is in fact a valuable effect of insulin here.

You can always tell when someone is undergoing chemotherapy treatments, because they typically lose their hair and are oftentimes very sick and nauseated. Have you ever wondered why? The reason is simple. The cells of patient's hair follicles and the cells which line the stomach and intestines have one common denominator: They are **rapidly dividing cells**. So are cancer cells. Chemotherapy drugs like to attack rapidly dividing cells, indiscriminately. However, in a tumor, not all the cancer cells are in this rapidly dividing stage all at once. The fact of the matter is that they take turns.

So when insulin joins up with the IGF receptors on those cancer cells, it stimulates growth in many of the cells that are not in this growth phase. It literally "turns on" cells and makes them active. Then, the chemotherapy administered, after insulin has been injected, actually targets the cells that are "active" and thus more susceptible to the chemotherapy. The end result, which is a beautiful thing for a cancer patient, is that the insulin renders more of these cells susceptible to chemotherapy attack.

How does it work? Basically, during IPT, a small dose of insulin is given to the patient that opens the cell membranes and induces hypoglycemia (low blood sugar), making the patient dizzy and weak. Remember, as Dr. Ayre stated, cancer cells have **16 times more** insulin and IGF receptors than normal cells. By inducing hypoglycemia, we can cause the cancer cells to open their receptors at a rate of 16 to 1, thereby allowing us to selectively target cancer cells! It typically takes about half an hour to induce hypoglycemia. Then, the cancer cells think they are going to be fed some sugar and open up their cell "doors."

However, at this point, we pull the "bait and switch" on the cancer cells, as low doses of traditional chemotherapy are administered intravenously. The cancer cells gobble up the chemotherapy, thinking it is sugar, and are killed via much lower doses than typical chemo. In an article appearing in the *European Journal of Cancer and Clinical Oncology* (Vol. 17, 1981), Dr. Oliver Alabaster of the Cancer Research Laboratory at George Washington University showed that insulin could increase the effectiveness of a certain chemotherapy agent (methotrexate) by as much as **10,000 times** and therefore could produce significantly greater results against cancer.

But what would happen if we add DMSO to the IPT equation? According to Dr. Ross Hauser, MD, *"Most medications do not adequately pass the blood-brain barrier. The blood-brain barrier retards the entry of many compounds into the brain, including chemotherapeutic agents. Theoretically, if there was a way to increase the transport of substances into the central nervous system and through the barrier, the efficacy of treatment would be greatly enhanced."* (Treating Cancer With Insulin Potentiation Therapy, p. 84)

On his website www.caringmedical.com, Dr. Hauser also states, *"Various substances can be used to optimize the cancer-killing effects of chemotherapy, in addition to insulin, dimethyl sulfoxide (DMSO)."* What Dr. Hauser is saying is that the DMSO binds to some types of chemotherapy, and then insulin opens up the membranes of the cancer cells to the chemotherapy. DMSO/IPT is a potent "double whammy" combination of treatments, especially for brain cancer.   While combining DMSO with IPT cannot be done at home, it is possible to find an IPT clinic and convince them to combine DMSO with IPT. In Dr. Hauser's book, he lists the types of chemotherapy drugs that bind to DMSO. This treatment should be extremely potent and have no side effects, since virtually all of the chemo drugs will wind up inside the cancer cells.

IPT has virtually no side effects. There is certainly no hair loss, no going home to shiver in bed for a couple of days, and no severe vomiting. Occasionally, some nausea is encountered for a few hours after the first couple of treatments, but this is also easily managed. IPT is tough against tumors while being very gentle for the patient, who continues to live a normal, vital lifestyle while being treated. Treatments last a little over an hour, so most patients are able to continue to work at their customary vocations while undergoing these weekly treatments. But why doesn't your doctor know about this effective, less expensive, less damaging protocol? The answer is simple: The FDA hasn't approved it, except as an "experimental procedure."

Why doesn't your oncologist know about this if it has been around for 60 years? It's not because it hasn't been documented to Big Medicine and Big Pharma – there are numerous published studies in professional journals. But remember, if you are ever in doubt, just **follow the money trail**. Let's put on our "math hats" here and figure out which treatment is more lucrative – traditional chemo or IPT. Well, since IPT uses only 1/10 of the expensive chemo drugs, I guess we found our answer, didn't we?

A conventional cancer patient on traditional chemotherapy will produce hundreds of thousands of dollars of revenue for the Cancer Industry. Such a simple and effective treatment like IPT would severely cut into their profits, wouldn't it? Sadly, as we have seen over and over, **profits** take precedence over **principle**. As a result, IPT is still being ignored as a much more effective cancer treatment alternative to traditional chemotherapy.

IPT has been in existence as a therapy since 1930, and has been used successfully as a treatment for cancer since January of 1946. IPT was initially developed in 1930 for the treatment of chronic degenerative disease by Donato Perez Garcia, Sr., MD. Over the years, his son (Donato Perez Garcia II, MD) and his grandson (Donato Perez Garcia III, MD) continued using this therapy successfully for several thousands of patients. Dr. Donato Perez III, who trademarked the current name of this treatment, IPTLD® (Insulin Potentiation Targeted Low Dose), now runs a clinic in Tijuana, Mexico. You can learn more about Dr. Perez and his clinic at www.iptldmd.com and you can contact him at drdonato3@iptldmd.com.

Another top notch physician who uses IPT is Dr. Richard Linchitz who runs Linchitz Medical Wellness in Long Island, New York. His website is www.linchitzwellness.com. Dr. Frank Shallenberger also uses bio-oxidative therapies and IPT at his clinic in Nevada. His IPT technology is top-of-the-line, and his website is www.antiagingmedicine.com.

LIFE ONE

LifeOne is a very specialized combination of natural herbal ingredients in liquid form bound in a specifically designed liposomal base. This liposomal base allows the full advantage of the active herbal ingredients to remain intact, without them being broken down in the digestive tract. This liposomal carrier enables the herbal active constituents to exert full effect on the immune system, malignancies and viruses. The active ingredients in LifeOne include the following natural herbs and ingredients:

> Chrysin – a flavonoid derived from Passion Flower that has anti-oxidant capabilities and increases Tumor Necrosis Factor
> Coriolus versicolor – an anti-viral Chinese mushroom with cancer fighting effects which stimulates the immune system and inhibits invasion of cancer cells
> Diindolymethane – a phytochemical found in cruciferous vegetables which has an anti-estrogen effect on cancer cells
> Resveratrol – an antioxidant in grapes which prevents platelet clumping, and blocks resistance to insulin, inhibits abnormal estrogen action and blocks viral replication and growth
> Tumeric extract (curcumin) – antioxidant which strongly blocks inflammation, inhibits insulin resistance, inhibits metastasis in the body, and has beneficial effects on HIV viral reproduction
> Quercetin – a flavonoid that brings about programmed death of cancer cells (apoptosis)
> Green Tea Extract – contains Epigallocatechin which is a primary cancer fighting agent and antioxidant
> Selenium Methionine – an organic form of selenium which is an antioxidant, has cancer fighting effects in the body, stimulates the immune system, and helps restore selenium values which are low in cancer and AIDS patients

LifeOne provides the ammunition necessary for the body to recover from cancer, AIDS, and other immunodeficiency diseases. In the first month of LifeOne therapy it is common for weight to drop and for blood pressure to fall. The weight loss is explained by improved endocrine function with falling levels of estrogen production (reversing the excess estrogen common in most people). With less available estrogen, insulin sensitivity is restored and the body begins to burn glucose normally.

LifeOne's mechanisms of action involve mobilization of killer lymphocytes to attack malignant cells, as well as killing many harmful viruses, and repairing the damaged immune system (which is always seen in cancer patients). It accomplishes this by stimulating production of killer lymphocytes and other lymphocytes that increase antibody production. LifeOne has two US patents as an immune healing product. Clinical trials of LifeOne in patients with cancer and HIV have been carried out in Venezuela and Mexico, respectively.

The standard recommended dose of LifeOne is two tablespoons (one ounce) three times daily for 25 to 30 days. The dose is then reduced to one tablespoon (one half ounce) for 11 months. Cancer patients who have **not** had chemotherapy and radiation may experience a sense of well being and increased energy within four or five days of starting LifeOne. According to the late Dr. Jim Howenstine, *"LifeOne has been able to cure an extremely wide variety of cancer cell types. Invitro testing has shown it to be effective on 7 out of 7 cancer cell types tested, including two types of breast cancer, colon cancer, prostate cancer, cervical cancer, ovarian cancer and acute Promyelocytic leukemia."* www.newswithviews.com/Howenstine/james62.htm

Unlike other natural cancer therapies, LifeOne has undergone extensive testing including invitro testing on several cancer cell lines. These tests demonstrate the effectiveness of the product against various cell lines at varying concentrations. Dr. Valerie Beason did this testing while she was working at the NIH and NCI. The tests showed that LifeOne did indeed kill all seven cancer cell lines tested, even though the cancer cell types were diverse. Equally important, it also showed that it did not harm normal cells.

LifeOne also underwent animal testing done by Dr. Joe Demers. His first test subjects were two ferrets that had developed malignant adrenal tumors. After both recovered fully his testing went on to include dogs and other animals. Due to his success, in his book, A Holistic Approach for the Treatment of Cancer, he now recommends LifeOne as his first treatment of choice for cancer in animals. In conjunction with Dr. Demers work with small animals, Dr. Toots Banner tested LifeOne on horses, with great success. Animal testing proceeded for several years and proved LifeOne to be the most effective and safest therapy available for animals according to test results of these two veterinarians.

Even though the invitro testing showed LifeOne to be effective against all seven cell lines tested, clinically it has also shown itself to be equally effective in patient treatment against hepatic cancer, renal cancer, glioblastoma multiforma, invasive ductal cell carcinoma, oligodendroglioma, lung cancer, and small cell lung cancer as well as bladder, colon, ovarian, pancreatic, melanoma, sarcomas, and brain tumors.

All testing done on LifeOne was independently done with no physicians or veterinarians paid for their research. These participating physicians did the research because they were actively looking for better methods of treatment. Can you see a difference in this approach as opposed to the bribery and corruption that characterize Big Pharma's drug testing?

One very strong proponent of LifeOne is Dr. Paul La Rochelle, who is an orthopedic surgeon as well as an oncological surgeon. Dr. LaRochelle has used LifeOne on countless patients diagnosed with stage four cancers, from breast to liver and many others. He has never failed to bring the cancer under control using LifeOne. He feels the biggest problem in treating cancer is not the cancer, but the lack of knowledge on the part of the physician. *"Finding the initial cause of the immune system's failure takes training that is simply not offered in today's medical schools. It is more complex than suggesting taking a pill for a symptom."*

Patients who have been given chemotherapy or radiation before starting LifeOne often have a slower response than others, but the slow response can be expedited by utilizing De Aromatase in conjunction with LifeOne. De Aromatase is also extremely beneficial for use in estrogen sensitive cancer cell lines. It is a natural product used for hormonal balancing for both men and women, which improves the function of the endocrine system (pituitary gland, hypothalamus, adrenal glands, and thyroid).

Factors that hinder prompt response to LifeOne include: elevated blood sugars, undiagnosed and or untreated bacterial and fungal infections, organ damage from chemotherapy and radiation therapy, poor compliance with the low glycemic diet, unrecognized adrenal insufficiency and abnormal hormone function – most commonly hyperestrogenemia – with the lack of adequate testosterone and progesterone.

The initial phase of LifeOne therapy always causes an inflammatory reaction wherever cancer cells are present, since it stimulates killer lymphocytes to attack cancer cells. In approximately 80% of patients, this causes no symptoms. In persons with brain tumors, tumor tissue pressing on nerves and in situations where a tumor mass is occluding swallowing or respiration, this inflammatory response needs to be blunted. This is easy to accomplish with physiologic doses of hydrocortisone or cortef. This reaction generally can begin as early as the third or fourth day of LifeOne use.

In persons who have healthier immune systems this may last for 14 to 18 days. Individuals who have more severely damaged immune systems may not begin this reaction until 10 to 14 days of LifeOne therapy have been completed. Delayed appearance of the inflammatory reaction can be a clue that a more intensive investigation for immune damaging problems is needed. Immune problems frequently include unsuspected or misdiagnosed fungal, mycotic and bacterial infections. Because of potential interference with the proper function of LifeOne, the developer of LifeOne believes that it is usually advisable to postpone detoxification until the 12-month course of LifeOne has been completed.

According to Dr. José Benavente, *"For a comparison with the LifeOne Formula, TAXOL, the number one chemotherapy ingredient in the world, is derived from a single natural ingredient that comes from the bark of the Pacific Yew tree which is then chemically reproduced in pharmaceutical laboratories and it no longer has anything natural about it. The LifeOne Formula contains more than 8 active natural ingredients obtained from around the world, all of which work synergistically in a liposomal delivery system to produce an unequalled attack against cancer. The complete story and history of the LifeOne Formula can be found at* www.healthpro.com.dm.

He continues, *"I encourage you to go to this website and pour over the vast amount of information they have available on this amazing product. The LifeOne Formula was originally conceived, manufactured, and patented as an immune system enhancer, and that is its sole intended use. The body's immune system is every person's most important weapon in the war against cancer."*

A knowledgeable health care practitioner is needed to monitor this therapy. The website where you can view the LifeOne protocol, research, testing, and ingredients is www.healthpro.com.dm.

If you want to purchase LifeOne, you can call the US distributor at 407-619-4959. Ask for Bo and he will take your order. He is a good friend of mine and will take excellent care of you.

OLEANDER

In the early 1960s, a Turkish doctor named H. Zima Ozel discovered a group of rural Turkish villagers who were amazingly healthy and disease free, compared to other similar villagers. When he investigated further, he found that the healthy villagers were all taking a folk remedy that had been used in the Middle East for over two millennia. This remedy was based on a common plant referred to in the Bible as the "desert Rose," or more commonly to most of us, the oleander plant. This plant is a highly toxic plant when ingested raw, but the source of a wonderful remedy when properly prepared.

The term *"oleander"* refers to two plant species, Nerium oleander (common oleander) and Thevetia peruviana (yellow oleander). Both species contain chemicals called "cardiac glycosides" that have effects similar to the heart drug digoxin, which can be toxic. However, virtually every substance a person puts in their mouth is toxic if taken in high enough doses. Sugar is toxic if you eat too much of it. So is processed salt.

Let's get back to our oleander history lesson. After his discovery, Dr. Ozel applied for a patent. In his patent application, he mentioned several case studies as well as one study which included 494 patients. Here is a quote from the patent application: *"Between January 1981 and December 1985, 494 patients with inoperable, advanced malignant diseases were tested with NOI (injections of oleander). All malignancy had previously been diagnosed at various specialized medical institutions in Turkey and abroad. The malignancies of these patients had progressed to a state where they could no longer benefit from existing anti-tumor therapies. These 494 cases included examples of almost all varieties of malignancies and were found in various organs."*

These 494 patients experienced improved quality of life as well as regression of cancer, while reporting no notable side effects. The best results were said to be in prostate, lung, and brain cancers. Even sarcomas showed stabilization. Could it be that the oleander plant, when prepared in the correct manner and administered correctly, is **preferentially toxic** to cancer cells? If you remember, it is widely accepted that there are numerous natural substances that are toxic to cancer cells but harmless to normal cells. In fact, there are many natural substances that fit into this category. For example, purple concord grapes have more than a dozen such substances. One of the goals of alternative cancer researchers is to find substances that are toxic enough to kill cancer cells, but not so toxic that they kill normal cells.

This is where oleander comes into the equation. As I have mentioned, oleander is toxic. It should always be handled with gloves. There are many other safety warnings when dealing with the oleander plant. Rest assured, it is very toxic ... to **both** cancer cells and normal cells. But when we are able to dilute it in the appropriate proportions, then it is still toxic to cancer cells but harmless to normal cells! This level of dilution and toxicity is now well-known.

Tony Isaacs has written what is, by far, the best eBook on oleander, entitled Cancer's Natural Enemy. If you plan on using this protocol, please visit www.rose-laurel.com and purchase this eBook. It is very inexpensive and very informative. In an email from Mr. Isaacs to Webster Kehr, he stated, *"I have heard nothing but good reports from those who have been using oleander soup or the oleander extract available now at Takesun do Brasil. Cancers gone, cancers in remission, tumors shrinking, etc. And the reports out of South Africa, where the government has embraced the mixture of oleander plus agaricus blazei murrill, pau de arco and cat's claw extract combo (80% oleander) is that every single patient is doing well. HIV-AIDS halted and stabilized or even apparently reversed. And not one single report to date of a serious side effect or adverse reaction to oleander extract. It is a good feeling to be able to help someone."*

There is a chapter in the eBook titled "The Anti-Cancer and Disease Protocol," which details an extremely effective program for anyone who wants to have the maximum chances of beating cancer and disease. This chapter includes information on cleaning and detoxification, diet, nutrition, building a strong immune system, and cancer-fighting supplements.

The simple and honest truth is that oleander works incredibly well. The remedy can be used alone, with other immune-boosting supplements, and even with prescription medications and conventional treatments such as the "Big 3." From testimonials that I have read, I have learned that combining oleander with chemo or radiation will either eliminate or greatly lessen virtually all of the deleterious side effects, including hair loss!

There are two ways to take the oleander cancer treatment. The highly preferred way is to take it as a capsule or extract, since they have already been mixed to be at a safe level for humans but are at a toxic level for cancer cells. You can also purchase oleander capsules and extract at www.sutherlandiaopc.com. Charlene and I take a couple of these capsules every day as a "preventative."

The second way to take this product is to make the "oleander soup" yourself. **BEWARE:** If you choose to make your own soup, even though the dilution factor is now well established, you should read and re-read <u>Cancer's Natural Enemy</u> several times **before** you begin processing a real oleander plant, since the oleander plant is toxic. Even a small amount of the raw material, if ingested, can cause **death**.

PROTOCEL™ (ENTELEV™/CANCELL™)

Entelev™ was originally conceived and developed by Jim Sheridan of Michigan, who was a chemist, attorney, and devout Christian. He began working on his formula back in the 1930s and continued perfecting it until the 1990s. Initially, Sheridan called his product by the scientific name KC49. However since he believed that the basic idea of his formula was a gift from God, Sheridan eventually renamed his formula "Entelev," which was taken from the Greek word "entelechy" meaning *"that part of man known only to God."* It was eventually renamed Cancell™ and is currently resold as Protocel™.

In this chapter, I will use the term Protocel™ to represent the line of products which includes both Entelev™ and Cancell™. Even as a young man, Jim was a devout Christian and constantly prayed for God to direct his steps and give him the ability to use his intellect for the good of all mankind, and even had early aspirations to find a cure for cancer. Little did he know that his prayers would be answered and his dreams would be realized.

A devout Christian, Sheridan credited his formula in part to his advanced studies in chemistry and in part to a dream which he believed came from God. He refused any financial compensation, claiming Entelev™ was *"a gift from God to all his children."* Mr. Sheridan spent his whole life researching, improving the formula, and trying to bring it to the suffering people of the world. When he could not get his formula approved, he gave the product away for free. Such altruism is rarely seen.

What is it and how does it work? Protocel™ is the world's most effective free radical scavenger (antioxidant). It is designed to specifically target anaerobic cells in the body by interfering with the production of ATP energy in all of the cells in your body, which in turn lowers the voltage of each cell by between 10% and 20%. The reason that I say that Protocel™ targets anaerobic (*i.e.*, cancer) cells is simple. All the cells of our body have a specific voltage, or electrical charge.

Healthy cells have a very high voltage, while unhealthy (anaerobic) cells have a very low voltage, due to the fact that they produce energy via fermentation. The slight reduction in voltage causes anaerobic cancer cells to shift downward to a point below the minimum that they need to remain intact, thus the cells basically self-destruct and break apart, or "lyse" into harmless proteins. The healthy cells of the body typically have such a high normal voltage that the slight reduction in voltage caused by Protocel™ does not harm them.

Let's back up a bit, shall we? The process by which our cells produce and distribute energy is called cellular "respiration" or "metabolism." Most people think of respiration as breathing, but every living cell in the body is technically involved in respiration, because the term "respiration" also refers to a chemical reaction in a cell which involves oxygen and which provides energy to the cell. Crucial to the respiratory system of each cell in our body is a process called "reduction oxidation," also referred to as the "redox" system.

According to Jim Sheridan, "*This system can be thought of as a ladder, with a different chemical reaction taking place on each step...the bottom steps of the ladder involve relatively simple or 'primitive' respiratory reactions. The primitive reactions at the bottom of the ladder take place without oxygen being present. The higher respiratory reactions require the presence of oxygen. Generally, for reduction you move down the ladder. For oxidation you move up the ladder.*"

The scientific basis for Protocel™ is to place a long-term drain of power on cancer cells. Now, cells undergo short-term drains of power all the time. Back in the 1990s, I was a competitive bodybuilder. Working out with weights causes short-term drains of power to the cells, then the cells nicely recover. But when a cell undergoes a long-term drain of power, despite the fact that the cell is overloaded, respiration will continue, but the balance of the respiration system will eventually be affected. For instance, smoking cigarettes causes a long-term drain of power to the cells in the lungs. This type of condition is called a chronic condition in which the cells work constantly and never rest.

A long-term drain of power causes the cell to move slowly down the rungs of the respiratory ladder. As long as there is a drain of power, the cell's movement down the ladder slowly continues. However, when it reaches a point, which is about 85% of the way down from the top of the ladder, the cell does not fall any further down the ladder and the cell remains "in balance." This is the lowest the cell can go on the respiratory ladder and still have significant similarities to a normal cell and is also the highest point on the ladder that the cell has similarities to a primitive cell. Sheridan called this point the "critical point" of the respiratory ladder.

The critical point is the dividing line between differentiated (normal) cells and primitive cells and is the point at which a cell turns cancerous. Once pushed down to the critical point, the cell wants to stay in that new steady state at the 15% point on the ladder. The problem with having a cell in steady state at the critical point is that the body doesn't really recognize the cell, thus it does not know how to deal with it. If the cell were still healthy, it would know how to recharge itself. If the cell were further down the ladder, the body would know how to get rid of it through natural processes. But the cancer cell is walking the line, straddling the fence between normal cells and primitive cells.

One of the chemicals which reduce respiration is catechol. The natural catechols have many different oxidation reduction potentials. Protocel™ was designed to take advantage of the fact that the cancer cell is *"straddling the fence"* by acting like a catechol, inhibiting respiration at the critical point and effectively forcing the cell to move further down the respiration ladder; so it is completely into the primitive stage. Once the cell is entirely in the primitive stage, the body recognizes it and will attack and dispose of it naturally. In some places (like the brain) the body will form a crust like membrane around the primitive cells. There will be the tumor but it is dead and enclosed. In other places (skin cancer) the body will effectively digest it in a process called lysis (self-digestion).

But won't a decrease in cellular respiration also damage normal cells? Plain and simply, the answer is "**no.**" Remember, normal cells are working well within their potential to produce energy as they are near the top of the respiration ladder. Since normal cells work at such a high level of the redox system, if their respiration potential is reduced somewhat, it is no real problem for them.

According to James Sheridan, *"No special diet is required ... However, do not take mega doses of vitamins C and E while taking Entelev/Cancell. The chemical make up of these two vitamins shifts the point on the Oxidation-Reduction ladder where Entelev/Cancell works. Since Entelev/Cancell was designed to hit hardest at the 'critical point,' any shift will reduce the effectiveness of Entelev/Cancell."* http://alternativecancer.us/how.htm#diet

Based upon the fact that this protocol's success hinges upon pushing cancer cells further down the respiration ladder, it is clear that you should not use this protocol in conjunction with products that are intended to increase the production of cellular energy.

Products to avoid include co-enzyme Q10, selenium, alpha lipoic acid, creatine, IGF, spirulina, chlorella, and super algae.

Remember: If you choose this treatment, you **must** follow the guidelines of which supplements, foods, and other alternative treatments you can combine with Protocel™. Many people report noticeable results in three to five weeks. In about two months, most people see results. I have heard it said that Protocel™ does not actually *"kill"* the cancer cell per se, but rather enables the body to rid itself of the cancer cells via normal means such as lysis. However, after a long conversation with Tanya Harter Pierce, I believe that Protocel™ actually does kill the cancer cells. Regardless of the exact cancer cure mechanism, be patient, as this can take a while.

According to Webster Kehr, *"If the Protocel treatment becomes less effective over time, there are a couple of possible reasons. First, is there something you are eating (including supplements) or drinking that is interfering with Protocel? Check this very, very carefully ... Second, there may be a more complex problem. The reason Protocel may become less effective is because Protocel may not be able to kill the Multiple-Drug Resistant (MDR) cancer cells (especially if the patient has been on chemotherapy). If you think this is the reason you should immediately add Paw Paw to your treatment. The Paw Paw will not only kill MDR cells, it will also enhance the effectiveness of Protocel in other ways."*

In the 1970s, the NCI started funding Dr. Jerry McLaughlin at Purdue University to find botanical substances that had cytotoxic (cancer killing) potential. He tested and screened over 3,500 species of plants, and found that the acetogenin compounds of the Annonaceae family had the most potential. It is these acetogenins that he found to drastically reduce the ATP production of the cells' mitochondria. He worked with the various species of this family, including the Paw Paw and Graviola. Using some very sophisticated chemical modeling techniques, he found and isolated over 50 acetogenins in Paw Paw and 28 in Graviola.

These acetogenins, which are basically long chains of carbon atoms, effectively reduce the growth of blood vessels that nourish cancer cells and also inhibit the growth of MDR cells. Both Paw Paw and Graviola can be used to enhance the effectiveness of Protocel™ as they both block ATP production, thus reducing the voltage of the cell until it basically falls apart via apoptosis. However, according to Dr. McLaughlin, Paw Paw is much more effective than Graviola. Tests were done under the direction of Dr. McLaughlin on two leading Graviola products, and these test showed that Paw Paw had between 24 and 50 times the cytotoxic potency of Graviola.

The combination of Paw Paw or Graviola with Protocel™ is a powerful "cancer-fighting" cocktail. In order to maximize the effectiveness of this cocktail, they should be taken every six hours, on the hour, twenty-four hours a day, seven days a week. As I mentioned earlier in this chapter, It has been theorized that Paw Paw and Graviola (like Protocel™), were not as effective if they were combined with certain antioxidants. Currently, it is still up for debate.

To be safe, it is recommended that you not take vitamin C and vitamin E with these products, since these two antioxidants do increase ATP and would thus negate their effectiveness. In 1997, Purdue University reported that Graviola's acetogenins *"not only are effective in killing tumors that have proven resistant to anti-cancer agents, but also seem to have a special affinity for such resistant cells."*

It's important to note that Protocel™ is a trademarked name for the formulas. Protocel 23™ is the trademarked name for Entelev™, and Protocel 50™ is the trade name for Cancell™. The name Protocel™ was developed shortly before Mr. Sheridan's death.

I must give credit to Tanya Harter Pierce for her amazing research on Protocel™. Much of the information in this chapter comes directly from her research, phone conversations, and emails. I cannot say enough good things about her book <u>Outsmart Your Cancer</u>. It was an excellent source of information on the Protocel™ treatment protocol. If you choose to use Protocel™, then you must purchase her book. It is "required reading" and is available at the following website: <u>www.outsmartyourcancer.com</u>.

SODIUM BICARBONATE (DR. TULLIO SIMONCINI)

Despite the fact that I disagree with the underlying premise of this treatment (*i.e.,* that cancer is a fungus), I must include it in this chapter, since there have been multitudes of cancer patients that have been completely cured using this protocol. Some of this information comes from Vicente Estoque, and I thank him for his research.

Dr. Tullio Simoncini is a Roman doctor who has a unique approach to treating cancer: he uses sodium bicarbonate, a chemical compound with the formula $NaHCO_3$. Of course, you may have long forgotten high school chemistry, and you may not be familiar with sodium bicarbonate . . . but I'll bet you've heard of baking soda!

Baking soda is commonly used as an antacid for short-term relief of an upset stomach, to correct acidosis in kidney disorders, to "alkalinize" urine during bladder infections, and to minimize uric acid crystallization during gout treatment. But according to Simoncini, sodium bicarbonate is unstoppably effective when it comes to cancer tissues. Simoncini's baking soda treatment is based on the theory that "cancer is a fungus," which is also the title of his book. While I disagree with his premise, namely that cancer is a fungus, he certainly has had excellent success with this protocol.

Perhaps the success is due to the fact that baking soda floods the cancer cells with a shockwave of alkalinity and oxygen, thus reversing the hypoxia which is always associated with cancerous tissue. Or perhaps it works because a comparison of cancer tissue with healthy tissue indicates that cancerous tissue always has a much higher concentration of toxic chemicals and pesticides than normal tissue, and sodium bicarbonate possesses the property of absorbing heavy metals, dioxins, and furans. Perhaps it's a combination of the two. Or perhaps there **is** a fungal link to cancer.   In any event, regardless of the cancer kill mechanism, there is no doubt that thousands of cancer patients credit Simoncini's sodium bicarbonate treatment with saving their lives.

The most important side effects of this treatment are thirst and weakness, unlike traditional treatments such as chemotherapy. According to Dr. Simoncini, *"Chemotherapy, in fact, destroys everything. It is a given fact that it dramatically exhausts the cells of the marrow and of the blood, thus allowing a greater spreading of the infection. It irreversibly intoxicates the liver, thus preventing it from building new elements of defense, and it mercilessly knocks out nerve cells, thus weakening the organism's reactive capabilities and delivering it to the invaders. This is mainly because it is not clear how it affects the colonies, and because by strongly debilitating the organism such intervention makes the invasion of the mycetes faster and more ferocious."*

Dr. Simoncini believes that the best way to try to eliminate a tumor is to bring it into contact with sodium bicarbonate, as closely as possible, using oral administration for the digestive tract, enemas for the rectum, douching for the vagina and uterus, intravenous injection for the lung and the brain, and inhalation for the upper airways. Breasts, lymph nodes and subcutaneous lumps can be treated with local perfusions. The internal organs can be treated by locating suitable catheters in the arteries (of the liver, pancreas, prostate, and limbs) or in the cavities (of the pleura or peritoneum). Simoncini theorizes that the sodium bicarbonate destroys the fungal colonies at the heart of cancerous tumors.

He also has reported on cases of brain tumors (both primary and metastatic) that stop growing after therapy with a 5% sodium bicarbonate solution. He also reports success with prostate cancer, intestinal cancer, stomach cancer, bladder cancer, breast cancer, cancer of the spleen, liver cancer, lung cancer, oropharyngeal cancer, peritoneal carcinosis, pancreatic cancer, and other cancers.

According to Dr. Simoncini, this protocol can be self-applied in certain types of cancer (oral, esophagal, stomach, rectal, intestinal) if the cancer is limited to the organ and has not metastasized. However, he does recommend the supervision of a doctor in these cases. In all other cases, the assistance of a doctor is mandatory to administer the infusions, etc.

There are numerous correlations and similarities between cancer and fungal infections. There are 400,000 species of fungi, out of which 400 are pathogens. In 1990, Elizabeth Moore-Landecker revealed fungi and their mycotoxins are able to cause genetic variations and mutations. The fact that mycotoxins (fungal toxins) can cause cancer is not up for grabs.

The American Cancer Society Textbook of Clinical Oncology states, *"Mycotoxins are genotoxic carcinogens, and exposure begins in utero and in mother's milk, continuing throughout life; these conditions favor the occurrence of disease."*

Dr. Doug Kaufman has noted many similarities between cancer and fungus. Let's have a look at some fascinating facts which he points out:

> Both cancer cells and fungi can metabolize nutrients anaerobically (without oxygen)
> Both cancer cells and fungi must have sugar in order to survive and will die in the absence of sugar
> Both cancer cells and fungi produce lactic acid
> Both cancer cells and fungi can be impacted by antifungal medicines

In his book, The Germ that Causes Cancer, in total agreement with Dr. Simoncini, Kaufman hypothesizes that cancer is a deep-rooted fungal infection that our immune system fails to recognize. He also believes that antibiotics, many of which begin as fungi, can contribute to the development of cancer. He hypothesizes that perhaps many cases of cancer are actually misdiagnosed and are in reality fungal infections or overgrowths. Fungal infections not only can be extremely contagious, but they also go hand in hand with leukemia (**every** oncologist knows this). For example, in 1999, Dr. Meinolf Karthaus watched three different children with "leukemia" suddenly go into remission upon receiving a triple antifungal drug cocktail for their secondary fungal infections.

According to Dr. Simoncini, *"My methods have cured people for 20 years. Many of my patients recovered completely from cancer, even in cases where official oncology had given up."* So, what is his cure rate? Dr. Simoncini gives the following statistics: *"If the fungi are sensitive to the sodium bicarbonate solutions and the tumor size is below 3 cm, the percentage will be around 90%, in terminal cases where the patient is in reasonably good condition it is 50%."*

Dr. Simoncini has a heart that really loves people, and his desire is to cure everyone from cancer. His intentions are quite noble – he is a man of honor and integrity. I believe it is fitting to conclude this section with a quote from Dr. Simoncini: *"My deep wish is to make this therapy available to all humanity. It is my firm hope that soon, the fundamental role of fungi in the development of neoplastic disease is acknowledged, so that it is possible to find, with the help of all existing forces of the health establishment, those anti-mycotic drugs and those systems of therapy that can quickly defeat, without damage and suffering, a disease that brings so much devastation to humanity."*

Dr. Simoncini can be reached at t.simoncini@alice.it and his website is www.cancerfungus.com.

ULTRAVIOLET BLOOD IRRADIATION THERAPY ("UVBI")

Considerable research into the use of ultraviolet (UV) light for treatment of disease was initiated in the 1870s. One of the first researchers to experiment with UV light was Niels Ryberg Finsen, who won the Nobel Prize for Medicine and Physiology in 1903 for his UV treatments of 300 people suffering from Lupus in Denmark.

Another maverick to experiment with light therapy was Kurt Naswitis, who directly irradiated the blood with UV light through a shunt in 1922. Then beginning in the 1920s and continuing through the 1930s, Seattle scientist Dr. Emmett Knott sought to harness the known bacteriacidal properties of UV rays in order to treat infectious blood diseases. Ultraviolet Blood Irradiation Therapy ("UVBI") is a scientifically accurate name given to what has previously been called PhotoBiologic therapy, Photophoresis, and Photoluminescence (among other names).

UVBI has been used for many years to deactivate bacteria, viruses, fungi, toxins, and other invading organisms. This therapy is performed by irradiating (with UV light) a calculated portion (100-125 mL) of the patient's blood for between 10 and 30 minutes, then reintroducing the blood back into the body. This irradiated blood then emits photonic energy to the rest of the blood, which stimulates a series of favorable reactions and generates an oxidative rich environment. This in turn deactivates toxins, increases oxygen availability, stimulates the immune system, decreases blood viscosity, inhibits clot formation in the main circulation, and improves blood circulation by way of vasodilatation (*i.e.*, the widening of blood vessels). UVBI also decreases platelet aggregation and stimulates singlet oxygen, which creates an oxidative environment promoting self-destruction of abnormal cells (cancer) via apoptosis.

Central to understanding the action of UVBI was the 1922 discovery by Alexander Gurvich that all living cells regularly emit **biophotons.** A photon is a single particle of light. Biophotons are the smallest physical units of light that are stored in and used by all biological organisms (including you). Vital sun energy finds its way into your cells via the food you eat, in the form of these biophotons. For reasons discussed below, red blood cells (erythrocytes) are peculiarly sensitive to light and will respond to it by emitting biophotons that in turn stimulate other red cells to do likewise. Bacteria and viruses are more vulnerable to biophotonic emissions than are normal cells.

Early researchers noted that UVBI has a "dual effect" on the immune system: normal doses stimulate leukocytes while excess doses destroy various leukocytes. The first effect is the basis of the immune response explanation of the beneficial effects of UVBI. The second suggests a reason why UVBI seems so effective against autoimmune diseases. In autoimmune disorders, it appears that the metabolically active T-cells and other immune cells absorb much greater numbers of biophotons than ordinary body cells, and this destroys them, slowing down or stopping the disease. Thus, UVBI can therefore be both "immuno-stiumulatory" and "immuno-suppressive" depending on which sets of cells are under discussion. Likewise, an initial dose of UVBI can stimulate a cell but repeated doses can eventually inhibit it or destroy it.

UVBI also oxygenates and improves the characteristics of the blood. This happens quickly following transfusion of treated blood and can transform clumps of red blood cells into free-flowing blood within minutes. Blood oxygenation might be connected with the fact that UVBI creates a small amount of **ozone** in the blood. Certain special characteristics of the red blood cells as well as their sheer numbers (25 trillion in adults) make them especially effective as agents of UVBI, which is considered primarily a red blood cell immunotherapy. The stimulation of red blood cells turns them into a "third arm" of the immune system. It is also possible that the fragments of bacteria, virus, and cells that are destroyed by UVBI act as a kind of "vaccine" in the plasma, enhancing the immune response. UVBI also reverses the suppression of the detoxifying function of the liver.

Dr. Emmett Knott, a pioneer in this therapy, together with his associates, sought to explain exactly how UVBI treatment obtains its therapeutic effect. They and subsequent researchers have identified two possible modes:

1. the ultraviolet treatment of the blood destroys or alters viruses and bacteria in the extracted blood in such a way as to provoke a reaction by the immune system upon its return to the body which, in turn, destroys most or all of the other bacteria or virus in the body; and

2. the treatment of a small fraction (5%) of the blood then spreads throughout the entire volume of the blood upon returning to the body, and the induced secondary emissions destroy viruses, bacteria, and activated white blood cells (leukocytes).

In the November 2, 2007, issue of *Science Daily*, there was an interesting article which spotlighted scientists at Newcastle University (Colin Self and Stephen Thompson) who have developed a cancer fighting technology utilizing UV light to activate antibodies which specifically attack tumors. According to Professor Colin Self, "*We have a means of being able to illuminate an area to turn on the immune system to kill cancer in that area. I would describe this development as the equivalent of ultra-specific 'magic bullets.' This could mean that a patient coming in for treatment of bladder cancer would receive an injection of the cloaked antibodies. She would sit in the waiting room for an hour and then come back in for treatment by light. Just a few minutes of the light therapy directed at the region of the tumour would activate the T-cells causing her body's own immune system to attack the tumour.*" www.sciencedaily.com/releases/2007/10/071030080626.htm

According to Dr. William Campbell Douglass, author of a book about light therapy called <u>Into the Light</u>, UVBI has brought about remarkable results in both prompting cancer remission and extending the lives of patients who have been diagnosed with cancer. At the Yale Cancer Center, Dr. Richard L. Edelson has developed a highly successful method of fighting Cutaneous T-Cell Lymphoma (CTCL) using a variation on UVBI. He calls his version "trans-immunization therapy." In his variation, the entire blood supply is treated, rather than just a small sample of the blood. Dr. Edelson's treatment (while highly successful) is also very expensive, and he only treats CTCL with it. The good news, though, is that there is every reason to believe that small samples of blood treated by UV light can be just as effective as treating the entire blood supply.

In the words of Dr. Robert Rowen, MD, *"If you give that blood a clean slate, you inactivate the organisms with the ultraviolet, and give it back to the body, the body can now see the antigen structure of those organisms, or in other words, the three dimensional structure. It knows that those organisms are there, but the organisms happen to be dead, so they're not going to hurt you. Your body can then see those organisms and mount a much more efficient immune response."*

UVBI should be a part of a multi-pronged approach to treatment. It's an ideal adjunctive therapy for cancer in that it adds oxygen to the body, cuts pain, reduces inflammation, and decreases infections. Lifestyle, immune system, nutrition, and detoxification all go hand-in-hand with UVBI. And don't forget, UVBI is much safer than the "Big 3."

VITAMIN B$_{17}$

When Dad died back in 1996, I began my cancer journey. The first alternative cancer treatment which I discovered was Vitamin B$_{17}$, also known as Laetrile. I saw a video of a champion arm wrestler named Jason Vale who had been cured of cancer by eating the seeds from apples and apricots (which contain vitamin B$_{17}$) and read lots of good information on his website. The logic and science of how and why vitamin B$_{17}$ kills cancer cells was fascinating to me. Laetrile therapy is based upon the theory that cancer is a result of a nutritional deficiency combined with the trophoblast theory.

In the 1940s, Dr. Ernst T. Krebs, Sr. and his son (Dr. E.T. Krebs, Jr.) and other doctors were involved in researching Beard's thesis on the trophoblast theory of cancer, and they affirmed that he was correct. In 1949, the elder Krebs wrote a paper on the pregnancy toxemias and the role of the pancreas and trophoblast. The following year, Dr. Krebs and his son published a paper The Unitarian or Trophoblastic Thesis of Cancer, in the Medical Record (Vol. 163, No. 7, July 1950).

In the following years, the father and son team investigated co-enzymes and the possibility that cancer results from a vitamin deficiency disease. In the early 1950s, they theorized that cancer was caused by the lack of an essential food compound in modern-man's diet, identified as part of the nitriloside family which is found in over 1200 edible plants. Krebs learned of the kingdom of Hunza in the Himalayan Mountains of Northern Pakistan, who were said to be "cancer-free." Doctors Krebs knew that they ate huge quantities of apricots, but they did not believe that the fruit contained any cancer fighting substances. Until they learned that the Hunzakuts also eat the pits of the apricot seeds, which are one of the richest sources of nitrilosides!

Nitrilosides are especially prevalent in the seeds of apricots, peaches, apples, millet, bean sprouts, buckwheat, and other fruits and nuts, including bitter almonds. Dr. Krebs was able to extract certain glycosides from plants which contained nitrolosides, and eventually applied for a patent for the process of producing a metabolite form of these glycosides for clinical use. He named it *"Laetrile."* (**LAE**-vo-mandeloni**TRILE**-beta-glucuronoside).

It took several years and actual clinical testing around the world before a model was proposed rationalizing the utility of Laetrile in the prevention as well as the treatment of cancer, when it received the name *"Vitamin B_{17}."* Now, it is important to remember that a vitamin is a co-enzyme, which basically means that it must be associated with an enzyme in order for the enzyme to function optimally. We know that the pancreatic and other enzymes are reliant upon several essential co-factors and co-enzymes. Let's remember this co-enzyme information as we learn a little bit more about the Hunzakuts.

The Hunzakuts consume between 100-200 times more B_{17} in their diet than the average American, due mainly to eating the seeds of apricots and also lots of millet. Interestingly, there is no such thing as money in Hunza. A man's wealth is measured by the number of apricot trees he owns. And the most coveted food is the pit of the apricot seed, one of the highest sources of B_{17} on earth. Visiting teams of doctors found the Hunzacuts to be cancer free. One of the first medical teams to study the Hunza was headed by world-renowned British surgeon Dr. Robert McCarrison. Writing in the AMA Journal January 7, 1922, he reported: *"The Hunza has no known incidence of cancer. They have an abundant crop of apricots. These they dry in the sun and use largely in their food."*

But why haven't you heard of vitamin B_{17}? It seems so simple! Well, the fact of the matter is that the Cancer Industry has suppressed this information and has even made it illegal to sell B_{17}. Big Medicine has mounted highly successful "scare" campaigns based on the fact that vitamin B_{17} contains quantities of "deadly" cyanide. This is patently false. Studies show that vitamin B_{17} is harmless to healthy tissue.

Here's why: Each molecule of B_{17} contains one unit of hydrogen cyanide, one unit of benzaldehyde and two of glucose (*sugar*) tightly locked together. In order for the hydrogen cyanide to become dangerous it is first necessary to unlock the molecule to release it, a trick that can only be performed by an enzyme called beta-glucosidase, which is present all over the human body only in minute quantities, but in huge quantities at only one place: **cancer cells.**

Thus the hydrogen cyanide is unlocked only at the cancer site with drastic results, which become utterly devastating to the cancer cells since the benzaldehyde unit unlocks at the same time. The cancer cells get a double whammy of cyanide and benzaldeyhde! Benzaldehyde is a deadly poison in its own right, but when it teams up with cyanide, the result is a poison 100 times more deadly than either in isolation. **The cancer cells are literally obliterated**!

But what about danger to the rest of the body's cells? Another enzyme, rhodanese, always present in far larger quantities than the unlocking enzyme beta-glucosidase in healthy tissues, has the ability to completely break down both cyanide and benzaldehyde into a thiocyanate (a harmless substance) and salicylate (which is a pain killer similar to aspirin). Interestingly, malignant cancer cells contain no rhodanese at all, leaving them completely at the mercy of the two deadly poisons. This whole process is known as selective toxicity, since only the cancer cells are specifically targeted and destroyed.

Now remember that I earlier referred to vitamin B_{17} as a co-enzyme and said that this therapy is based, in part, on the trophoblast theory of cancer? The trophoblast theory focuses on the importance of pancreatic enzymes (trypsin, chymotrypsin, and amylase) to digest the protective coating around cancer cells. **Here's the connection between this theory and vitamin B_{17}**: In the presence of certain inhibitors in our blood, trypsin is inactivated and must be acted upon by hydrogen cyanide to become active again. On this basis, vitamin B_{17} acts as a co-enzyme to trypsin, since it provides hydrogen cyanide, a harmless molecule, which reactivates the trypsin which is necessary to digest the protective coating of cancer cells. Fascinating, isn't it?

The hundreds of clinical studies conducted by many competent physicians around the world, including those directed by Dr. Emesto Contreras at the Oasis of Hope Hospital in Mexico, give us complete confidence that B_{17} therapy poses no threat to normal cells. This is **bad** news for the Cancer Industry. Apricot seeds are cheap...real cheap...not nearly as expensive as their latest chemotherapy drug cocktail.

The longest and most famous laetrile tests ever performed were run for nearly five years at the USA's most prestigious cancer research center, Memorial Sloan-Kettering Cancer Center in New York. Dr Kanematsu Suguira, the preeminent cancer researcher in America, headed the team of researchers. At the conclusion of the trials, on June 15, 1977, they released a press statement. The press release read; *"Laetrile was found to possess neither preventative, nor tumor-regressent, nor anti-metastatic, nor curative anticancer activity."*

So that is it then, right? **Wrong**. When a journalist asked Dr. Sugiura *"Do you stick by your belief that laetrile stops the spread of cancer?"* He replied, *"**I stick**."* He was then asked why Sloan-Kettering was against using laetrile to fight cancer. Sugiura answered *"I don't know. Maybe the medical profession doesn't like it because they are making too much money."*

Dr. Lloyd Schloen, a biochemist at Sloan-Kettering, also performed test on laetrile, but he had also included proteolytic enzymes to his injections and reported **100% cure rate** among his albino mice. This data had to be buried. Sloan-Kettering took action quickly. They performed their own tests which were designed to contradict Dr. Schloen's findings. They then changed the protocols of the tests and amounts of laetrile to make certain that they failed. Not surprisingly, the tests failed, and that is what they reported. They couldn't let the word out that laetrile had been proven to be a natural, effective cure for cancer. This would have spelled economic disaster for the Cancer Industry.

The most effective method of B_{17} treatment has been six grams, intravenous once a day, usually given for three weeks. You should also add **zinc**, since it is the transportation mechanism for B_{17} in the body. Biochemists and researchers have found that you can give massive doses of B_{17} to a patient, but if the patient was deficient in zinc, none of the B_{17} would get into the tissues of the body. Also important with B_{17} therapy are **pancreatic enzymes**, which form the first layer of defense the body has against cancer. If you have a low supply of these digestive enzymes then it will be difficult for B_{17} to work. Also, emulsified vitamin A is usually used as an additional supplement to B_{17} therapy. And laetrile therapy is best used in conjunction with a very strict nutritional regimen, oftentimes with a raw foods diet. If you want to take B_{17} as a preventative, Dr. Krebs suggested a minimum level of 50 milligrams per day for normal, healthy adult.

We purchase vitamin B_{17} from Medicina Alternativa: www.tjsupply.com or CytoPharma: www.cytopharma.com. Over the past decade, we have purchased B_{17} from both companies and both have proven to be reliable sources. A bottle of one hundred pills (100 milligrams per pill) is right around $20.

Lastly, here's a b**it of trivia:** the bitter almond tree, a wonderful source of nitrilosides, was banned from the United States in 1995.

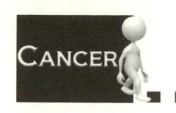

CHAPTER 7
FIVE STEPS & SEVEN TOXICITIES

> "THERE IS NOTHING MORE DIFFICULT TO TAKE IN HAND, MORE PERILOUS TO CONDUCT, OR MORE UNCERTAIN IN ITS SUCCESS THAN TO TAKE THE LEAD IN THE INTRODUCTION OF A NEW ORDER OF THINGS BECAUSE THE INNOVATOR HAS FOR ENEMIES ALL THOSE WHO HAVE DONE WELL UNDER THE OLD CONDITIONS & LUKEWARM DEFENDERS IN THOSE WHO MAY DO WELL UNDER THE NEW."   – PRINCE MACHIAVELLI

This chapter is a synopsis of Dr. Rashid Buttar's cancer treatment methodology, and most of the information was provided directly by Dr. Buttar himself. Dr. Buttar understands what is going on with the Medical Mafia and also understands the fundamental issues creating disease, such as heavy metal and other toxicities. More importantly, he understands what needs to be done to bring a person back to health.

5 STEPS IN TREATING CANCER

Step 1 – Clean
Detoxify the biological system (long term)

This step is the initial and primary step of cleaning up the biological system. Heavy metals along with the persistent organic pollutants (POP's) are increasing in our bodies. As a result of a chronic lack of good nutrition and an over abundance of the above mentioned toxicities, changes begin taking place within the physiological system as described with an analogy of a volcano of various toxicities erupting and causing massive burden on the immune system.

Eventually, this process leads to an increase in cell mutations and cancer oftentimes is the result, since the protective antioxidant pathways are unable to keep up with the increasing rate of cell mutations. Apoptosis (programmed cell death) which is responsible for the self destruction of abnormal, unhealthy cells begins to become suppressed, allowing cancer cells to grow unchecked. This is what begins to happen in the picture of cancer.

Step 2 – Optimize
Reconfigure the physiologic environment (re-establish)

This step is the most lengthy and most difficult of the five steps. This step includes all therapies designed to make the patient's internal biological system "unfriendly" to cancer, such as proper nutrition, supplementation (vitamins, minerals, herbs and antioxidants), autohemotherapy, hydrogen peroxide, hyperthermia, and hyperbaric oxygen or other treatments that increase oxygenation. It also includes supporting the adrenal system, the optimization of the gastrointestinal system, and supporting the mental aspects (spiritual, emotional and psychological) that are so vital in cancer treatment. Also critical in this stage is the **restoration of hope**.

Step 3 – Repair
Rebuild and stimulate the immune system (immune modulation)

This step focuses on rebuilding and repairing the patient's compromised immune system. Dr. Buttar has a very precise regimen which utilizes highly specific immune modulating poly-peptide analogs to accomplish this goal. It is important to remember that if cancer exists in the body, by definition the immune system is damaged. Therefore, it becomes essential to repair the immune system and "upregulate" it to the point that it can begin to naturally address the issue of the cancer on its own.

Step 4 – Identify
Target acquisition of the cancer (AARSOV)

This step is used as a specific method of acquisition of the cancer by the now repaired and reinitiated immune system that was previously damaged and not functioning properly. Dr. Buttar refers to this technique with the acronym "AARSOTA," which stands for "*Autogenous Antigen Receptor Specific Oncogenic Target Acquisition.*" Essentially, it's a method by which the body is enabled to identify the cancer as being foreign and allows the immune system to move against the cancer.

As an example, human chorionic gonadotropin (HCG) and alpha feto protein (AFP) are non-specific markers of cancer, but they are also markers of pregnancy. The fetus is growing inside a woman's body but is foreign. Why doesn't the immune system fight against the fetus? Because these markers (HCG and AFP) allow the body to know that this growing organism should not be attacked. However, cancer cells are able to mimic a fetus by releasing the same markers. Dr. Buttar developed AARSOTA as a means to overcome this "cloaking" device that cancer uses to fool the immune system into leaving it alone. The AARSOTA allows the body's immune system to identify the "signature" of the cancer and begin fighting it.

Step 5 – Maintain
Sustain changes achieved with the first four steps

Oftentimes, cancer patients revert to their old habits and fail to follow through on the important aspects of their cancer protocol; thus, the cancer returns. The changes initiated in the first four steps must be sustained; otherwise, the cancer will come back. Dr. Buttar's fifth step focuses on maintaining the progress which has been accomplished in the first four steps and keeping the cancer at bay...permanently.

THE 7 TOXICITIES

According to Dr. Buttar, *"My experience having worked with several thousand patients from all over the world has taught me that the vast majority of toxins come from seven major sources. I speak from firsthand knowledge when I say that if these seven toxicities are effectively addressed and removed — with 'effectively' being the key operative word here — the vast majority of oxidative stress is eliminated."*

He continues, *"When this occurs, chronic disease, by definition, simply cannot exist. It becomes impossible for chronic disease to set up house in a body where the oxidative burden is minimal or nonexistent because the cause (toxicities) are no longer present to induce the increased burden of oxidative stress leading to chronic disease."*

On the following pages, I will review and briefly explore these seven toxicities.

Toxicity 1 – Heavy Metals

Heavy metals include mercury, lead, antimony, nickel, cadmium, tin, arsenic, uranium, as well as a host of others. In addition to causing significant oxidative damage, heavy metals are "doubly dangerous" because they have the ability to displace many of the essential minerals your body needs to function properly. These minerals include, among others, for example, magnesium, copper, manganese, zinc, and selenium. Adding insult to the injury, heavy metals and (mercury in particular) wreak additional havoc on the endocrine system, which regulates hormonal levels. And as if it couldn't get any worse, some people may even have an additional issue due to alleginicity (having an allergic reaction) to the metal in question.

Dr. Buttar is the Chairman of the American Board of Clinical Metal Toxicology, so it's his responsibility (along with the rest of the executive board) to help establish educational guidelines for doctors on the dangers of heavy metals, how to identify the presence of heavy metals, and how to remove them safely and effectively from their patients. It's also his responsibility to keep up-to-date on the latest research regarding heavy metals and chronic disease. Much of this research is published on Toxline, a search engine that is associated with the National Library of Medicine's website. Toxline is under the auspices of the Agency for Toxic Substances and Disease Registry (ATSDR), which is a subdivision of the Centers for Disease Control (CDC).

A simple Toxline search on "mercury" reveals 358 studies linking mercury with heart disease, 643 linking mercury with cancer, and 1,445 linking mercury to neurodegenerative disease (such as autism, Alzheimer's, etc.). Keep in mind, mercury is just one of the many heavy metals known to have serious health issues. The example used in these search criteria was looking just at "mercury." The search criteria were not looking for all metals contributing to these disease processes. Those who argue against chronic heavy metal toxicity as a valid concern in clinical medicine have compromised their own integrity, and their motives have become highly suspect. The simple facts scream the truth that anyone can easily confirm themselves if they would simply open their eyes and put aside their bias!

I chose mercury for this example because it causes some of the worst damage in the human body and is considered to be the second most toxic element known to man, according to the Environmental Protection Agency (EPA). Only uranium is considered to be more toxic. For instance, whenever we hear of a mercury spill in a high school, the students are evacuated, hazmat teams are rushed in, and the immediate area is bordered off as a "hazardous spill area." No one is allowed to return until the Occupational Safety and Health Administration

(OSHA) has cleared the building. This, by the way, is when inorganic mercury has been spilled, in actuality the least toxic version of the metal.

Toxicity 2 – Persistent Organic Pollutants

The second category of toxins is known as the persistent organic pollutants (POP's) because they tend to "persist" in the body and are extremely difficult to eliminate. Some of these POP's can continue on for generations, being passed from mother to daughter and affecting both sexes while still in utero. Many of these include insecticides from the 1950s and 1960s. While they may no longer be allowed or used, their effects are still causing birth defects in children two generations later.

In 2000, the World Health Organization Congress met in South Africa to discuss the implications of the 12 most deadly organic compounds and pollutants, affectionately named "the Dirty Dozen." There was a concerted effort for industrialized countries to reach an agreement to begin removal of these dangerous elements from the environment because the Dirty Dozen had now clearly been implicated in the causation of numerous disease processes. These deadly organic compounds and pollutants include DDT, PCB's, dioxin, chlordane, furans and a number of other insecticides.

Even if all industrialized countries immediately stopped using these substances, these POP's have already gotten a monumental head start. For example, the "newest" toxic chemical in the Dirty Dozen was introduced in 1957, over 50 years ago, and the oldest has been in use since 1913, almost 100 years ago. These POPs exist in pesticides, insecticides, varnishes, cleaning solutions and virtually every product in an aerosol can, a bottle underneath your kitchen sink or in your garage right now. Be careful when using any chemical product, no matter how safe the manufacturer claims it to be.

In 2005, the Environmental Working Group put out a report by Jane Houlihan and Timothy Kropp, PhD, titled "Body Burden: The Pollution in Newborns." The placental cord blood of newborn babies was tested for 413 different industrial chemicals and found to be positive for 287 of these substances, which included PCB's, mercury, DDT, dioxin, fluorinated hydrocarbons, organophosphates, and many other categories of POP's. This blood was obtained on these infants' very first day on the planet! What are the full implications of these and similar toxicities being passed from mother to infant?

Toxicity 3 – Opportunistics

The third toxicity represents the opportunistic infections, which include bacteria, viruses, parasites, yeast and a host of other critters. I call them the "opportunistics" because these organisms need an opportunity before they can set up house in the body. The right environment must be created in order for them to survive and thrive. This third class of toxicity is actually heavily dependent on the first and second toxicities, because heavy metals and POP's suppress the immune system and render the body vulnerable to opportunistic pathogens. Opportunistics are the only class of the seven toxicities that modern medicine has done a reasonably fair job of addressing with antibiotics, antivirals, antifungals and so on. However, medical professionals have miserably failed to establish why there are so many more infectious pathogens today than in years past. No one has considered the first and second toxicities as the cause of the rampant increase in opportunistic infections, further contributed by drug resistance from the overuse of antibiotics and other medications.

Moreover, the problem of why one person gets a particular infection and another one doesn't, has never been addressed. The answer is because of the variance in people's immune systems due to differences in the type and amount of toxic burden that everyone is carrying, which cause the decline in the immune system. The problem, even though these drugs work, is that if you don't address the underlying cause of the immune suppression, the problem (infection) will recur. The first and second toxicities, which are responsible for the drop in immunity, are ignored by traditional medicine. You can beat back these infections with drugs for a while, but once the drugs are stopped, the problem **always** comes back. Unless the immunosuppressive cause is removed, these issues continue to recur like a bad dream. This is why conditions like yeast infections in women and jock itch and athlete's foot in men are persistent and are an indication to look much deeper.

Toxicity 4 – Energetic Toxicity

The first three toxicities discussed are objectively measurable, but the remaining four are a bit more esoteric. Energetic toxicity includes all the high-powered energy waves that pass over, under and through our bodies every day. In modern society, our bodies are bombarded by energetic toxicity from things we can't see, including electromagnetic radiation (from power lines and microwaves) and ambient radiation (from cell phones, military radar systems, TV's, and computer screens). And this fourth toxicity is increasing at a stunningly rapid exponential rate.

The level of ambient cell phone radiation we are exposed to is just one example of energetic toxicities. What possible implications could cell phones have regarding toxicity? Dr. George Carlo, an attorney and researcher from the Science and Public Policy Institute, conducted a study on cell phone radiation and cancer back in the 1980s, long before the explosion in cellular usage. The study was actually sponsored jointly by the federal government and a cell phone manufacturer. The goal was to prove that cell phone radiation did not cause cancer, but unfortunately, his data proved just the opposite.

Dr. Carlo explained to Dr. Buttar (in person) that from 1984 to 2004, the first billion cell phones entered the global market. It took only the next 18 months (not 20 years) for the second billion to appear. Less than one year later, the third billion cell phones flooded our airwaves. As a result, ambient cell phone radiation has increased 500,000% in the last decades in the average urban area. In his book <u>Cell Phones: Invisible Hazards in the Wireless Age</u>, Dr. Carlo reported that the rate of death from brain cancer was higher among handheld phone users. Because the cell phone company sponsored the research, they claimed ownership of the data and prevented its release. But Dr. Carlo wrote several books on the subject that revealed the health and environmental impact of this particular toxicity.

Some readers may be familiar with the increasingly frequent news stories about the drastic reduction in the population of honeybees over the last several years. In fact, the bee populations are rapidly disappearing on four of the five continents. The reasons have been attributed to parasites, pestilence, and insecticides. But in actuality, it has to do with a naturally occurring mineral called magnetite and how the ambient cell phone radiation affects this mineral. Bees have magnetite in their intestinal tracts. Humans have it in their brains. Birds have it in their beaks. Magnetite helps orient us by aligning with Earth's magnetic grid and allows for direction finding. It accounts for the ability of animals and birds to find their way back home from thousands of miles away and helps to explain how certain species find their way back to their nesting grounds and follow specific migratory patterns.

The magnetite in the intestinal tracts of the bees, when aligned with Earth's magnetic grids, allows the bees to find their way back to their hives. However, the incredible increase in ambient cell phone radiation prevents the magnetite from aligning correctly with Earth's magnetic grid, so the bees get disoriented and never make it back to the hive. The result is that the bee populations are rapidly diminishing.

Another example is homing pigeons, which have magnetite in their beaks, as do most birds. Racing homing pigeons is an ancient and very upscale sport that challenges birds in races of up to 600 miles. As recently as a few years ago, the number of pigeons that kept on course and finished the race was 85%, but today, an average of only 15% make it back alive.

Imagine the catastrophic impact of the disappearance of honeybees. Bees pollinate an immense amount of our food supply. Without bees, most food won't grow. The USDA estimates that about one-third of the total human diet is derived from insect-pollinated plants and the honeybee is responsible for 80% of this pollination. A study from Cornell University in 2000 concluded that the direct value of honeybee pollination to US agriculture is more than $14.6 billion, and that was a decade ago!

Before I move on to the next toxicity, there's one last thing I want to mention in this discussion of the fourth toxicity, and that is the use of microwave ovens. Just know it's **not** a natural way of heating food. The cancer patients Dr. Buttar has tested for energetic toxicity exposures have the highest levels of microwave radiation exposure of all the various types of energetic pollution. I personally have not used a microwave since 2005 and don't even have one plugged into the wall at either my home or office. I hope that will convince you to throw your microwave oven out. Toaster ovens and convection ovens are fine, however.

Toxicity 5 – Emotional/Physiological Toxicity

Whether you know it or not, your cells have their own intelligence. They also have memory that's completely independent of your conscious intellect. Athletes and dancers know what "muscle memory" is. When you train over and over and it comes time to compete, your body remembers all the actions that are needed, automatically, without your even having to think. Similarly, therapists who deal with trauma and posttraumatic stress disorder often use physical interventions instead of "talk therapy" because that is where those memories are stored, within the body, like muscle memory.

The link between physical health and mental health is not even up for debate anymore. For example, every patient suffering with cancer I have seen did not begin to recover until they had addressed their emotional issues. Only those who were able to successfully come to terms with and release their anger, to forgive and choose to love unconditionally have a chance of winning the battle.

Dr. Ryke Geerd Hamer, a German oncologist whose son tragically died in a hunting accident in 1978, has done some remarkable work in this arena. He and his wife were intensely grief-stricken with the loss of their son. Eventually, Dr. Hamer himself developed testicular cancer and his wife developed breast cancer, from which she passed away. He ultimately discovered there was a psychological/emotional link to all cancers and eventually healed himself. Tens of thousands of people have read his books and credited their remissions to his work.

Negative emotion is one of the most toxic and dangerous forms of oxidative stress because it's insidious and often suppressed. These emotions fester like an abscess, corrupting the good and rotting away the love. They hide from us even when we think we've dealt with them, and they lurk in our subconscious creating more discourse and pain. Be brave and go to those scary places! It may be the missing link in treating your disease.

Toxicity 6 – Food Toxicity

The sixth toxicity isn't about the chemicals or additives in our food. Those would be included in the first two toxicities. The sixth toxicity involves the genetic modification of food, the manipulation and irradiation of what we do to the substances we consume, and the immunologic issues that surround modern food production. The concerns are that these forms of food manipulation are very new and unexplored and we simply don't have any idea of their implications for human physiology. The ramifications could be disastrous.

Who wants to take the risk of consuming these items and then waiting to see what the effects are 20 years down the line? Genetic modification of food manipulates the actual essence of these food substances by altering the DNA. When ingested and incorporated into our bodies, this altered DNA is now becoming part of our own essence. The altered DNA has the potential of damaging or, even worse, of becoming incorporated into our own genetic code.

The DNA in corn, soybeans, and other produce has already been genetically modified, but the question is, what will it do to the DNA inside of you when you consume it?

In addition, your body may not recognize this genetically modified substance as food, since it has been altered from its original genetic state. Anything foreign to the body is an antigen, to which the body will make antibodies, thus potentially giving rise to a host of new autoimmune diseases. There are just far too many unanswered questions. The easiest rule of thumb is to completely avoid genetically modified organism (GMO) produce and irradiated produce. Remember, if it was changed in any way from its original, God-given form, it doesn't belong in your body. It goes back to the same advice: **God given = Good ... Man-made = Madness**.

<u>Toxicity 7 – Spiritual Toxicity</u>

Dr. Buttar's seventh toxicity is called "spiritual toxicity." His belief is that a person has spiritual toxicity any time they feel someone does not have the right to believe something that contradicts their own personal doctrine. Their rigid personal beliefs cause this toxicity, according to Dr. Buttar.

While I agree with Dr. Buttar that all people have the right to believe whatever they want, this does **not** mean that all beliefs are equally **accurate**. I am a Christian and the Bible clearly teaches that there is only **one** way to heaven, and that is through repentance and belief in Jesus Christ as Lord and Savior. Those who place their faith in another "savior," though they may be completely sincere, are sincerely wrong. Jesus says it Himself in John 14:6: "*I am **the** way, **the** truth, and **the** life. No man comes to the Father but through me.*"

I want to thank Dr. Buttar for his assistance with this chapter. To learn more about Dr. Buttar and his innovative approaches to treating cancer, autism, and other diseases, please visit <u>www.DrButtar.com</u>.

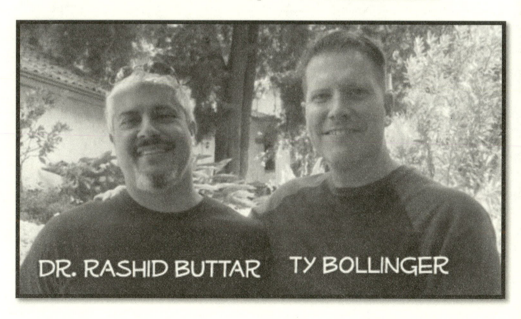

DR. RASHID BUTTAR   TY BOLLINGER

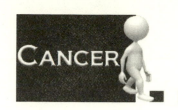

CHAPTER 8
3 COMMON CANCERS & "CACHEXIA"

> "MAMMOGRAMS INCREASE THE RISK FOR DEVELOPING BREAST CANCER & RAISE THE RISK OF SPREADING OR METASTASIZING AN EXISTING GROWTH."
> —DR. CHARLES B. SIMONE

There are multitudes of various types of cancers, and the purpose of this book is not to address specific cancers, per se, but rather to educate the reader on the particular non-toxic alternative cancer treatments that work on the majority of advanced cancers. With this being said, I have addressed three common cancers in this section of the book: breast cancer, skin cancer, and prostate cancer. This chapter concludes with a section on the "cachexia cycle."

BREAST CANCER

Each year, over 225,000 women will be diagnosed with breast cancer and almost 25% of these women will die of the disease. The USA has one of the highest breast cancer rates in the world. Fifty years ago, only one in twenty women was diagnosed with breast cancer. Now, the number is one in seven. Since it is so common among women, I have devoted an entire section of the book to breast cancer.

Every October begins the media blitz known as National Breast Cancer Awareness Month. Pink ribbons abound and the message you keep hearing is, *"Get Your Mammogram!"* High profile companies like Avon and Revlon have joined ranks along with the Dallas-based Susan G. Komen Foundation's "Race for the Cure." One of the many mottos of the Breast Cancer Awareness Month is *"Early Detection is Your Best Protection."*

So, I guess we're all ready to wave our pink ribbons, put on those jogging shoes, and hit the roads, right? Wait a minute! Before we all get swept away in an emotional whirlwind, we need to look at a few facts about breast cancer. First of all, who profits from breast cancer? I know it sounds cynical, but hey, this entire book is focused on cutting through the propaganda and getting to the truth. And truth is oftentimes obscured by the emotions of the disease. So, let me ask you a question. Did you know that the primary sponsor of Breast Cancer Awareness Month is AstraZeneca? This Big Pharma player masterminded the initial event in 1985.

AstraZeneca is the company that manufactures the controversial and widely prescribed breast cancer drug, Tamoxifen. In his book, Indicted: Cancer Research, Dr. Tibor J. Hegedus writes: *"Tamoxifen is given to women with breast cancer to block the entrance of estradiol into the tumor cells dependant upon this hormone to stimulate growth. When the hormones are blocked from reaching their primary targets, they are forced to travel to other organs."* This, in turn, stimulates proliferation of cells in the lining of the womb and in certain cases causes endometrial cancer!

Remember the section on what causes cancer? Remember Dr. Stephen Ayre's quote on Insulin Growth Factor? According to L.R. Wiseman, a pathologist at the Royal Victoria Infirmary, *"Tamoxifen stimulates cell proliferation by sensitizing cells to proliferative effects of IGF."* In her article entitled *"Tamoxifen, Tears, and Terror,"* Betty Martini writes, *"IGF is a hormone designed to make things grow up, calves and babies; it also stimulates and accelerates cancer in sensitized women, those taking Tamoxifen. One of the reasons for the uproar in Monsanto marketing the bovine growth hormone which is injected into cows is the outrageous increase in IGF which will yield a firestorm of cancer from the milk. A chemical company is selling us a gasoline named Tamoxifen to put out the fire."* www.holisticmed.com/toxic/tamoxifen.shtml.

In his book Milk: The Deadly Poison, Robert Cohen states *"The single most disturbing aspect of rBGH from a human safety standpoint, concerns Insulin-like Growth Factor (IGF), which is linked to breast cancer."* According to Dr. Samuel Epstein, *"IGF is not destroyed by pasteurization, survives the digestive process, is absorbed into the blood and produces potent growth promoting effects."* Epstein says it is highly likely that IGF helps transform normal breast tissue to cancerous cells, and enables malignant human breast cancer cells to invade and spread to distant organs.

Do you get the picture? Can you imagine anyone using both the rBGH milk and Tamoxifen? In a 1994 article, Betty Martini wrote *"Tamoxifen has been tested and retested for more than 15 years. The testers admitted fraud, many contraindications were just ignored, test results were limited in duration and after-effects not tallied, though women sickened and died from them. The tests didn't prove the stuff works, so they're doing them over again, with your money. They'll keep testing until they can figure a way to rig the results in favor of healthy women buying the poison for a disease we don't have, but the drug will give it to us!"*

In April 1996, the World Health Organization declared Tamoxifen to be a carcinogen, but AstraZeneca continues to market this toxic drug. On May 16, 2000, the *New York Times* reported that the National Institute for Environmental Health Sciences listed substances that are known carcinogens. Tamoxifen was included in that list! Taking a carcinogen to stop the spread the cancer is like playing "Russian Roulette" with a fully loaded machine gun! The journal *Science* published a study from Duke University Medical Center in 1999 showing that after two to five years, tamoxifen actually **initiated** the growth of breast cancer!

It is less known that AstraZeneca also makes herbicides and fungicides. One of their products, the organochlorine pesticide, Acetochlor is implicated as a causal factor in breast cancer. Millions of tons of toxic substances are now released into the environment each and every year. Yet only three percent of the 80,000 chemicals in use have been tested for safety. (Sharon Batt, "Cancer, Inc", *Sierra Magazine,* September-October 1999, p. 36) These toxic time bombs are found in our water, air, and soil.

Why is there such a deafening silence when it comes to environmental toxicity, carcinogens found in herbicides, pesticides, plastics, and other toxic chemicals that are known to cause cancer...especially breast cancer? According to Dr. Robert Rowen, MD, *"by the time a cancer is detectable; almost 100% of people have circulating cancer cells in their bloodstream. Hence, it's really a joke to cut the tumor out, and an absolute lie for the surgeon to say 'We got it all.' The only answer to cancer is prevention. But, that, too, is difficult. We are so awash in a sea of poisons that even unborn babies are marinating in up to 200 different man made toxic chemicals. Our foods are sprayed with them. Monsanto is condemning us to GMO Frankenfood with the blessing and protection of our own government. Our soils are depleted of minerals and the Standard American Diet (SAD) makes all but a few of us dangerously nutritionally depleted. Most all of us are at risk of eventually hearing the 'C' word."* www.secondopinionnewsletter.com

Did you know that the American Cancer Society was founded with the support of the Rockefeller family in 1913? Members of the chemical and pharmaceutical industry have long held important positions on the ACS board of directors. Could that have any bearing on the curious silence concerning environmental causes of cancer? Just a thought....

Sadly, breast cancer has become the darling of corporate America. Companies use the pink ribbon to sell their products and boost their image with consumers as they boost their bottom line. Meanwhile, breast cancer rates continue to rise every year. There can be many contributing factors to breast cancer, and this chapter is by no means comprehensive, but I have focused on three main causes of breast cancer: **1) Mammograms, 2) Antiperspirants**, and **3) Bras.** You might find this list quite startling but you will begin to understand as I outline the role each of these plays in breast cancer development.

CAUSE #1: MAMMOGRAMS

Breast cancer is the leading cause of death among American women between the ages of 44 and 55. Massive campaigns exist to encourage women to have annual mammograms to "prevent" breast cancer by "early detection." But what if, rather than preventing breast cancer, mammo-grams actually caused breast cancer? Dr. Charles Simone (former NCI associate) asserts: *"Mammograms increase the risk for developing breast cancer and raise the risk of spreading or metastasizing an existing growth."*

You see, a mammogram is nothing more than an x-ray picture of your breast that can reveal tumor growths otherwise undetectable in a physical exam. Like all x-rays, mammograms use doses of ionizing radiation to create this image, thus more breast tissue is exposed to cancer causing radiation each year. Radiologists then analyze the image for any abnormal growths. Is mammography an effective tool for detecting tumors? Many physicians say **"no."** In a Swedish study of 60,000 women, 70% of the tumors detected by mammograms turned out to be false positives. These "false positives" are not only emotional and financial strains on the victims, but they also lead to many superfluous and invasive biopsies. (Lidbrink, E., et al. *British Medical Journal*, February 3, 1996, pp. 273-276)

According to Dr. Russell L. Blaylock, one estimate is that annual radiological breast exams increase the risk of breast cancer by 2% a year. So over ten years the risk will have increased 20%. In his book, The Politics of Cancer on page 539, Dr. Samuel Epstein states, *"Regular mammography of younger women increases their cancer risks. Analysis of controlled trials over the last decade has shown consistent increases in breast cancer mortality within a few years of commencing screening. This confirms evidence of the high sensitivity of the premenopausal breast, and on cumulative carcinogenic effects of radiation."*

In 1995, the British medical journal *The Lancet* reported that, since mammographic screening was introduced in 1983, the incidence of ductal carcinoma in situ (DCIS), which represents 12% of all breast cancer cases, has increased by **328%,** and **200%** of this increase is due to the use of mammography. Why, then, does conventional medicine keep recom-mending mammograms?

Do the math: a $150 mammogram for all 70 million American women over 40 is a whopping **$10 BILLION** per year industry. According to Dr. James Howenstine, *"This industry supports radiologists, x-ray technicians, surgeons, nurses, manufacturers of x-ray equipment, hospitals etc. and will not be allowed to disappear by curing and preventing breast cancer."* In an article from the July 2006 issue of the *Journal of Clinical Oncology,* researchers showed that the radiation from mammograms actually causes breast cancer. In a study of 1600 European women, researchers found that women who had at least one mammogram were 54% more likely to develop breast cancer than those who never had one.

In the words of Mike Adams, *"If you were an evil genius who wanted to design and manufacture a **cancer-causing machine**, it would be difficult to beat the present-day mammography machine. It exposes human tissue to high-powered radiation that, if repeated often enough, practically guarantees cancer will eventually develop. In one sense, it's sort of a 'slow suicide machine' that takes years (or decades) to complete its work on your body. But before you die, you get to spend your life savings on 'treatments' that will leave you bankrupt just before they leave you dead. That's the whole point of the cancer industry, after all: To maximize profits from cancer. Mammography is a key piece of the puzzle in accomplishing precisely that. But at the same time, it's a 'perfect weapon' for generating lucrative repeat business."*

Mike continues, *"If you're an oncologist, the best way to ensure you'll have a cancer patient to treat at age 55 is to start exposing them to radiation at age 40 (or earlier). It's sort of like a diabetes clinic offering free candy to children: At some point, after they eat enough processed sugar, they'll come back as repeat customers suffering from diabetes. Mammography is, by any honest assessment, **pure quackery**. It's no more accurate at detecting tumors needing acute treatment than just waving your hand over someone and guessing whether they have a tumor that needs treatment. In fact, waving your*

hand over someone is a lot less harmful, so it's actually better."
www.naturalnews.com/027537_mammograms_cancer_industry.html

In my opinion, mammograms are nothing more than a clever tool aimed at recruiting new patients (via scare tactics and fear) into the highly profitable world of "cancer treatments." **Beware:** any time you threaten to take away "repeat customers" from the Cancer Industry (especially in the "bread and butter" field of mammography), you're in for a dog fight.

COUNTERTHINK

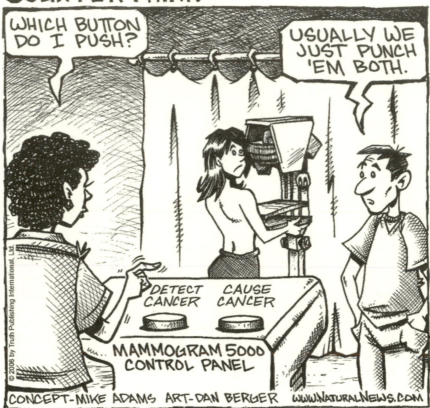

Thanks to Mike Adams and *www.NaturalNews.com* for the cartoon above.

There is a superior alternative: **advanced thermography**. This procedure does not use mechanical pressure or ionizing radiation and can detect signs of breast cancer years earlier than either mammography or a physical exam. Thermography is able to detect the possibility of breast cancer much earlier, because it can image the early stages of angiogenesis. Angiogenesis is the formation of a direct supply of blood to cancer cells, which is a necessary step before they can grow into tumors.

Thermographic breast screening is brilliantly simple. Thermography measures the radiation of infrared heat from a woman's body and translates this information into anatomical images. Normal blood circulation is under the control of the autonomic nervous system, which governs unconscious body functions. To screen for breast cancer, a thermographer blows cool air over a woman's breasts. In response, the autonomic nervous system reduces the amount of blood going to the breast, as a temperature-regulating measure. However, the pool of blood and primitive blood vessels that cancer cells create is not under autonomic control and is unaffected by the cool air. It will therefore stand out clearly on the thermographic image as a *"hot spot."*

According to Dr. Robert Rowen, MD, *"Before tissue degenerates into cancer, the body's metabolic rate around the site increases. A unique aspect of cancerous tumor growth is a process called neo-angiogenesis (new blood vessel growth). As the cells multiply, they need an increase blood supply to bring in nutrients and remove waste. The increase in circulation gives off heat. An infra-red type camera can detect this heat, giving the patient and doctor an opportunity to take action long before a tumor develops. This makes thermography a tremendous weapon in the fight against breast cancer!"* http://www.secondopinionnewsletter.com/

CAUSE #2: SHAVING & ANTIPERSPIRANTS

Research shows that one of the leading causes of breast cancer could be the use of antiperspirants. The human body has a number of areas that it uses to purge toxins from the body; these are behind the knees, behind the ears, the groin area, and the underarms. The toxins are purged from the body in the form of sweat (perspiration). The main problems with antiperspirants is that, as the name clearly suggests, they prevent you from perspiring, thus inhibiting the body from purging toxins from the underarm area.

Where do the toxins go? Well, that's the problem. These toxins do not just magically disappear. Instead, the body deposits them in the lymph nodes below the arms since it cannot sweat them out. This causes a high concentration of toxins and leads to cancer. Numerous clinical studies, dating back decades, have shown that nearly all breast cancers occur in the upper outer quadrant of the breast. This basic observation has now become textbook fact. Guess what...this is precisely where the lymph nodes are located!

In 2004, Dr. Kris McGrath, a Chicago allergist, performed a study published in the European Journal of Cancer Prevention which he claims is the first to find a connection between antiperspirants, underarm shaving, and cancer. He studied 400 Chicago-area breast cancer survivors and found that women *"who performed these underarm habits more aggressively"* had a diagnosis of breast cancer 22 years earlier than the non-users and theorized that substances found in deodorants, such as aluminum chlorohydrate, were entering the lymphatic system through nicks in the skin caused by shaving. www.nbc5.com/health/2747353/detail.html

There are several excellent brands of aluminum free deodorants available now. However, be sure that the deodorant you choose does not contain parabens. Parabens are used as preservatives, and on the label they may be listed as methyl paraben, ethyl paraben, propyl paraben, butyl paraben, isobutyl paraben or E216. Here's why: researchers have also found traces of parabens in every sample of tissue taken from 20 different breast tumors. Studies suggest that parabens (found in underarm deodorants and other cosmetics) can seep into the tissue after being applied to the skin. This finding concerns researchers since parabens have been shown to be able to mimic the action of estrogen, which can drive the growth of human breast tumors.

Men are much less likely to develop breast cancer prompted by the use of antiperspirants, because the antiperspirant is more likely to be caught in the underarm hair, rather than directly applied to the skin. However, women who shave their underarms increase the risk of cancer by causing barely visible nicks in the skin, which allow the chemicals to enter easily into the body through the underarms.

CAUSE #3: WEARING A BRA

The connection between bras and the development of breast cancer was reinforced in a study conducted on the Fiji Islands. In 1997, medical anthropologist Sidney Singer compared the incidence of breast cancer in two groups of women in Fiji. Half of the women wore bras and the other half went without. The diet, environment and lifestyle of both groups were the same. Singer discovered that those who wore bras had the same rate of breast cancer as American women. Those who went bra-less experienced practically no breast cancer whatsoever.

In their book entitled <u>Dressed to Kill: The Link Between Breast Cancer and Bras</u>, Dr. Sydney Singer and his wife, Soma Grismaijer, presented some startling statistics:

➢ Women wearing a bra 24 hours a day had a **3 in 4** chance of developing breast cancer.

➢ Women wearing their bras more than 12 hours a day, but not to bed, had a **1 in 7** chance of developing breast cancer.
➢ Women wearing bras less than 12 hours a day had a **1 in 152** chance of developing breast cancer.
➢ Women who rarely or never wore bras had a **1 in 168** chance of developing breast cancer.

Why? According to Dr. David Williams, *"Wearing a bra at least 14 hours a day tends to increase the hormone prolactin, which decreases circulation in the breast tissue. Decreasing circulation can impede your body's natural removal of carcinogenic fluids that become trapped in the breast's sac-like glands (lymph nodes). These glands make up the largest mass of lymph nodes in the upper part of your body's lymphatic system."* www.shirleys-wellness-cafe.com/breastcancer.htm

Apparently, the restrictive nature of bras inhibits the lymphatic system (our internal network of vessels and nodes that flushes wastes from the body) from doing its job. The mammary glands are filled with lymphatic vessels that move from the breast, through the auxillary lymph nodes under the armpit, over the collar bone, to the thoracic duct. This is how the breast drains toxins and keeps its internal environment clean. However, if something impedes the cleansing process, an imbalance occurs and the estrogen by-products become destructive molecules called free radicals that begin cellular damage which leads to breast cancer.

The correlation between bras and breast cancer is **four times greater** than smoking is to lung cancer! Pushup bras are said to be the most restrictive. If you cannot discontinue wearing a bra, consider wearing one as little as possible, and use a bra that allows some breast motion, without cutting tightly under and along the outer edges of the breasts where the milk ducts are located.

Now get the picture in your mind of the topics just discussed; we have a constricted lymphatic system causing a toxic backup in the mammary glands, which (in some cases) gets presented annually to a clinic to get squished and assaulted with X-rays. This sounds like a perfect scenario to produce cancer, doesn't it?

Dr. Lorraine Day was diagnosed with invasive breast cancer and had a lumpectomy of a small tumor. But the tumor soon recurred, became very aggressive and grew rapidly. As a physician, Dr. Day was well aware that physicians are more afraid of cancer than patients are, because doctors know that chemotherapy, radiation, and surgery are not the answer to cancer. She used alternative treatments to treat her cancer.

SKIN CANCER

Skin cancer is usually associated with a limited set of risk factors connected to ultraviolet (UV) radiation. These include excessive sun exposure (especially during adolescence), red or blonde hair, and fair skin. More than 1.5 million skin cancers are diagnosed yearly in the USA alone. According to the Skin Cancer Foundation, as of 2006, about one in five Americans and one in three Caucasians will develop skin cancer in their lifetime. Skin cancer is the most common of all cancers, representing one out of every three new cancers.

There are two main types of skin cancer:

1. Skin cancer in moles (malignant melanoma)
2. Non-melanoma skin cancer (basal cell carcinoma and squamous cell carcinoma)

Melanoma is the most serious form of skin cancer. Melanoma is a malignant tumor that originates in melanocytes, which are cells that produce the pigment melanin that colors our skin, hair, and eyes and is heavily concentrated in most moles. If you have melanoma which has metastasized to other parts of the body, then you need to seriously consider a strong advanced cancer treatment. Once metastasis has occurred with melanoma, it is very serious and usually deadly, especially if treated with the "Big 3." The treatments mentioned in this chapter are not applicable to malignant melanoma that has metastasized. Let me repeat myself. The treatments mentioned in this chapter are **not** applicable to malignant melanoma that has metastasized!

There are two non-melanoma skin cancers: **basal cell carcinoma** (BCC) and **squamous cell carcinoma** (SCC). BCC is a cancer that begins in the deep basal cell layer of the epidermis (the outer layer of the skin). It is the most frequent type of skin cancer and is six to eight times more common than malignant melanoma. BCC is a slow-growing cancer, and it never spreads to other parts of the body. SCC begins in the squamous cells of the epidermis and is not as common as BCC; however, it grows much faster than BCC especially when located near the eyes, ears, mouth, or the pubic area. Chronic overexposure to sunlight is the cause of almost all BCCs and SCCs, which occur most frequently on exposed parts of the body (the face, ears, neck, scalp, shoulders, and back). Occasionally, they develop in non-exposed areas.

The external treatment of skin cancer with "escharotic" pastes and salves actually seeks out and destroys cancer cells. Escharotic pastes and salves are caustic compounds that are applied externally on the skin over the skin cancer. They successfully erode the tissue and eventually destroy and remove the underlying tumor.

The two most respected and well-known authorities in the use of the escharotic approach were American doctors J. Weldon Fell and Frederic E. Mohs. Dr. Fell was a faculty member at New York University and later was one of the founders of the New York Academy of Medicine. In the early 1850s, he moved to London and built up a very successful cancer treatment practice based on escharotic therapy using bloodroot (sanguinaria canadensis) and zinc chloride as the foundation. Bloodroot is one of the most beautiful eastern North American woodland herbs and was commonly used to treat cancer by the Native Americans.

Dr. Frederic Mohs called his approach "chemosurgery" and used an adhesive paste. His was more an integrative approach that combined the use of the escharotic paste with surgical tumor removal. His contribution was enormous as he put the procedure on a very sound, scientific footing, with a tremendous amount of research. He wrote a medical text entitled Chemosurgery: Microscopically controlled Surgery for Skin Cancer which was last published in 1978. The medical "soundness" of his approach was underscored in a 1990 report that stated he had a verifiable and documented 99% success rate in his treatment of skin cancers!

The cancer-killing concoction of zinc chloride, bloodroot, and other substances was recreated in the 20th century and named "*Cansema Black Topical Salve*." Cansema is a topical ointment that, when applied to skin cancer, kills the cancer cells and creates an "eschar" (a pus formation). The body then expels the scab and leaves a pit in the skin. Over the next few weeks, the pit heals over, usually leaving a slightly discolored area where the lesion was removed. Typically, this area will heal over within a period of several months, making it difficult to tell that a cancer was removed from the site.

During the summer of 2008, I had a couple of places on my face (one on my nose and the other between my eye and ear) which I suspected were BCC. No matter what I did, they wouldn't go away. I used Cansema on them for about a week, and they both fell off. In 2011, I used Cansema to take care of a large BCC on my leg. Cansema is now called "*Amazon Black Topical Salve*" and we purchase it from Alpha Omega Labs. Their website is www.HerbHealers.com. **Warning**: Do **not** take the salve internally.

Another excellent salve is called "*Two Feathers Healing Formula*" and is found at http://www.healingformula.net/. It is manufactured by the same Native American family that has made the formula for over a hundred years. It contains a combination of several herbs that are blended, in perfect harmony, in an age old fashion using a curing technique. These herbs and method of formulation make the compound safe to use internally, where 90% of the healing takes place, and can also be applied topically, safely, as a drawing salve.

Another treatment for skin cancer is called *"PDQ! Herbal Skin Cream"* which is all natural and comprised of a proprietary blend of herbs and other organic matter (tree bark, leaves, and roots). I have personally spoken to a couple of folks who used this to completely cure their skin cancer. An ingredient in common eggplant has been shown to cure skin cancer. The extract is called *"solasodine glycoside"* (aka BEC5) which binds to cancer cells and causes them to rupture. Dr. Bill Cham first discovered BEC5 in an Australian weed (Devil's Apple); then he discovered it was in eggplant as well. He documented that over 70,000 Australians have cured their skin cancer with BEC5.

In a double blind, placebo-controlled study at the Royal London Hospital, doctors found that approximately 78% of patients using a topical preparation of BEC5 saw their skin cancers healed. And follow-up research showed that once the cancer was gone, it didn't come back! This stunning success was topped only by the fact that, unlike chemotherapy, BEC5 does **not** kill healthy cells. It targets and eliminates only cancer cells, which means that instead of *destroying* your immune system, BEC5 actually helps *strengthen* it.

Vitamin C is another viable treatment for skin cancer. When vitamin C comes into contact with skin cancer, it hardens the tumor and forms a crust, such that the scab falls off in a couple of weeks or so depending on how big the tumor is and how aggressive you get with the vitamin C. The solution is made by adding 1/8 teaspoon of pure vitamin C crystals to one teaspoon of water (a ratio of 1:8). If you add any more vitamin C, it will not dissolve. This should make enough solution to last all day. If more is made than is needed you should store it in a closed container in the refrigerator.

The treatment is to apply the mixture (using a cotton swab or Q-Tip) to the tumor. This should be done two or three times a day. It is best to put a bandage or other cotton covering over the tumor after each treatment, if possible. Since vitamin C (ascorbic acid) is also anti-infective and is used topically and intravenously for burn patients, you would be curing the cancer and fighting infection at the same time. You can find the recommended form of vitamin C crystals at the Life Extension Foundation's website: www.lef.org/newshop/items/item00084.html.

Another alternative cancer treatment for skin cancer is silver. It can be purchased from many vendors. I used to have a colloidal silver generator and made my own colloidal silver, so I am very familiar with this product. The best silver, in my humble opinion, is "Sovereign Silver," which is manufactured by Natural Immunogenics Corporation. Their website is http://www.natural-immunogenics.com/.

PROSTATE CANCER

Approximately 190,000 men in the USA will be diagnosed with prostate cancer this year. Prostate cancer is a common cancer in men, and the probability of getting prostate cancer rises with age. Prostate cancer may get a lot of press, but consider the numbers: American men have a 16% lifetime chance of receiving a diagnosis of prostate cancer, but only a 3% chance of dying from it. That's because the majority of prostate cancers grow **slowly**. In other words, men lucky enough to reach old age are much more likely to die *with* prostate cancer than to die *from* it.

According to conventional cancer "wisdom" (and I use that term loosely), prostate cancer is generally "detected" by high PSA levels and/or by surgical biopsies, and it is "treated" by surgically removing the prostate gland and/or with radiation. You see, the pattern of conventional medicine is to use "diagnostic tests" to loop the unsuspecting public into the esoteric "treatment" which frequently causes cancer rather than actually treats it. Coupled with the fact that the average conventional physician is "drunk and high" on the propaganda of Big Pharma and follows the "test" protocol dutifully and blindly, most cancer patients don't stand a chance.

In the case of prostate cancer, the "test" protocol is the prostate-specific antigen (PSA) test. The annual bill for PSA screening is at least $3 billion! If your PSA is high, then your doctor will order a biopsy or operation. The problem is that a biopsy or the prostate "removal" operation can **cause** a dormant cancer to spread through the rest of the body. The PSA test is known as the "gold standard" for detecting prostate cancer. But is it really? Does a high PSA equal prostate cancer? This is an important question, because a high PSA leads most men straight to biopsies, then to "the knife," and then straight to incontinence and impotence. Of course, let's not forget that these procedures will guarantee billions of dollars for your doctor and the Medical Mafia.

According to recent articles in the *New York Times* and *Washington Post*, the PSA test is essentially worthless. You see, the PSA test simply reveals how much of the prostate antigen a man has in his blood, which is a marker of inflammation. However, infections, benign swelling of the prostate, and over-the-counter drugs (like Ibuprofen) can all elevate a man's PSA level, but **none** of them signals cancer.

Dr. Thomas Stamey of Stanford University was one of the original boosters of the PSA test. At a 2004 conference, he stated, *"PSA no longer has a relationship to prostate cancer. The PSA test is not relevant any more. You might as well biopsy a man because he has blue eyes."* In fact, the PSA test has been such a dismal failure in detecting prostate cancer, its inventor (Richard J. Ablin) has been speaking out against his own discovery for more than a decade! Most recently, in a March 2010 edition of *The New York Times*, Ablin wrote, *"The [PSA] test is hardly more effective than a coin toss. As I've been trying to make clear for many years now, PSA testing can't detect prostate cancer...The test's popularity has led to a hugely expensive public health disaster."*

Conventional oncologists are quick to take credit for the increasing survival rate of men diagnosed with prostate cancer as a result of the PSA test and "early detection," but they don't bother to mention that nearly every one of those men would have survived just fine anyway – only without the incontinence and impotence caused by the treatments. According to Dr. David Williams in the June 2009 issue of *Alternatives* newsletter, *"The fact is that nearly every man who makes it to age 50 will die **with** prostate cancer, but very few die **from** it."*

In 2009, *The New England Journal of Medicine* published results from the two largest studies of the PSA screening (one in Europe and one in the USA). The results of the American study show that over a period of seven to ten years, screening did **not** reduce the death rate in men 55 and over. The European study showed a slight decline in death rates, but also found that 48 men would need to be treated to save one life. That means that 47 men will now be unable to function sexually or stay out of the bathroom for over half an hour. That's incredible. http://content.nejm.org/cgi/content/full/NEJMoa0810696

What can you do to proactively prevent prostate cancer? Primarily, you should try to be physically active and walk or rebound as often as possible, since the movement of the muscles and organs in the pelvic area increases circulation to the prostate gland. Another excellent exercise is "air bicycling" while lying on your back. From a dietary perspective, you need to lay off the meats, dairy, and alcohol, and eat plenty of fruits and veggies. Saw palmetto and turmeric are excellent herbs for the prostate, and lycopene (from cooked tomatoes or watermelon) is essential. Also, try eating a handful of walnuts and pumpkin seeds each day and plenty of hot peppers (which contain capsaicin). Lastly, be sure to drink lots of water.

An excellent supplement for the prostate is called "Super Beta Prostate™" and is available at www.newvitality.com. It contains many essential minerals (including zinc, copper, iodine, chromium, and selenium) which improve prostate function, and it also contains beta-sitosterol, which has been shown to support healthy urinary flow, healthy urinary function, and healthy prostate functioning.

Another excellent prostate supplement is called "Pros-Food™" and is available at www.healthresources.net. It contains ten optimal nutrients for prostate health, including: zinc, copper, selenium, saw palmetto, stinging nettle, pumpkin seed, pygeum, beta-sitosterol, red clover, and lycopene.

Some of this prostate information was published in the June 2009 issue of *Alternatives* newsletter by Dr. David Williams. In my opinion, the PSA test is the "male" equivalent of mammograms for females, since it results in so many "false positives" and actually causes more cancer than it prevents. According to Dr. Williams, conventional prostate cancer treatment is the "billion-dollar scam."

On a side note, a large body of evidence demonstrates that PSA is not a "prostate-specific" antigen at all. As a matter of fact, PSA has been shown to be expressed in many forms of female tissues. The breast is a major female organ able to produce PSA.

THE "CACHEXIA CYCLE"

Cancer's main devastating effect on the body is cachexia, which is basically the "wasting away" of the body characterized by weight loss and eventual debilitation. According to the National Cancer Institute, "*It is estimated that **half** of all cancer patients experience cachexia, the rapid loss of a large amount of weight along with fatigue, weakness, and loss of appetite. Cachexia is a serious problem among many patients who have advanced cancer.*" Dr. Harold Dvorak, former chief of pathology at Beth Israel Hospital in Boston, states "*In a sense, nobody dies of cancer. They die of something else – pneumonia, failure of one or another organ. Cachexia accelerates that process of infection and the building-up of metabolic poisons. **It causes death a lot faster than the tumor would**, were it not for the cachexia.*"

Cachexia is caused by the inefficient glucose burn resulting from **an**aerobic respiration. The cancer cell ferments the glucose and produces lactic acid, then the liver converts the lactic acid back to glucose (a process called "gluconeogenesis"), which also consumes enormous amounts of energy. Thus, the cancer cells convert glucose to lactic acid, and the lactic acid travels to the liver. The liver converts the lactic acid back to glucose, which then travels back to the cancer cells, and so on. This cachexia cycle consumes an enormous amount of energy and may cause the body to start "eating" its own muscles and bones in order to feed the cancer cells.

Dr. Joseph Gold was a research scientist for NASA, a United States Air Force officer, and a medical doctor. When he completed his distinguished military career, he embarked on a mission with one goal, to answer the question: *"Is there a chemical way to inhibit gluconeogenesis and stop cachexia?"* In 1969, Dr. Gold heard biochemist Paul Ray deliver a paper explaining that hydrazine sulfate could shut down the enzyme necessary for the production of glucose from lactic acid. Many would say that this was *"pure luck"* or *"coincidence,"* but I would say that it was ***"Divine Providence!"*** He immediately tested hydrazine sulfate on mice and found that, as he suspected, it inhibited gluconeogenesis, thus reversing the cachexia cycle. Voila! Gold had discovered a perfect way to starve the cancer.

In the early 1970s, Dr. Gold met with the National Cancer Institute in an effort to begin clinical testing on hydrazine sulfate. During this meeting, he gave them his research files, discussed the recommended dosages, and detailed a list of those things that should **not** be used during therapy, such as alcohol, sleeping pills, and tranquilizers. Dr. Gold explicitly warned the NCI that patients could die if they were taking tranquilizers. So, what happened? The NCI tested it, did not follow the protocol, purposely sabotaged the study, killed off all the patients, and issued a paper stating that it was *"worthless."*

So, what's the rest of the story? Instead of following the protocol of 60 milligrams of hydrazine sulfate per single dose, the hospital performing the study engaged in underdosing and overdosing patients. In some instances, patients were being given only between one and five milligrams per day. Others who were started on the correct dosage and were showing improvements were abruptly switched to between 90 and 100 milligrams per single dose, wiping out their good responses. Also, it turns out that none of the NCI patients were warned about the fact that tranquilizers were forbidden. Under pressure from the General Accounting Office (GAO) investigators, doctors who conducted one of the NCI trials admitted in a letter to the *Journal of Clinical Oncology* that virtually all (94%) of the subjects had taken tranquilizers while receiving hydrazine sulfate. Despite those admissions, the GAO still managed in its report to declare that the NCI's trials *"were not flawed."* That is absurd. It's kind of like stating that a car has a burned up motor, four flat tires, and no brakes, nevertheless it is ready for use on the highway.

According to Dr. Gold, the *"NCI's actions with respect to hydrazine sulfate, characterized by intimidation, coercion, steadfast opposition, and possibly clinical trial-rigging, are truly one of the most shameful, scandalous medical undertakings in this country's history, depriving vast numbers of people of their health, happiness, and lives."*

Every properly conducted, controlled clinical trial performed in accordance with internationally accepted standards of scientific conduct, without exception, has indicated efficacy and safety of hydrazine sulfate. The largest study of hydrazine sulfate, conducted on 740 cancer patients in the Soviet Union, found that it produced stabilization or regression of the tumor in 50.8% of the patients. http://alternativecancer.us/hydrazinesulfate.htm

Due to the fact that hydrazine sulfate inhibits gluconeogenesis, it causes tumors to stop growing, stop spreading, and oftentimes shrinking them and/or causing them to disappear. Webster Kehr accurately points out that the action of hydrazine sulfate is to stop the cachexia cycle in the liver; whereas cesium chloride stops the cachexia cycle at the cellular level.

Here is Dr. Gold's hydrazine sulfate protocol:

➢ A single 60 milligram capsule every day for the first 3 days (at or before breakfast)
➢ A single 60 milligram capsule twice a day for the next 3 days (at or before breakfast and before dinner)
➢ A single 60 milligram capsule 3 times per day each day thereafter (approximately every 8 hours beginning with breakfast)

This protocol is based on a patient weight of 120 pounds and above; for a patient below 120 pounds, half dosages have been reported effective. Generally it is reported that hydrazine sulfate is most effective when administered by itself (no other medications given for 30 minutes before or after administration of hydrazine sulfate) before meals. If adequate response is made on two capsules daily, patients have been reportedly maintained on this dosage schedule and not increased.

Best efficacy with hydrazine sulfate has been reported by maintaining daily treatment for 45 days followed by an interruption for one to two weeks, then reinstitution of treatment. In addition, it has been reported that there is an incompatibility of hydrazine sulfate with ethanol, barbiturates, and tranquilizers. Patients receiving hydrazine sulfate should thus avoid alcoholic beverages, tranquilizers, and barbiturates. Additionally, the cancer patient must maintain a low carbohydrate diet (*i.e.,* don't eat sugar). Remember, you are trying to starve the cancer, not treat it to a buffet dinner! Remember, **sugar feeds cancer.** So when the doctor tells the cancer patient (who is wasting away from cachexia) to eat whatever he can to put weight on, whether it be ice cream or candy, the doctor may as well have given him a gun with one bullet. The worse thing that a "terminal" cancer patient can do is eat whatever he wants.

Warning: Hydrazine sulfate is an MAOI ("Monoamine Oxidase Inhibitor") which inhibits an enzyme that breaks down monoamines (*i.e.,* serotonin, norepinephrine, and dopamine) that control our moods. However, MAOIs also metabolize the amino acid tyramine. Eating foods with tyramine can raise your blood pressure and heart beat and can cause a horrible headache. So, when you are taking hydrazine sulfate, do not eat foods containing tyramine such as aged, fermented, or pickled foods (*i.e.,* most cheeses, lunch meats, hot dogs, yogurt, wines, and beers).

Also off limits are lima beans, fava beans, lentils, snow peas, soybeans, yeast extracts/brewer's yeast, sauerkraut, bananas, avocados, canned figs, raisins, red plums, raspberries, pineapples, chocolate, caffeine, peanuts, almonds, and pumpkin seeds. This is not a comprehensive list. In general, any high protein food that has undergone aging should be avoided. Also, any over-the-counter cold or allergy remedy should also be avoided. Usage of vitamin C should be restricted to 250 mg/day, and vitamin B_6 should be avoided altogether.

Important: Hydrazine sulfate is frequently used with other alternative cancer treatments, which we will discuss later in the book, which may or may not have food/supplement/drug restrictions. Keep in mind that hydrazine sulfate also has a long list of prohibited foods. If you begin to get bad headaches, the chances are that you have eaten foods containing tyramine. You should check with your doctor or nutritionist if you have a question. To purchase hydrazine sulfate, please visit www.essense-of-life.com. I am aware that it is advertised for pets, but it is the highest quality. And please remember that hydrazine sulfate should be taken in exact doses because it is a drug. Overdosing can do more harm than good.

Another excellent treatment for cachexia is hemp, which has been shown to increase appetite and food intake. A 1970 survey showed that 93% of hemp users reported enjoying food more after they smoked and subsequently ate more, while numerous other studies have shown that hemp reduces nausea and vomiting.

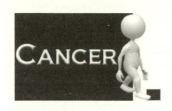

CHAPTER 9

FREQUENCY MATTERS

> "THE LIVING CELL IS ESSENTIALLY AN ELECTRICAL DEVICE."
> - DR. ALBERT SZENT-GYORGYI (NOBEL PRIZE WINNER)

Electromagnetic fields ("EMF") is a broad term which includes electric fields generated by charged particles, magnetic fields generated by charged particles in motion, and radiated fields such as TV, radio, microwaves, and other household appliances. Numerous experts are convinced that there is a direct link between EMF exposure and cancer.

On the flip side of the coin, **pulsed** electromagnetic fields ("PEMF") are a necessary for optimal cellular health, and there is compelling evidence that PEMF is a valuable therapeutic option for a wide range of human disorders. No longer should the doctor say: *"Take two aspirin and call me in the morning."* To be current and accurate, the saying should now be: *"Reduce your exposure to EMF, expose yourself to the appropriate PEMF, and then call me in the morning."*

THE DANGERS OF "DIRTY ELECTRICITY"

There is a relatively unknown factor that is quickly being recognized for its profound and insidious impact on our overall health. It has many forms and different names. It's called "dirty electricity" (aka "EMF"). The bottom line is you're putting your own life energy knowingly or unknowingly in the face of altering frequencies which ultimately may create the environment for disease. EMF is being recognized as a critical missing link for helping us understand the escalating levels for so many diseases today.

Everyone in our modern society is exposed to the EMF that surrounds all electric devices. Each and every one of your trillions of cells has its own optimal frequency for health; EMF has the capacity to disrupt that critical balance. The current information on EMF is blatantly obvious and can no longer be ignored. Leading experts in the field of EMF are already describing it as a *"hidden environmental crisis."* I describe it as *"the invisible elephant in the room."*

But public awareness is growing due to increasing media exposure of the dangers of EMF. Dr. David Carpenter, Dean at the School of Public Health, State University of New York believes it is likely that up to 30% of all childhood cancers come from exposure to EMF. Martin Halper, the EPA's Director of Analysis and Support states: *"I have never seen a set of epidemiological studies that remotely approached the weight of evidence that we're seeing with EMF. Clearly there is something here."*

Dr. George Carlo headed the wireless industry research team in the early 1990s and discovered definitively that EMF from cell phone use **does** cause a submolecular, electronic disturbance which creates an environment for diseases including cancer. The cell industry invested $28 million dollars into this research and when Dr. Carlo "spilled the beans" on this life threatening research, the cell phone industries shunned him and attacked his character. Dr. Carlo then compiled all his research in a book called <u>Cell phones-Invisible Hazards of the Wireless Age</u>.

It's estimated we are now being exposed to a **trillion** times more EMF than our grandparents were. These unnatural energy fields, especially those produced by alternating currents operating at 60 cycles per second (which Tesla warned us about), are suspected of causing sleep disorders, chronic pain, chronic fatigue syndrome, depression, anxiety, memory loss, tinnitus, respiratory problems, and a host of other health issues.

EMF has been scientifically linked to suppression of melatonin, breast cancer, prostate cancer, brain cancer, damage to the blood brain barrier, Alzheimer's disease, miscarriages, ALS (Lou Gehrig's disease), Multiple Sclerosis, hypertension, diabetes, thyroid problems, and asthma. As a matter of fact, epidemiological studies in Sweden by Maria Feychting showed that individuals exposed to high levels of EMF had 3.7 times the risk of developing leukemia compared to those not exposed. <u>http://en.scientificcommons.org/maria_feychting</u>

On the next page is a chart which shows the magnetic field readings (mG) found near common household appliances. This is the typical measure of EMF exposure.

Keep in mind that the recommended exposure limit is 1 (one) mG.

Living Room	6 in. away	1 ft	2 ft	4 ft
COLOR TVs		20	8	4
WINDOW AIR CONDITIONERS		20	6	4
CEILING FANS		50	6	1

Bathroom	6 in. away	1 ft	2 ft	4 ft
HAIR DRYERS	700	70	10	1
ELECTRIC SHAVERS	700	100	10	1

Bedroom	6 in. away	1 ft	2 ft	4 ft
DIGITAL CLOCK		8	2	1
ANALOG CLOCK		30	5	3
BABY MONITOR	15	2	-	-

Laundry/Utility	6 in. away	1 ft	2 ft	4 ft
ELECTRIC CLOTHES DRYERS	10	3	-	-
WASHING MACHINES	100	30	-	-
IRONS	20	3	-	-
PORTABLE HEATERS	150	40	8	1
VACUUM CLEANERS	700	200	50	10
SEWING MACHINES	12 chest level	5 head level	-	-

Home Office	6 in. away	1 ft	2 ft	4 ft
PC MONITORS (Color)	20	6	3	-
FAX MACHINES	9	2	-	-
PENCIL SHARPENERS	300	90	30	30

Kitchen	6 in. away	1 ft	2 ft	4 ft
BLENDERS	100	20	3	-
CAN OPENERS	1500	300	30	4
COFFEE MAKERS	10	1	-	-
DISHWASHERS	100	30	7	1
FOOD PROCESSORS	130	20	3	-
GARBAGE DISPOSALS	100	20	3	-
MICROWAVE OVENS	300	200	30	20
MIXERS	600	100	10	1
ELECTRIC OVENS	20	5	1	-
ELECTRIC RANGES	200	30	9	6
REFRIGERATORS	40	20	10	10
TOASTERS	20	7	-	-

What practical measures should we take to create a healthier environment? The hidden environmental crisis is no longer invisible. We are not going back to living in simple dwellings or living without modern conveniences. But we should certainly make ourselves much more aware of the very real threat to our health that EMF poses to all of us each and every day. The goal is to simply acknowledge the problem, identify the sources of the problem, seek out the solutions to the problem, and then better manage and avoid living in harm's way.

"PEMF"

While EMF can be dangerous, pulsed electromagnetic fields ("PEMF") are a known and scientifically proven noninvasive healthy lifestyle necessity. The positive effects of PEMF applications have been known for decades and are the subject of numerous scientific works. PEMF works like a "cellular battery charger." Basically, in layman's terms, the low-frequency pulses create a brief, intense voltage around each cell. The mitochondria (within the cell) then grab some of this energy. This, in turn, makes the cell more efficient at producing ATP and delivering oxygen throughout the body. In other words, PEMF works like a "spark plug" for energy production in the cell.

PEMF is vitally essential to our health and wellbeing. Just ask the Russian Space Agency. In April 1961, Soviet cosmonaut Yuri Gagarin made history when he orbited the earth with his 1 hour and 48 minute flight. Gagarin was the first to experience space sickness from the exposure to zero magnetic fields due to the absence of the earth's magnetic fields. Yuri had air, water, food, light, limited movement and the very best that Russian technology at that time could provide. This was competition at the highest level and every consideration was taken to achieve the highest level of success. This experiment was the first demonstration of the profound importance of an unknown essential for life: PEMF. Since that flight, PEMF devices have been used in every space suit and space station.

Why does the body need the magnetic field of the earth? It is a vital source of energy to all living things on this planet. Valerie Hunt, Ph.D. (who did research on energy fields at UCLA) closely duplicated the zero magnetic field scenario that Yuri Gagarin experienced in his historical flight. She had a "mu" metal cage built so that she could put subjects in for observation. Mu metal has the unique ability to block out magnetic fields of the magnitude of the earth's magnetic field and the electromagnetic pollution, which surrounds us. Two individuals were placed in the room and connected with EEG, EMG, and ECG devices to measure effects on the body in the absence of environmental magnetic fields. To her amazement, in just a few minutes they began to sob and said they felt like they were falling apart emotionally. In a few more minutes, they were beginning to lose coordination, muscle control, and she had to pull them out to avoid affecting the heart muscle. All this occurred within just a matter of minutes!

Research indicates poor cell membrane performance is either cause or a dominant cofactor in most chronic and autoimmune disease. According to Nobel Prize winner Otto Warburg, healthy cells exist with a trans-membrane potential (TMP) of between 70 and 90 millivolts. Due to the constant stresses of modern life and a toxic environment, cell voltage tends to drop as we age or get sick. As the voltage drops, the cell is unable to maintain a healthy environment. If the electrical charge of a cell drops to 50 millivolts, a person may experience chronic fatigue. If the voltage drops to between 15 and 30 millivolts, the cell often can become cancerous.

PEMF makes it possible to raise the critically low TMP of cancer cells and therefore to reduce one of the critical factors of tumor growth. Effects that are seen when the TMP is increased include: enhanced cellular energy (ATP) production, increased oxygen uptake, changes in entry of calcium, movement of sodium out of the cell, movement of potassium into the cell, changes in enzyme and biochemical activity, and changes in cellular pH.

According to Marcel Wolfe, a holistic lifestyle research educator, *"PEMF research proves routine neurological, physiological and psychological repair. When the frequency is spot-on, absolutely NOTHING compares, not far infrared, not laser, not ultra sound. PEMF Research has repeatedly proven BETTER physiological repair in far less time than any other type of care while indicating absolutely no adverse reactions. It is important to remember that this energy is sub-threshold, meaning that the users generally will not feel the application. When frequency and exposure duration are adequate the results can be astounding."*

There are over 1,000 clinical studies and over 7,000 research papers validating the therapeutic benefits of PEMF. In an August 6, 2007, *Science Daily* article entitled "Electric Fields Have Potential As A Cancer Treatment," it was reported that low-intensity electric fields can disrupt the division of cancer cells and slow the growth of brain tumors. So here is the $64,000 question. Does frequency matter? According to Marcel Wolfe, *"Frequency **does** matter. Frequency is not just a piece of the health puzzle it is the glue that holds it all together and the major means necessary for communication to make it all happen."* Hence the quotes from Albert Einstein: *"Frequency is everything;"* and *"frequency trumps chemistry."*

THE "MRS 2000+"

Due to our current lifestyle, our bodies are constantly deficient in energy that can only be provided by exposure to beneficial PEMF. And the need for healthy sources of energy will only increase over time. One important piece of equipment, in my opinion, is a PEMF device. The "MRS 2000+" (MRS stands for **M**agnetic **R**esonance **S**timulation) is one of the most effective devices I have researched in the area of PEMF. It is the top selling PEMF system worldwide used by thousands of world class professional and amateur athletes and almost half a million home unit users and millions of clinical users. The MRS 2000+ has been around since the mid 1990s with hundreds of clinical studies and case studies that have been documented.

Most importantly, it is the closest PEMF experience to that of nature. That is, the earth's magnetic field is at 40 uT (microtesla), and the MRS uses intensities very close to this strength. Without going into too much detail, the naturally occurring pulsed field on the earth is the "Schumann resonance," and the first two major harmonics are 7.83 and 14.2 HZ. The MRS 2000+ uses these harmonics plus millions of frequencies in this range, plus it contains a "biorhythm clock" so you run the appropriate program for the time of day. That is, you get energizing frequencies in the early part of the day and more relaxing frequencies in the evening. Also, the full body pad is much thicker, softer, and more comfortable than other mats. While this does not affect the quality of the field, it does give a more enjoyable experience.

I want to thank Marcel Wolfe for his contributions to the information in this chapter. Mr. Wolfe is a lifestyle research educator who has worked in the holistic health field for over 20 years. Since the mid 1980s, he has studied the full spectrum of frequency technologies such as color and light therapy, static magnets, tachyon, negative ion generation, multiwave oscillators, and Rife generators. Mr. Wolfe is a specialist in the field of PEMF's, and he continues to lecture for corporations, organizations, and health expos around the world. If you decide to purchase an MRS 2000+ or would like more information on PEMF, I strongly recommend that you contact him. His phone number (in Canada) is 416-256-7981.

PART 3

DETOX

DIET

NUTRITION

SUPPLEMENTS

&

GMO

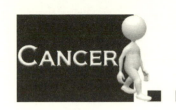

CHAPTER 10
SPOILED ROTTEN

> "THERE IS ONE MAJOR CAUSE OF DISEASE, AND THIS IS ACIDOSIS (LOW PH). DO YOU KNOW THAT ITS MAJOR CAUSE IS PUTREFACTION OF FECAL WASTE REABSORBED INTO YOUR SYSTEM? THIS CAUSES TOXEMIA WHICH MEANS DIRTY BLOOD . . . THE ONLY WAY FOR YOUR BLOOD TO BECOME TOXIC IS BY REABSORBING YOUR OWN TOXIC FECAL WASTE FROM THE LARGE INTESTINE."
> —DR. DARRELL WOLFE

This chapter, entitled "Spoiled Rotten," is devoted entirely to cleansing (detoxification), which is in reality the most important yet overlooked part of a cancer treatment protocol. Let me repeat myself: **Cleansing** is the most important yet overlooked part of an effective cancer treatment/prevention protocol. According to Dr. Darrell Wolfe, *"The 'intestinal well-being' of the average person amazes me as I walk through the busy crowds of downtown this morning. As a health practitioner of 25 years I shake my head at the obvious. For a society so advanced and in search of health breakthroughs, why can't we see, feel, or smell the obvious? We are the nation of the **spoiled rotten**."*

What exactly does Dr. Wolfe mean by the above statement? Statistics show that the average person is overweight, and 25% of us are carrying around an extra 25 pounds of not just weight, but toxic waste. It is truly amazing how many men look like they are pregnant! Have you ever wondered how a man's belly could get so huge? Especially when the rest of his body is relatively thin? Well, what we are really dealing with is the large intestine (which is a muscle) that lacks tone, has fallen down, and bulges out of the abdomen, filled with stagnant waste material. Did you know that the average person has around 10 pounds of fecal matter putrefying (*i.e.*, rotting) within his/her body? As Dr. Wolfe so aptly stated, many of us are "**spoiled rotten**."

WHAT IS CLEANSING/DETOX?

Detoxification is the process of clearing toxins from the body or neutralizing or transforming them, and clearing excess mucus and congestion. A poor diet, poor digestion, a sluggish colon, reduced function in the liver, and dismal elimination from the kidneys all lead to increased toxicity and a lack of oxygen at the cellular level.

As I have mentioned numerous times throughout this book, the lack of oxygen at the cellular level creates the perfect environment for anaerobic microbes such as bacteria, parasites, viruses, and fungi to rapidly propagate. These microbes can be many, many times smaller than our body's cells, so our cells literally become infected by these microbes and eventually cause our cells to either die, or "morph" into cancer cells.

Once the body (specifically the liver, gallbladder, kidneys, and bowels) loses its ability to process all the toxins and pollutants we are bombarded with every day, the body's oxygen supply dwindles, the immune system begins to collapse, the body's pH becomes more and more acidic (*i.e.*, acidosis), and we have the perfect breeding ground for deadly microbes and parasites. These microbes are the end result when our body's immune system has lost the ability to protect its cells from carcinogens.

These viruses, bacteria, parasites, and fungi act as the actual catalyst for cancer and nearly all other diseases. By "hijacking" a healthy aerobic cell, these bacterium and virus invaders start exhausting the cell's oxygen and energy supply, until the cell either dies or mutates into an anaerobic cell. This anaerobic cell (*i.e.*, cancer cell) now relies on fermenting sugar to produce energy. The battle with cancer is truly fought at the cellular level, in an effort to cleanse the body of microscopic invaders while radically changing the body's internal terrain back to a healthy one. This is why cleansing is so vitally important to all of us.

DEATH BEGINS IN THE COLON

According to Dr. Darrell Wolfe, *"Your body is a temple for your spirit and emotions to find balance in the physical plane, but it must be in a healthy state in order accomplish that balance. That healthy state is delivered to you along an amazing assembly line know as the digestive tract. It starts at the mouth and goes down the esophagus to the stomach and then to the small intestine, which is twenty feet long.*

In total we are looking at thirty to thirty-two feet of intestines. That's a long way for your food to travel. Everything has to be digested in its proper time. The process of eating and digestion is a work of art, simple and effective."

He continues, *"Improper eating throws all sense of discipline and rules out the window causing grief, and eventually disaster to your body. Most people are only conscious of the first five inches of the process, only aware of the taste and texture from the mouth to the throat. So what we have is five inches of delight followed by thirty feet of misery."*

At the time of the writing of this fifth edition, my children are twelve, eleven, six, and three years old. They run around all day long, and they almost **never** get tired. Why do you think they have so much energy? Yes, they are young, but most importantly, they are **not toxic**. They have not had 40+ years of absorbing toxic waste migrating from stagnant fecal debris in their large intestine polluting their blood, lymph, organs, and tissue cells.

Do you have really bad breath? If you do, it is **not** caused solely from what you ate at breakfast! It could also be a result of what you ate last month...or last year! Remember that hot air rises, and it is rising from your abdomen and out through your mouth. *Does anyone have a mint?* Don't be fooled...mints, toothpaste, and mouthwash are only temporary measures which mask the symptoms and never get to the real root cause, which is your own toxic "internal manure pile."

Why do people use underarm deodorant and perfumes? To hide the truth. The truth is they stink. Why does body odor increase as we age? The answer is – we are **spoiled rotten**. We rot from the inside out. You should know that almost all deodorants and perfumes are toxic and harmful to your body, even some of the so-called natural products. As I discussed earlier in the book, many underarm deodorants may be a contributing factor to lymph problems and breast cancer.

Why do many people avoid going to the bathroom in public? Because of the foul stench they leave behind. Imagine walking into your own house and being confronted by a rank smell and not knowing where it was coming from. You would not rest until you found it. I'm sure you wouldn't spray deodorizers through the house to mask the odor. However, even if you change your diet and start eating properly, you will never have vibrant health if you don't clean out your personal *"sewer pipes."* Perhaps the most important statement in this entire chapter is this: you will not have rotting if you understand the art of cleansing.

However, most people do not want to talk about their putrefying fecal matter. They stick their head in the sand hoping it will go away. A toxic colon is the breeding ground for disaster.

According to Dr. Darrell Wolfe, *"There is one major cause of disease and this is acidosis (low pH). Do you know that its major cause is putrefaction of fecal waste reabsorbed into your system? This causes toxemia which means dirty blood. Let me pose a question to you. Do you believe that you could have systemic candida, chronic fatigue, headaches, sore throat, skin disorders, heart disease, gout, arthritis, sinus problems, even cancer - without your blood being dirty and toxic? The list of illnesses is endless. The only way for your blood to become toxic is by reabsorbing your own toxic fecal waste from the large intestine."*

Is it any wonder that we oftentimes hear the phrase, *"Death Begins in the Colon"?*

THE "DOMINO EFFECT"

Let me talk about the "domino effect." What is the major cause of toxemia (dirty blood)? Absorption of toxic fecal waste from the large intestine (colon). So if you can get the large intestine operating properly, you won't absorb the fecal toxic waste. That is not the case with 99% of the population. When the blood becomes overburdened by these deadly toxins and poisons, the liver has to pick up the overload. Your liver already does over 500 different functions for the body and now must pick up the slack and handle the toxic waste from the large intestine. The liver works overtime until it becomes chronically fatigued, and then the body starts experiencing an array of negative side effects. So, it's off to the doctor's office, and he tells you that you're OK and that this is just *"normal for your age."*

In reality, it's not normal. What has happened is that the liver had to do much more than its share because of the toxic blood situation caused by the encrusted fecal waste in the large intestine. Now the liver must pass on this burden of toxic waste caused by a sluggish large intestine (colon) to the kidneys. But the kidneys aren't so happy about taking on this extra burden. They already felt the added pressure for the last few years due to the colon being dysfunctional prior to the liver plight. Nevertheless, the kidneys do their best, but as time goes on, chronic low back pain sets in due to these unwanted toxic poisons. Other symptoms are showing from the over-worked kidneys like sweaty palms, bags under the eyes, frequent urination, and bladder infections. The kidneys are now taking the brunt of this toxic waste. Where does it go from here? To the holding tank called the bladder.

This is what Dr. Wolfe calls the "domino effect." First toxic colon, then the blood, liver, kidneys, bladder and now the lymph system become toxic.   So, the million dollar question is this: How do we get our internal sewer system back in order?   The answer is . . . **CLEANSING and DETOX!**

THERE IS AN ORDER

If you detoxify the blood with a clogged liver, where do the toxins go? So, you must detoxify the liver **before** you detoxify the blood. Next, if you detoxify the liver, but forget about your toxic colon, it will just get clogged again. Because of our fast-food American diets, our colons are, for the most part, stuffed with toxins that are straining our immune systems. Therefore, first you should cleanse the colon, then rid your body of parasites, then cleanse the kidneys, then the liver and gall bladder, then the rest of the body and the blood. This is the most intelligent order to follow.

This sequence is highly recommended by many natural health practitioners and medical doctors alike.

1) Colon cleanse
2) Parasite Cleanse
3) Kidney Cleanse
4) Liver/Gall Bladder Cleanse
5) Blood Cleanse

Step One: The Colon Cleanse

In the words of Henry Wheeler Shaw: *"A good reliable set of bowels is worth more than any quantity of brains."* I agree wholeheartedly with Mr. Shaw! The Royal Society of Medicine did a major study and found that a dysfunctional large intestine (aka colon, bowels) is the major contributor to 85% of all disease and illness. A dysfunctional colon is the major fuel to the fire of all illness and disease, including cancer. And until this organ gets your full attention and cooperation, not only will you not prevent or reverse illness, you will remain sick and tired of being sick and tired.

Dr. John Harvey Kellogg, famous surgeon and the father of Kellogg's Corn Flakes, believed that the colon was the origin of most health problems, hence his creation of a bran cereal to aid in colon function. He maintained that 90% of disease is due to improper functioning of the colon.

Did you know that your large intestine is often referred to as the "mother of all organs"? It is the first organ developed in the fetus. Why? Because it is the most important. Without a proper waste disposal (sewer system), life would cease to exist before it even gets started. Just picture the disaster we would face if our cities' sewer systems backed up into our streets and homes. But isn't that exactly what has happened with the "internal sewer system" of many people today, as we have become breathing cesspools of toxic bacteria, gases, viruses, fungi, and worms, living off stagnant, rotting waste? We are **spoiled rotten**.

Americans have the third highest incidence of colon-rectal cancer in the world (behind Scotland and Argentina). It is now killing more Americans than ever before in history. Many people think it's a dirty subject, and some think it's embarrassing. But cancer and death are worse, so let's talk about preventing it. According to the U.S. Health Service, over 90% of Americans are walking around with clogged colons. The saying "you are what you eat" is categorically correct and all the more reason to cleanse and detoxify the body. When the bowels are impacted, problems arise such as constipation, hemorrhoids, diverticulitis, ulcerative colitis, colon cancer, and a plethora of other ailments.

According to Dr. Richard Schulze, *"The first step in everyone's health program should be stimulating, cleaning and toning all the elimination organs, and the bowel is the best place to begin."* Dr. Schulze states that cleansing the colon (bowel) happens in three steps. First, get the bowel regular (one bowel movement per meal). Next, clean the toxic, putrid waste from the pockets, bends and folds of the colon. Finally, keep the colon clean through daily maintenance. www.risingstarlc.com/schulze.htm.

Dr. Schulze readily admits that after 20 years of clinical experience, he's found that 80% of all maladies, whether arthritis, acne, multiple chemical sensitivity, or cancer were cleared up within two weeks of cleaning the bowel. One of the best colon cleanses on the market today was created by Dr. Schulze and is called Intestinal Corrective Formula (#1 and #2). You can find it at www.herbdoc.com. Another excellent colon cleansing formula (which I personally use) is called Aloe Ease and can be found at www.newvitality.com.

Many people mistakenly believe that a two to four week cleanse is sufficient to restore their health. They are wrong. Daily maintenance of the digestive tract is imperative and necessary to re-establish and preserve your wellbeing. The goal should be colon regeneration and maintenance. If you've ever done a colon cleanse, you probably felt great for about a month but then you went back to normal. What happened? Your internal sewer system got backed up again, didn't it? The key is to keep the colon clean and not get clogged up again.

Not only must we cleanse, but we must re-establish a strong immune system in the digestive tract with the proper friendly bacteria (flora). Without this friendly flora being present, life as we know it would not exist. Most people have had the friendly bacteria in their digestive tract destroyed due to harsh chemicals, tap water, poor diet, antibiotics, and other toxins. Soil based organisms (SBO's) have the highest integrity of all friendly bacteria for the proper re-establishment of a healthy digestive tract.

Remember, the "golden rule" for effective digestion (i.e., a clean colon) is **never** to mix a protein and a starch. Meat requires protein enzymes for digestion and potatoes require starch enzymes. When these enzymes are put together they neutralize each other and your food putrefies (rots).

Step Two: The Parasite Cleanse

Most people believe parasites are only a serious problem in third world countries, but nothing can be farther from the truth.

Scientists have identified over **300** types of parasites thriving in the USA today, including but not limited to the following: pinworms, tapeworms, hookworms, ringworms, whipworms, roundworms, and heartworms. The USDA tells us that the average cubic inch of beef contains up to 1,200 larvae. It is estimated that over **90%** of Americans suffer from parasites and don't even know it. When symptoms appear, the worms/parasites have probably been in your system for over a decade!

According to Dr. Hazel Parcells, *"Make no mistake about it, worms are the most toxic agents in the human body. They are one of the primary underlying causes of disease and are the most basic cause of a compromised immune system."* www.frequencyrising.com

Parasites are scavenger organisms living within us, aiding many serious health ailments to develop, including cancer. Parasites thrive in the intestinal tract, liver, pancreas, and brain where they become "obese" when fed their favorite diet of sugars, processed and junk foods, toxins, and excessive carbohydrate consumption. The danger of these uninvited visitors exists in that they become extremely toxic and even deadly, as waste materials are expelled into the host body, their eggs hatch and larvae grow in tissue all over the body.

Parasites have three main goals/effects within the human host:

> ➢ Grow fat on your nutrition
> ➢ Drink your blood
> ➢ Overload you with their waste, which is then reabsorbed into your bloodstream, weakening the entire immune system function

Dr. Hulda Clark died in 2009, but prior to her death, she was one of the most knowledgeable people in the world on parasites. Clark earned a doctorate in biophysics and cell physiology, and she wrote three best-selling books: <u>The Cure for All Cancers</u>, <u>The Cure for All Diseases</u>, and <u>The Cure for HIV and AIDS</u>.

Dr. Clark discovered that there seemed to be two predisposing factors involved with every case of cancer she encountered:

1. the presence of a parasite (the human intestinal fluke) also referred to as "Fasciolopsis buski," and
2. the presence of various solvents and toxins within the body (including isopropyl alcohol) which, combined with the parasites, set up the needed conditions for the onset of cancer.

Dr. Clark was best known for a device which she called *"the Zapper,"* which kills pathogens in the body.

One interesting similarity between Dr. Clark's theories and other theories on cancer relates to mycotoxins (fungal toxins). Earlier in the book, I mentioned Dr. Doug Kaufman and Dr. Tullio Simoncini, both of whom hypothesize that cancer is a deep-rooted fungal infection that our immune system fails to recognize. In parts of Africa, aflatoxin (the #1 mycotoxin) is considered the number one cause of liver cancer due to the eating of moldy food. The liver seems most susceptible to damage from aflatoxin when isopropyl alcohol is consumed in ordinary food stuffs, and the intestinal fluke enters the field, paving the way for cancer.

Dr. Clark recommends washing all foods with ozonated water, since ozone can render any toxin less toxic, kill all forms of molds, and eliminate parasite eggs found on garden vegetables. You simply fill the kitchen sink with tap water, drop in an air stone (a ceramic aerator at the end of a plastic tube which is attached to an ozonator), and bubble ozone gas through the water for 10 minutes, while the vegetables, grains, or beans soak. She has tested and verified that this cleans up this situation, making the food suitable and safe for consumption.

How do you get rid of parasites? Clark claims that three herbs can rid you of over one hundred types of parasites, without so much as a headache and without nausea. These "miracle" herbs are:

> ➢ Black Walnut Hulls (from the black walnut tree)
> ➢ Wormwood (from the Artemisia shrub)
> ➢ Common Cloves (from the clove tree)

These three herbs must be used **together**. Black walnut hull and wormwood kill adults and developmental stages of at least 100 parasites. Cloves kill the eggs. Only if you use them together will you rid yourself of parasites. If you kill only the adults, the tiny stages and eggs will soon grow into new adults. If you kill only the eggs, the million stages already loose in your body will soon grow into adults and make more eggs. They must be used together as a single treatment.

According to Dr. Clark, the killing of all parasites and their larval stages together with removal of isopropyl alcohol and carcinogens from the cancer patient's lifestyle will result in a remarkable recovery, generally noticeable in less than one week.

Upon a close analysis of Dr. Clark's protocol, perhaps some of its success results from the inclusion of wormwood. Artemisinin is an extract from the Artemisia (aka wormwood) shrub, and it has been shown to inhibit angiogenesis (the formation of new blood vessels). In the mid 1990s, two researchers at the University of Washington in Seattle (professors Henry Lai and Narendra Singh) began to study the use of Artemisinin in human patients. They found Artemisinin selectively targeted cancer cells while leaving normal breast cells and white blood cells unscathed.

Cancer cells collect and store iron because they need extra iron to replicate DNA when they divide. Therefore, the cancer cells have a higher concentration of iron than normal cells. According to Professor Lai, it is believed to work because when Artemisinin comes into contact with iron, a free radical damaging cascade ensues. When Lai and Singh tested the combination of Artemisinin with transferrin (an iron-enhancing molecule), the results were astounding. There was a 98% reduction in breast cancer cells within 16 hours! ("Selective toxicity of dihydroartemisinin and holotransferrin toward human breast cancer cells," *Life Sciences 70*, 2001)

Studies have shown that 100% of leukemia cells are destroyed with this combination in only eight hours, likely because of the fact that they more rapidly divide, have a higher iron concentration, and have higher percentages of transferrin receptors (which transport iron). Apparently, the more aggressive the cancer, the better that it may respond to this treatment!

Dr. Clark's parasite cleanse can be purchased at www.drclark.com. I am good friends with David Amrein, the Naturopath who runs the website and is also the President of the Dr. Clark Research Association. You can take the parasite cleanse along with your colon cleanse or after it, just as long as it is completed before you begin your liver cleanse. Just be sure that you don't skip the parasite cleanse. According to Dr. Ross Andersen, *"Other prominent physicians agree with me; that in human history, the parasite challenge is likely the most unrecognized of all endemic problems. Because they cannot be seen and rarely present immediate symptoms, they remain invisible as a cause or contributing factor to what can be a serious disorder."*

Step Three: The Kidney Cleanse

Why is kidney cleansing important? Every day, your kidneys process the blood and help to sift out waste products (like mercury, lead, arsenic, copper, and other toxins) and extra water. The waste and extra water become urine. The urine then flows to your bladder through the ureters. Your bladder stores urine until you go to the bathroom. When your kidneys become overloaded with toxins, diseases of the kidneys and bladder can happen as you are unable to discharge the waste and urine from your body. Crystals form in urine from various salts that build up on the inner surfaces of the kidney. Eventually these crystals become large enough to form kidney stones. A kidney cleanse is a procedure which is used to dissolve deposits inside the kidneys that can lead to kidney stones.

We now know that hard minerals (mainly from tap water) cannot be assimilated by our bodies; thus, they begin to build up in our kidneys and other organs, contributing toward many diseases, including cancer. According to Dr. Charles Mayo (of the Mayo Clinic), *"'Water hardness' is the underlying cause of many, if not all, of the diseases resulting from poisons in the intestinal tract. These (hard minerals) pass from the intestinal walls and get into the lymphatic system, which delivers all of its products to the blood, which in turn, distributes to all parts of the body. This is the cause of much human disease."*

There are hundreds of herbal recipes, and many different homeopathic remedies used for cleansing kidney stones. One popular way to cleanse kidney is to do a watermelon cleanse. Just purchase a few huge watermelons and eat them all throughout the day. Another popular kidney cleanse is celery seed tea. Just pour boiling spring water over a tablespoonful of freshly ground celery seeds and allow it to steep. Celery seed tea is very potent in case of kidney stones and chronic kidney diseases. Celery seeds have a direct action on the kidneys, increasing the elimination of water and speeding up the clearance of accumulated toxins from the joints. Celery seed tea is oftentimes combined with dandelion root to increase the efficiency of elimination by both the kidneys and the liver. However, if you are pregnant, do not drink celery seed tea since it is a uterine stimulant!

Probably the most popular kidney cleanse is Dr. Clark's kidney cleanse found here: http://curezone.com/clark/kidney.asp. Also, Dr. Schulze's kidney cleanse is available at www.herbdoc.com.

Step Four: The Liver & Gall Bladder Cleanse

I have heard it said, *"Don't tell your girl you love her with all your heart. Tell her you love her with all **your liver**."* That seems odd, doesn't it? But when you consider that the liver performs over 1,000 tasks daily and filters every drop of blood that flows through it, I guess you can see that it makes sense.

The liver produces chemicals to combat viruses and bacteria, supports phagocytosis (cell-eating), and produces antihistamines to neutralize substances that promote the growth of cancer. It is such a powerhouse that scientists estimate that up to 80% of the liver can be damaged without producing any symptoms! Plus, the liver regenerates itself every six weeks! In his 1994 article entitled "The Liver, Laboratory of Living," Dr. Leo Roy stated, *"No disease, especially degenerative diseases including cancer and AIDS, could survive longer than a few weeks in the presence of a healthy liver."* (*Immune Perspectives,* Summer 1994)

In his book, <u>The Liver And Cancer</u>, Dr. Kasper Blond of Vienna, Austria refers to the liver as the *"gateway to disease."* In the book, he states, *"No other stimulus is necessary (for the growth of cancer) than a metabolic toxin which has not passed the liver filter or has not been neutralized owing to liver failure."* He later states, *"Cancer of the lung is not caused by nicotine, but by the alimentary toxins having bypassed the liver filter."* Remember the baseball star Mickey Mantle? He was diagnosed with lung cancer while awaiting a liver transplant.

Do you see the connection?

There are many ways to clean and maintain your liver, but the best liver flush I have seen is the five day liver and gallbladder flush from Jon Barron. You can find it at www.jonbarron.org. Another good liver flush is from Dr. Schulze at www.herbdoc.com. Drink a quart of organic, unprocessed, apple juice each day for three days. You don't have to fast during this period, but it is recommended that you do fast. On the evening of the third day, drink eight ounces of organic, cold pressed, extra virgin olive oil. Stir it up (along with the juice of one lemon) and drink it down quickly. Then grab a small trashcan and lie in a fetal position, curled up on your right side for ½ hour. Keep the trashcan by your face just in case you vomit. The next morning, you should find a few small green or black objects in your stool. These are gallstones.

There is science behind the liver & gallbladder cleanse. Apple juice is high in malic acid, which acts as a solvent to weaken adhesions between solid globules. The organic olive oil stimulates the gallbladder and bile duct to contract and expel its contents. Dr Schulze claims our diets are just too sweet, that we must get some bitter herbs and greens to stimulate the bile flow. He recommends eating some parsley or kale (or any bitter herb/green) just prior to a meal to get the bile flowing. Beet juice, alfalfa juice, wheat grass juices are a delight for the liver. And as I've already mentioned, coffee enemas also stimulate the flow of bile.

Step Five: Cleanse your Blood

The blood stream is our *"River of Life."* We very seldom give even a second thought to the blood that is coursing through our bodies until we have had an injury and this precious fluid flows out before our eyes.

One of the first things we can do to improve the circulatory system is to clean out the channels through which the blood flows. Due to faulty digestion and the use of hard water, the walls of arteries, veins, and capillaries become coated with inorganic waste materials. This waste forms a lining that does not allow the cell structure of the veins and arteries to be fed properly, so these originally soft pliable tissues become hard and lose their elasticity. Then, like an "old" rubber hose, they cannot expand or contract with ease and they become, through weakness, ballooned out, or brittle and then break, as in varicosity. The heavy use of breads, pastries, and refined sugars leach out the calcium from the veins and arteries and when there is a calcium deficiency we have weakness, which allows malfunction.

When the colon, kidneys, and liver have deteriorated in their ability to keep the blood clean of waste, the blood then cannot perform its many functions adequately. Oxygen distribution to the cells of the body is curtailed, the immune system is busy with having to handle some of the excess contaminants in the blood, and degenerative disease is the end result. So, again, we are back to where we started...cancer is always associated with a lack of oxygen at the cellular level.

There are actually several ways to cleanse your blood. One of the most effective is to take digestive enzymes between meals or before bed. Within a matter of minutes the enzymes enter the bloodstream and begin cleaning the debris out of the blood and stimulating the immune cells. But I also recommend that you use an herbal blood cleanser to remove toxic residues from the blood so that it is hostile toward cancer and tumors. The great blood cleansing herbs are as follows: red clover, burdock root, chaparral, poke root, and sheep sorrel. These are the herbs you will find in the famous blood cleansing formulas such as Hoxsey tea, Essiac tea, and Dr. Schulze's formula. They literally drive tumors out of the body.

Jon Barron has an excellent blood cleanse available at his website: www.jonbarron.org. According to him, the best way to take this type of formula is as an herbal tincture, which concentrates the herbs up to 30 times. Take between four and twelve droppers full a day (depending on your need) in juice. Take rest days as needed, but finish the entire bottle. Repeat as often as needed.

NOTE: Much of this chapter was excerpted (with permission) from Dr. Darrell Wolfe's article entitled "Spoiled Rotten."

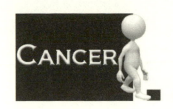

CHAPTER 11
NUTRITION IS ESSENTIAL

> "DON'T BOTHER LOOKING IN THE HISTORY BOOKS FOR WHAT HAS SLAUGHTERED THE MOST AMERICANS. LOOK INSTEAD AT YOUR DINNER TABLE...WE EAT TOO MUCH OF THE WRONG THINGS AND NOT ENOUGH OF THE RIGHT THINGS."   - DR. ANDREW SAUL

"FIGHT IT" OR "FUEL IT"

I have devoted several chapters to nutrition and diet, since one's diet is the most important piece of the cancer treatment puzzle. Let me reiterate: **diet** is the most important piece of the puzzle. Beginning on an alternative cancer treatment protocol is like putting wood into the fireplace (*i.e.*, your body). Once that wood catches fire and starts burning, the fire is going to kill the cancer cells that have colonized in your fireplace. However, eating a poor diet is like pouring water on that same fire. A bad diet will destroy many alternative cancer treatments. In fact, many scientific studies have proven that diet alone can cause cancer. So, if you want to reverse your cancer, then you must reverse your diet. Your diet is actually what "cures" cancer, since it builds the immune system and balances your "internal terrain."

The truth be told, many people have actually reversed their cancer by doing nothing more than changing their diet. The cancer diet is just as important as the cancer treatment. As I have compared many effective alternative cancer treatments to those that were less effective, it is evident that even a small "glitch" in the cancer diet can interfere with the effectiveness of the particular treatment. If the diet is fueling the cancer cells, then they are very resistant to most treatments. Just remember this: if the diet is not fighting the cancer, then it is fueling the cancer. There is no middle ground.

It is the diet (not the treatment) that will provide a long-term cure for cancer, since the diet builds the immune system and balances the internal terrain. Both of these things are essential to have long-term success in fighting cancer. Much too often people think they are cured of cancer when the tumor is gone or when the cancer cells are dead. They then revert to their old way of life, their old diet, their old vices, and the cancer returns. What we must remember is that some internal condition allowed the cancer to grow initially, and if that internal condition returns, due to poor diet, then the cancer will also return.

The human body is made from the most common elements found on earth. In Genesis, we read the story of the creation of the world and the Garden of Eden. We read in Genesis 2:7 that God *"formed man out of the clay of the ground and blew into his nostrils the breath of life."* What did God use to create Adam? God made him from the richest top soils on earth. I am 100% convinced that every element was present in the soil which God used to make Adam, and his fruits and nuts and grains and vegetables grew in these same soils. But then Adam fell, and so did our environment.

With the top soils in America having been depleted of 90% of their mineral value, the needless chemicals and hormones that are added to our soils and foods, and the processing that destroys the vitamins and digestive enzymes, making them more acidic, it's no wonder we have an epidemic of degenerative disease. In researching his book, <u>Nutrition Under Siege</u>, Alex Jack examined data published by the USDA ARS Nutrient Data Laboratory and concluded that a comparison of the data *"show(s) a sharp decline in minerals, vitamins and other nutrients in many foods since the last comprehensive survey published over twenty years ago,"* which he attributes to *"a steady deterioration in soil, air, and water quality."* These elements, which are now missing from the average American diet, are **crucial** to the maintenance of good health and to life itself.

A hundred years ago, cancer was virtually unknown, but today it seems like everyone has a relative who has died of this dreaded disease. What has changed? Have our bodies changed? Have our genetics changed? Or have we depleted our soils of essential nutrients? Have we changed what we put into our bodies? And have these foods we ingest, in turn, altered our internal terrain in such a way as to make us more susceptible to disease?

In his book entitled <u>Beating Cancer With Nutrition</u>, Dr. Patrick Quillin provides us with a tremendous analogy: *"Fungus grows on the bark of a tree due to the favorable conditions of heat, moisture and darkness. You can cut, burn and poison a fungus all you want, but as long as favorable conditions persist, it will return. Similarly, cancer develops in a human when conditions are right. Documented factors that favor tumor formation include toxic burden, immune suppression, malnutrition, mental depression and elevated blood glucose. . . Unless we correct these cancer inducers, cytotoxic therapies are doomed to failure.”* What Dr. Quillin is saying is that we need to focus on the cancer **causes** rather than **symptoms**.

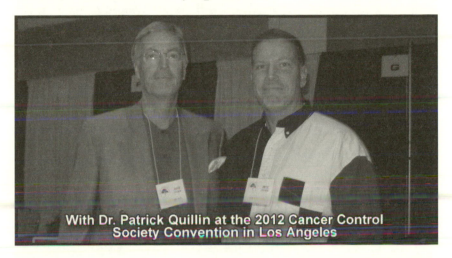

With Dr. Patrick Quillin at the 2012 Cancer Control Society Convention in Los Angeles

The lack of minerals and vitamins in the soil, the chemicals in our foods, drinking sodas, microwaving foods, eating junk foods, processed foods, foods contaminated with pesticides, and fake-foods are just a few of many dietary factors which have tainted our internal terrain, primarily altering our pH balance, and providing fertile soil for cancer to grow. Our acidic, junk-food, fast-food, empty-calorie diet is one of the primary villains in the rise of cancer.

As I mentioned, there is no middle ground. Either the food we eat is fighting cancer, or it is fueling cancer. Thus, the food we eat can be grouped into one of two categories:

1. Food that **fuels** cancer: Either by feeding cancer cells or preventing our immune system from killing cancer cells. These foods include the following: mycotoxins (toxic fungi), acidic foods, sodas, sugar, trans-fats, coffee, MSG, sodium nitrite, aspartame, processed foods, foods with pesticides, pasteurized milk & cheese, refined flours, fluoride, chlorine, etc.
2. Food that **fights** cancer: Either by killing cancer cells, balancing our pH, or preventing cancer from spreading through nutrients, enzymes, vitamins, and minerals. These foods include the following: spring water, apples and their seeds, apricots and their seeds, purple grapes and their seeds, raspberries, blueberries, strawberries, cantaloupe, carrots, broccoli, peppers, tomatoes,

avocados, garlic, lemons, limes, coconut oil, flax seeds, flax oil, raw walnuts, chlorella, spirulina, herbs, etc.

The key to a successful "cancer diet" is to eat foods that fight cancer and to avoid eating foods that fuel cancer. Simple, right? Not in 21st century America! A century ago, we didn't have much processed food. Families would eat fresh fruits and veggies, fresh bread, fresh nuts, fresh grass-fed beef, fresh eggs, and wash it down with mineral-rich well water or raw cow's milk. But today, the mom is just too busy to cook. So, for breakfast, everyone has a few donuts or muffins. Mom and Dad wash them down with coffee while the kids have a large glass of pasteurized chocolate milk. For lunch, it's a trip to the fast food restaurant for a cheeseburger and French fries with a soda and ice cream for dessert. And then dinner consists of pizza, chips, and beer or sodas, with a candy bar before bed.

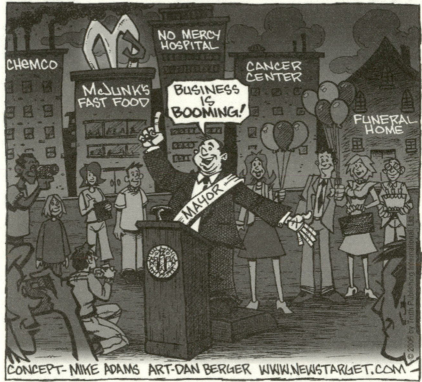

Thanks to Mike Adams and *www.NaturalNews.com* for the cartoon above.

Do you see a problem here? Unfortunately, the typical American diet contains about 95% of the foods that fuel cancer. These foods are highly acidic, thus causing an imbalance in our pH level. Let's take a look at French fries: we skin potatoes then slice them thin to expose their surface area, then we freeze them, then deep fry them in trans-fatty oil, and finally we glob on the salt. In the end, there is no fiber, no nutrition, and no minerals. There is nothing left but a wad of indigestible, highly acidic waste. Is it any wonder that some of us are barely making it from day to day? Our internal terrain is in horrible shape!

Not only are these foods acidic, but they are also deficient in enzymes. Since enzymes will make food spoil quickly, the best way to keep foods from spoiling and give them a longer "shelf life" is to remove or destroy the enzymes. But *"aren't enzymes important?"* you may ask. They absolutely are. An important role that enzymes play in the human body is in digesting food. But our processed foods today are missing these vital enzymes.

JUST JUICE IT!

One excellent way to get enzymes is to drink fresh squeezed fruit and vegetable juice. Since fruits and vegetables are juiced raw, the enzymes remain alive. Most people have compromised intestines due to eating junk food for years and years; thus, they have a difficult time absorbing nutrients. Juicing our plant foods is the equivalent of pre-digesting them, thus we are able to absorb more nutrients.

Fresh juicing may be the answer for those of you who just don't like to eat raw vegetables. I know that if you're used to hamburgers and fries, that the thought of eating a fresh salad with broccoli, carrots, cucumbers, beets, and celery may not be the most appetizing thought, so fresh juice is an excellent alternative to eating the recommended three to four pounds of fresh, raw vegetables per day. Juicing is simply the most practical way to meet your daily needs of fresh vegetables and fruit.

We try to juice frequently. Our juice usually includes organic carrots, beets, apples, celery, and cucumbers. The children love it. I usually drink about half of my juice and then add the pulp into the other half. The benefit of this is that it adds fiber to the juice, which serves as a fertilizer to healthy bacteria in the colon. Drink the juice **immediately** after juicing, since the nutrients and enzymes begin to deteriorate from exposure to oxygen and light.

A tremendous cancer fighter is wheatgrass juice. According to Webster Kehr, *"If we look at oxygen as a bullet to kill cancer cells, then we should look at wheatgrass as a shotgun blast at treating cancer. The number of ways it deals with cancer is incredible. First of all it contains chlorophyll, which has almost the same molecular structure as hemoglobin. Chlorophyll increases hemoglobin production, meaning more oxygen gets to the cancer. Selenium and laetrile are also in wheatgrass, both are anticancer. Chlorophyll and selenium also help build the immunity system. Furthermore, wheatgrass is one of the most alkaline foods known to mankind. And the list goes on."*

Wheat grass juice has been shown to cleanse the lymph system, restore pH balance, build the blood, and remove toxic metals from the cells. It also contains chlorophyll, which has a chemical structure similar to hemoglobin that helps transport oxygen in the blood.

PLANT FOODS & PHYTONUTRIENTS

When it comes to which foods offer the best cancer "medicine," nothing beats plant foods, due to the fact that they contain scores of enzymes and thousands of phytochemicals. "Phyto" means plant; thus, phytochemicals are plant chemicals, including vitamins and minerals. However, there are thousands of other phytochemicals other than vitamins and minerals which are contained in plants.

One well-known phytochemical is beta-carotene, which gives carrots and sweet potatoes their bright orange color. Beta-carotene is actually a member of a family of phytochemicals called carotenoids, which give fruits and vegetables their bright colors. Research indicates that phytochemicals lower our risk of cancer. It's important to keep in mind that only plants (fruit, vegetables, nuts, seeds, grains, & legumes) contain phytochemicals.

Plant foods, especially the green leafy vegetables, contain enzymes which enable the body to detoxify (cleanse) itself more efficiently and eliminate cancer causing substances. Green plant foods contain chlorophyll, which has a chemical structure similar to hemoglobin that helps transport oxygen in the blood. Plant foods are also loaded with antioxidants, which help protect the body against oxidation. As we discussed earlier, our cells use oxygen and glucose to produce ATP, our energy supply. However, free radicals are a by-product of this chemical reaction. Free radicals, also called oxidants, cause oxidation, which damages the cell walls. Oxidation is like rust on your car.

Sprouts are rich with vitamins, minerals, proteins, and enzymes and deliver them in a form which is easily assimilated and digested. Interesting, since sprouts are **live** foods, they will continue to grow slowly, and their vitamin content will actually increase after you harvest them. Compare this with store-bought vegetables and fruits, which start losing their vitamin content as soon as they're picked and often have to be shipped thousands of miles.

Sprouting is a very effective way to add raw foods to your diet. If you can supply a jar, some screen or netting, and rinse the sprouts twice a day, you can grow delicious, organic sprouts in less than a week. Growing your own sprouts means having your own private supply of fresh organic vegetables every day from a couple square feet of counter space. And seeds can multiply up to fifteen times their original weight. Excellent sprouting choices include alfalfa, almonds, broccoli, cabbage, fenugreek, garbanzos, lentils, mung, peas, radish, red clover, and sunflower seeds. Be sure to refrigerate your completed sprouts. Ideally you want to eat them right after you pick them. Those sprouts are still growing in your plate! **Now that's fresh!**

Honestly, the health benefits of regularly eating fresh plant foods are nothing short of miraculous. Based on the latest health research, there is no doubt that plant foods can reduce the risk of cancer, and even if you already have cancer, plant foods help you recover and stay healthy. There are literally thousands of studies telling us that plant foods reduce the risk of getting cancer and also prevent the recurrence of cancer.

We absolutely love raspberries, strawberries, blackberries, and blueberries. All of these berries contain a variety of phytochemicals and antioxidants. Berries are also rich in many vitamins and minerals, including zinc, calcium, and magnesium – minerals that most Americans lack. All of these berries also contain ellagic acid, a compound which prevents cellular mutations and is an anticarcinogen. Clinical tests also show that ellagic acid prevents cancer cells from inhibiting the p53 gene to cause cell apoptosis. Blueberries contain "epicatechin," which is why they are so potent at improving liver function, and they also contain "pterostilbene," which protects against colon cancer.

The children all enjoy eating cherries. Interestingly, cherries contain perillyl alcohol, which can induce tumor cell death. In 1999, Michigan State University scientists discovered that cherries' dark coloring material is an outstanding source of antioxidants known as "*anthocyanins*." In fact, the antioxidant activity of tart black cherries is greater than that of vitamin E, which is the "benchmark" antioxidant. Cherries also contain pain-relieving compounds (COX inhibitors) which are so effective that the FDA went out of its way to try to muzzle cherry growers, preventing them from linking to scientific studies on cherries! Finally, cherries contain surprisingly high levels of melatonin, a hormone previously thought to be produced only by the pineal gland in the brain. Melatonin is part of the body's natural way of regulating sleep which also has anti-cancer properties.

My children all love apples, and they have learned to eat the seeds as well. The seeds contain nitrilosides (vitamin B_{17}) which have been shown to kill cancer cells. Fresh sprouts are also a favorite of ours – they are a whole food. We eat them on sandwiches and salads. Sprouting grains and vegetables also increases their alkalinity. We also love to use fresh herbs, such as basil, cilantro, parsley, etc.

Two important things to remember about plant foods: 1) eat them **raw** since enzymes are destroyed at 112°, and 2) eat **organic** vegetables and fruits (if possible) since conventionally grown plant foods are laden with toxic pesticides. However, if you can't find organic produce, don't use that as an excuse to go back to pizza, French fries, burgers, and beer. Go ahead and buy the conventional produce and wash it well in warm, soapy water.

ESSENTIAL ENZYMES

In the previous chapters, we have learned about the importance of keeping our body's pH in an alkaline state. Now, let's review some basic nutrition science. The chemistry of digestion is really simple; with all the three major types of food being protein, carbohydrates, and fats. We digest these three types of food into their usable forms: proteins into amino acids, carbohydrates into glucose, and fats into fatty acids.

Most people believe that when you eat food it goes into a pool of stomach acid where it's broken down, nutrients absorbed in the small intestine, then passed out of the body through the colon. This is not exactly accurate. **God intended for us to eat enzyme rich foods and chew our food properly**. If we all did that, the food would enter the stomach laced with digestive enzymes. These enzymes would then "predigest" our food for up to an hour, breaking down as much as 75% of the food we just ate. Unfortunately, most of us don't eat a proper diet, and we definitely don't chew our food properly. Remember, the important thing is not how much food we eat, but rather how much food we **digest**.

What is an enzyme? I just knew you were going to ask that! An enzyme is a catalyst. But what's a catalyst? I remember my high school chemistry teacher, Mrs. Reed, who taught us the definition of a catalyst. Just in case you've had a momentary memory lapse, a catalyst is a substance which causes a chemical reaction to take place without, itself, becoming a part of that chemical reaction. There are numerous enzymes within the body that are responsible for the hundreds of chemical reactions which must take place in order to keep the body functioning normally.

But by themselves, enzymes are just pieces of the digestive puzzle. For enzymes to actually perform thousands of tasks, they need help from vitamins and minerals (co-factors). The enzyme and the co-factors orchestrate themselves in a complicated biochemical opus called a "complex." It is the enzyme complex that brings about the essential enzyme activity.

According to Dr. Tim O'Shea, *"Vitamins, minerals, and enzymes need each other, like the three legs of a stool. In the wacky marketplace of today's food supplements, it's like we're assaulted on all sides by people screaming '**Vitamins**!' others yelling '**Minerals**!' and others hollering '**Enzymes**!' as though each one alone were the Magic Bullet that can cure anything. The real ideas are cooperation, synergy, and co-factoring. Nothing exists in isolation in the body. An enzyme without co-factors has no enzyme activity. Enzymes are known to have very specific jobs to do. Their activity is compared to keys that must fit certain locks. Enzymes are long-chain proteins held together in very specific shapes by hydrogen bonds."*

He continues, *"Think of a ball of string which is held in a very weird shape by tiny strips of Velcro. If anything happens to the Velcro-like bonds, the enzyme protein unravels, losing its shape. Without the shape, the key can no longer fit the lock. Then it's no longer an enzyme - just another foreign protein. And what do foreign proteins cause in our body? Right - inflammation. Immune response. And that's exactly the meaning of auto-immune. The body now attacks itself because it senses there's an alien on board. Self has become not-self."* www.thedoctorwithin.com

If the bonds are broken, the enzyme collapses and can no longer do its specific job. Such a collapsed enzyme is said to be **denatured**. Free radicals, heating above 112°, processing, canning, genetic engineering, and fluoride are just a few things which can cause an enzyme to become denatured. Interestingly, the enzymes in raw food actually digest up to 75% of the food without the help of the enzymes secreted by the body.

There are three major classes of enzymes: metabolic enzymes (enzymes which work in blood, tissues, and organs), food enzymes from raw food, and digestive enzymes. There are also three main categories of digestive enzymes: proteases (for protein digestion), amylases (for carbohydrate digestion), and lipases (for fat digestion).

Without enzymes, there is no life. Organic raw fruits and vegetables are awesome. They contain enzymes, some contain nitrilosides, and they are chock full of vitamins and minerals. However, as I have mentioned, cooking vegetables destroys their enzymes. At 112°F, enzymes are destroyed. **A good rule of thumb is to eat it raw**: raw fruits, raw vegetables, and raw milk. Cooking destroys enzymes and so does pasteurization.

You see, pasteurization has its roots in the false germ theory of Louis Pasteur. God gave us pure milk in a natural raw form that is loaded with natural substances that boost our immune systems as well as give us many essential enzymes, vitamins, and minerals that keep our digestive systems and bodies working at the optimum levels of health. But the man-altered, pasteurized milk we buy at the store is a devitalized, enzyme deficient, "nutritionless" food. Unlike the propaganda we hear on television, pasteurized milk is incapable of rebuilding or maintaining bones and teeth as it is **not** a good source of calcium (since the enzyme phosphatase which is required to absorb calcium is destroyed during the pasteurization process).

Studies also have shown that lipase (an enzyme in milk which helps fat digestion) is totally destroyed by pasteurization, which also diminishes vitamin content, destroys vitamins B_{12} and B_6, kills beneficial bacteria, and is associated with allergies, increased tooth decay, colic in infants, growth problems in children, osteoporosis, arthritis, heart disease, and cancer. In the words of Dr. Timothy O'Shea, pasteurized milk is equivalent to *"liquid formica."*

America is an obese nation. The CDC states that one out of every three Americans is considered obese (*i.e.,* weighs 30% more than his normal weight). Ever wonder why? Well, part of it is that we are a nation of gluttons and sluggards. Self-control is considered passé. However, part of the reason for America's obesity is the fact that our diet typically is 90% cooked foods. Hog farmers learned a long time ago that hogs get fat twice as fast if they are fed cooked food. Cooking destroys what? You got it...**enzymes**.

MISSING MINERALS

There are six nutrient groups – water, vitamins, minerals, fats, proteins, and carbohydrates – all six groups are necessary for optimal health. Truth be told, when we look at most people's diet, minerals may be the "missing link." Many people think minerals and vitamins are the same, but they are not. The main difference is that vitamins are organic substances (meaning that they contain the element carbon) and minerals are **in**organic substances.

Four elements compose 96% of the body's makeup: carbon, hydrogen, oxygen, and nitrogen. The remaining 4% of the body's composition is mineral. There are several opinions about how many minerals are essential. Some say 14, some say 16, the debate is ongoing. However, everyone is in agreement that we all need small amounts of about 25-30 minerals (14-16 of which are considered to be "essential") to maintain normal body function and good health, but due to unwholesome dietary habits and also poor soil conditions, most of us are mineral deficient.

There are two groups of minerals: macrominerals and microminerals. Macrominerals (aka "major minerals") are needed in the diet in amounts of 100 milligrams or more each day. They include potassium, chlorine, phosphorus, calcium, magnesium, sulfur, and sodium. Macrominerals are present in virtually all cells of the body, maintaining general homeostasis and required for normal functioning.

Microminerals (aka "trace minerals") are micronutrients that are chemical elements. They include iron, molybdenum, chromium, copper, manganese, fluoride, iodine, zinc, and selenium. They are dietary minerals needed by the human body in very small quantities as opposed to macrominerals which are required in larger quantities. Remember, with minerals, more is not necessarily better. Excessive intake of a dietary mineral may either lead to illness directly or indirectly because of the competitive nature between mineral levels in the body, so be sure to follow the recommended daily doses.

In this section, I will briefly touch on magnesium, calcium, chromium, and zinc. I know that iodine is a mineral and so is selenium, but I have given these two minerals their own sections (later in the book) so I won't discuss them here.

Magnesium

Magnesium has an incredible healing effect on a wide range of diseases as well as in its ability to rejuvenate the aging body. Magnesium is essential for over 300 enzyme reactions (especially in regard to cellular energy production), for the health of the nervous system and brain, and also for healthy bones and teeth. Magnesium chloride (magnesium /chlorine compound) used transdermally has been shown to boost the immune system. For example, white blood cells destroy up to three times more microbes than before, after the intake of magnesium chloride. Magnesium chloride has also been shown to be effective with bronchitis, asthma, emphysema, and pneumonia. Regions with soil rich in magnesium have less cancer than those with low magnesium levels, according to epidemiological studies. Scientists from India have demonstrated how the incidences of tumors of the breast in rats can be reduced 88% by a single application of magnesium chloride, vitamin C, vitamin A, and selenium.

Magnesium is also essential in the area of detoxification, especially heavy metals. For instance, glutathione requires magnesium for its synthesis. According to Dr. Russell Blaylock, low magnesium is associated with dramatic increases in free radical generation as well as glutathione depletion. This is vital since glutathione is one of the few antioxidant molecules known to neutralize mercury. Without the cleaning and chelating work of glutathione (magnesium), cells begin to decay as cellular filth and heavy metals accumulate: excellent environments for deadly infections. www.naturalnews.com/023279.html

Calcium

In the October 13, 1998, issue of the *New York Times* is an article entitled "Calcium Takes Its Place As a Superstar of Nutrients" which reports from a study in the *Journal of the American Medical Association* that "*increasing calcium induced normal development of the epithelia cells and might also prevent cancer in such organs as the breast, prostate and pancreas.*"

Once the calcium has been broken down, its absorption into the body is totally dependent on the presence of vitamin D in the intestine, so be sure to get plenty of natural sunlight. No other mineral is capable of performing as many biological functions as is calcium. This remarkable mineral provides the electrical energy for the heart to beat and for all muscle movement. It is also the calcium ion that is responsible for feeding every cell, a feat accomplished by latching on to seven nutrient molecules and one water molecule, pulling them through the nutrient channel, detaching the load, and repeating the process. One common denominator which links all people who live past 100 years is that they all get massive amounts (*over 5 grams*) of calcium daily.

Another important biological job for calcium is DNA replication, which is the basis for all body repairs and is crucial for maintaining health and preventing degenerative disease. As important as all these and hundreds of other biological functions of calcium are to human health, none is more important than the job of pH control. It has been said that "*Calcium to acid, is like water to a fire.*" Calcium quickly destroys oxygen robbing acid in the body fluids.

Chromium

Research at the USDA has revealed that chromium plays a very important role in amplifying insulin response in diabetics. In 1977, the first published case of a chromium-diabetes link showed that the severe diabetic symptoms that developed in a woman while on long-term IV feeding were alleviated by supplemental chromium. According to Dr. Walter Metz, the USDA researcher who identified chromium as the fundamental component of the glucose tolerance factor (GTF), "*often 50% or more of the subjects in various studies improve following chromium supplementation.*" The body needs GTF to metabolize sugar. Scientists have found that eating foods high in simple sugars stimulate chromium loss through the urine. In addition, refined carbohydrates are devoid of chromium and other imperative trace minerals.

While glucose transport is the primary role of insulin, chromium's main function is increasing insulin's **efficiency** in regulating blood sugar levels. Research indicates chromium helps open the door to the cell membrane, allowing glucose to enter. This occurs when chromium is converted into GTF, which supports the functions of insulin in the body. According to Dr. Scott Whitaker, author of the best-selling book MediSin, "*without a doubt, using food grade chromium GTF will eliminate diabetes within 6 weeks along with cod liver oil and a diet that has eliminated all processed grains and refined sugars.*" Anyone with diabetes who uses insulin should consult with a healthcare provider about chromium supplements, since the insulin dosage may have to be adjusted.

Zinc

The role of zinc in a wide range of cellular processes (including cell division and proliferation, immune function, and defense against free radicals) has been well established. Zinc is the most abundant trace element in cells, and increasing evidence emphasizes zinc's important role in both genetic stability and function. Zinc is found in over 300 enzymes, including copper/zinc superoxide dismutase, which is an important antioxidant enzyme, and in several proteins involved in DNA repair. Zinc also helps to protect cellular components from oxidation and damage. Zinc deficiency can lead to immune dysfunction and impairments in growth, cognitive function, and hormonal function. Vitamin B_{17} (laetrile) along with zinc, magnesium, selenium, and vitamins A and B cause the body's defense mechanism against cancer to be built up, thus deterring cancer growth within the body. In addition, zinc is the transportation system for the disbursement of laetrile in the body, thus building up the immune system against cancer. There is a reciprocal connection between zinc and copper. If blood zinc levels are too high the copper levels will be too low. For instance, people who live in areas with "soft water" tend to be zinc deficient since their copper levels are typically high due to leeching from the copper plumbing.

VITAL VITAMINS

All vitamins are required for many of the natural processes of the human body, and are, in fact, essential to life. Because the body cannot synthesize vitamins on its own, they must be supplied through diet or by taking supplements. Vitamins are either "water-soluble" (water is required for absorption and are excreted in urine) or "fat-soluble" (requires fat for absorption and are stored in fat tissue).

There are **nine** different "water-soluble" vitamins: vitamin C and eight B vitamins – thiamine (B_1), riboflavin (B_2), niacin (B_3), pantothenic acid (B_5), pyroxidine (B_6), biotin (B_7), folic acid (B_9), cyanocobalamin (B_{12}). There are **four** different "fat-soluble" vitamins: vitamins A (Beta Carotene), D, E, and K. Each of these vitamins has a unique role and function in our bodies. For example, vitamin A promotes eyesight and helps us see in the dark, while vitamin K helps blood to clot. Vitamins are vulnerable to heat, light, and chemical agents, so cooking, food preparation, processing, and storage must be appropriate to preserve vitamins in food.

Ideally, we should be able to obtain adequate levels of essential vitamins through our diet. However, due to modern farming techniques, food processing methods, and the effects of cooking, our food is often stripped of vitamins by the time it reaches our plates. Supplements may offer a sensible solution to this problem. It is important to note, however, that most vitamins require the presence of other nutrients to be utilized properly by the body. For this reason, it may be best to obtain vitamins from a whole food supplement or a multiple vitamin-mineral formula, rather than taking supplement forms of individual nutrients.

DIET & DISEASE

One of the major issues I have with most physicians is that they know virtually **nothing** about nutrition. Some medical schools teach on nutrition for a couple of weeks, but most doctors have never had a course on nutrition. According to Dr. Phillip E. Binzel, *"My biggest problem (at first) was understanding nutrition. In four years of medical school, one year of internship, and one year of...residency, I had not even one lecture on nutrition."*

Just take a look at most doctors and you will realize that they are generally very unhealthy people. Dr. Neal Pinckney states, "*I found out that doctors typically aren't given much training in nutrition and that some so-called nutrition experts are not well qualified in that field. A large sample of physicians was asked how much training they got in nutrition in medical school. The average was less than three hours, with many having only one hour or less. That's out of nearly 3,500 hours of medical training. The truth is that doctors may get their nutrition information from the same newspapers and TV programs we do, and unless they have taken extra training in nutrition, they may not know much more about nutrition than the rest of us.*"

Dr. Patrick Quillin is an expert at the relationship between diet and disease. He is dead on accurate when he preaches that we need to focus on the **cause** of disease rather than treating the symptoms: "*Mrs. Jones might be suffering from metastatic breast cancer because, in her case, she is still hurting from a hateful divorce of 2 years ago, which drives her catecholamines into a stress mode and depresses her immune system; she goes to bed on a box of high sugar cookies each night; she has a deficiency of fish oil, zinc, and vitamin E; and she has an imbalance of estrogen and progesterone in her body. Her oncologist may remove the breasts, give her Tamoxifen to bind up estrogen, administer chemo and radiation; but none of these therapies deals with the underlying causes of the disease. And it will come back unless these driving forces for the disease are reversed.*" www.patrickquillin.com

Our bodies are like cars. If we put high quality fuel into our car, the engine will run smoothly and quietly, it will perform better, and it will last longer. However, if we start filling the tank with diesel fuel, jet fuel, kerosene, rubbing alcohol, or lamp fuel, then we are bound to have some serious problems with the car's engine. Eventually, our car will begin to make funny noises, overheat, and eventually won't even start when we turn the key. A good car mechanic would quickly diagnose the problem: low quality fuels are causing engine problems. A bad car mechanic would tell you that there is no correlation whatsoever between the fuels you put in the car and the performance you get out of the car.

Unfortunately, when it comes to diagnosing "engine problems" in our bodies, many (not all) doctors are like bad car mechanics. They just don't see the relationship between proper fuel (nutrition) and optimal performance (good health). Case in point: My good friend, Chris Wark (http://www.ChrisBeatCancer.com) was diagnosed with stage 3 colon cancer at 26 years old, and agreed to surgery. Following surgery, Chris asked his surgeon what type of diet he should be eating. To his surprise the surgeon replied, "*...just don't lift anything heavier than a beer.*" According to Chris, "*The first meal the hospital served me two days after my colon surgery was a sloppy joe; that didn't strike me as* *a very healthy meal after having a third of my large intestine removed!"*

Because the cancer had spread to his lymph nodes, doctor's prescribed chemotherapy which they said would give him a 60% chance of living an additional 5 years. But Chris says that "poisoning" his way back to health did not make sense to him. He asked about alternatives to chemotherapy, but his doctor replied that there were none and *"if you don't do chemotherapy you are insane."* Chris and his wife went home and began praying to God for guidance. About a week later, he found a package on his doorstep. It was a book entitled <u>God's way to Ultimate Health</u>, written by George Malkmus who was also diagnosed with colon cancer as a young man and healed it over 40 years ago by eating a raw vegan diet and by juicing. Chris said it was very clear that he needed to heal his body by "overdosing with nutrition" instead of by using toxic chemotherapy. And that's exactly what he did! Today, over ten years later, Chris is the picture of health, thanks to his healthy diet and "nutritional overdosing." I was priviledged to speak with Chris at the "Healing Strong" conference in Atlanta in September of 2013. He is an inspiration to me.

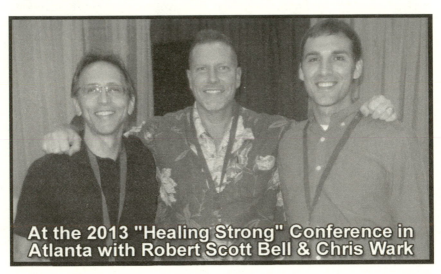

At the 2013 "Healing Strong" Conference in Atlanta with Robert Scott Bell & Chris Wark

Bottom line: Most doctors know next to nothing about nutrition. Of course, this is merely a broad generalization, so please don't think that I'm "bashing" all doctors. Many of my good friends are doctors and I believe that most doctors have good hearts and noble intentions. I'm merely stating the obvious – that most doctors who have minimal knowledge of nutrition. This being so, it is important to learn as much as possible about this subject, since you will probably not obtain much solid nutritional information from your doctor.

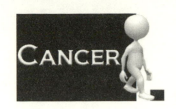

CHAPTER 12
FANTASTIC FOODS & SUPER SUPPLEMENTS

> "LET FOOD BE YOUR MEDICINE AND MEDICINE BE YOUR FOOD."   -HIPPOCRATES

Have you ever heard someone say that taking nutritional supplements is useless and will only give you *"expensive urine?"* If I only had a nickel for each time I have heard that! It kills me when I hear someone say something this naïve. A statement like this reveals a profound ignorance of the medical literature on the value of supplements.

The truth is that a percentage of most supplements **is** excreted in the urine, but this does not mean that they are worthless. The important factor is **not** whether you excrete some of the various nutrients, but rather what these nutrients do on their way through your body. Let's look at water. Of course you excrete much of the water that you consume. If you didn't, you would look like the Pillsbury Dough Boy! You excrete some through the urine, some through sweat, and some as vapor in your breath. The fact that you excrete it does not mean that you do not need to drink the water! Have you ever heard someone say that you don't need to drink water because you're just going to excrete it anyway? That would be ludicrous to say, wouldn't it?

The fact of the matter is that the most expensive urine in the world is created by taking multiple overpriced prescription drugs, **not** vitamins and supplements. With more than 40% of the American population now on prescription drugs, the drug content in human urine is now so high that trace amounts of antidepressants and high cholesterol drugs (such as Prozac and Lipitor) can be found in public water supplies! Compared to prescription drugs, supplements are cheap prevention, and the truth is that they are essential to a well-balanced, cancer-fighting, optimally-nutritious diet.

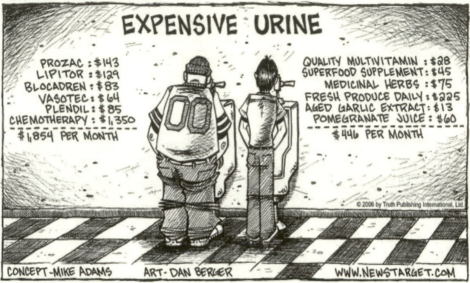

Thanks to Mike Adams and *www.NaturalNews.com* for the cartoon above.

Thomas Edison is quoted as saying, *"The doctor of the future will no longer treat the human frame with drugs, but rather will cure and prevent disease with nutrition."* If he had replaced both instances of the word *"will"* with *"should,"* then he would have been correct. Doctors **should** cure and prevent disease with nutrition. Unfortunately, most doctors still believe that drugs are the answer and completely overlook proper nutrition and supplements.

ALGAE (CHLORELLA & SPIRULINA)

Chlorella is a *"miracle whole food"* which gets its name from the amount of chlorophyll it possesses. It is single cell algae and actually contains more chlorophyll per gram than any other known plant. Chlorophyll is one of the greatest food substances for cleansing the bowel and other elimination systems, such as the liver and the blood, and it also is instrumental in transporting more oxygen to the body and the brain. In addition, the *"mysterious"* Chlorella Growth Factor (CGF) speeds up the healing rate of any damaged tissue, including cancerous tissue.

In addition to amplifying the immune system's response to cancer cells, chlorella acts as a preventative measure against cancer by raising blood levels of the protein albumin. According to <u>Earl Mindell's Supplement Bible</u>, "*Numerous studies have documented that a low albumin level is a marker for serious illnesses such as cancer and heart disease. They point to test-tube studies confirming that raising albumin levels can both prevent cancerous changes and extend the life span of human cells.*"

In a Japanese study, scientists placed lab mice on a chlorella regimen for ten days and then injected the mice with three types of cancer. Amazingly, over 70% of the mice injected with chlorella did **not** develop cancer, while 100% of the untreated mice **did** develop cancer and died within 20 days. In his book <u>Treating Cancer with Herbs</u>, Dr. Michael Tierra writes, "*I recommend chlorella to all cancer patients regardless of any other green drink they might use … It is virtually a complete food in itself. It acts as both a powerful nutrient and a detoxifying food.*"

Chlorella also helps in balancing your body's pH level, helps remove toxic heavy metals, and contains a wide array of vitamins, minerals, and enzymes. It also stimulates the production of red blood cells and even eliminates bad breath. And it is safe for children. In a study conducted on identical twins, the one given chlorella grew much faster, healthier, and had fewer sicknesses than the twin who was not given chlorella.

Spirulina is a blue-green algae found in alkaline, warm-water lakes. It contains concentrations of nutrients unlike any other single grain, herb, or plant. Spirulina is around 70% complete protein, with all essential amino acids in perfect balance, and also provides high concentrations of many other nutrients, chelated minerals, trace elements, and enzymes. Spirulina contains the essential fatty acids (linoleic and alpha-linolenic), gamma-linolenic acid, and arachidonic acid. Spirulina is virtually the only vegetarian source of vitamin B_{12}, which is needed for healthy red blood cells. It also has substantial amounts of chlorophyll, although not as concentrated as chlorella, and it has been shown to boost the immune system. Perhaps most importantly, lab studies have shown that spirulina polysaccharides can work to repair damaged genetic material; thus, spirulina possesses important antineoplastic (cancer-fighting) attributes.

Some scientists speculate that the "manna" of the wandering Israelites, which God provided for them each morning, and was described as tasting "*like wafers made with honey,*" may have been a form of dried, dormant spirulina. Of course, this is pure speculation, but it's an interesting theory, nonetheless.

The ability of spirulina to grow in hot and alkaline environments ensures its sanitary status, as no other organisms can survive to pollute the waters in which spirulina thrives. Unlike the stereotypical association of micro-organisms with "scum" and "germs," spirulina is actually one of the cleanest, most naturally sterile foods found in nature. Its adaptation to heat also assures that spirulina retains its nutritional value when subject to high temperatures during processing and shelf storage, unlike many plant foods that rapidly deteriorate at higher temperatures.

If you want more information on chlorella and spirulina, I strongly recommend the online book entitled <u>Superfoods for Optimal Health: Chlorella and Spirulina</u>, written by Mike Adams, the "Health Ranger." It is available for free here: <u>www.chlorellafactor.com</u>. Mike also has an amazing product called "Clean Chlorella" which is available for purchase at <u>http://store.naturalnews.com/</u>.

ALOE VERA (GLYCONUTRIENTS)

We all know what the aloe vera plant is, right? It's that funny looking plant that looks sort of like a cactus without the thorns. Growing up, around my house, we **always** had a huge aloe vera plant. As soon as anyone got sunburned, Mom would cut off one of the thick leaves and apply it to the burn. By the next day, the burn would be greatly improved, since aloe soothes the skin, hydrates it, nourishes it, and accelerates the regeneration of new skin tissue.

But aloe vera is not only beneficial for soothing sunburns, but it's also used in the treatment of frostbite and different types of burns, including burns resulting from chemicals and radiation exposure. It has been used for thousands of years to treat wounds as well as for wound-cleaning and also has an analgesic (pain-relieving) effect due to its content of magnesium and salicylic acid. Also high in vitamin C and selenium, aloe vera is considered to be an antioxidant.

Before I continue with the healing benefits of aloe vera, let me review some basic terminology which will help you better understand the following information:

➢ A saccharide is a sugar.
➢ A glycan is a chain of saccharides.
➢ A monosaccharide is a single sugar molecule (like glucose).
➢ A disaccharide is a chain of two sugar molecules (like lactose which is composed of glucose and galactose).
➢ An oligosaccharide is a chain of sugars that is from three to 20 molecules long.

> A polysaccharide is a chain of sugars that can range from 10 to thousands of sugar molecules long and wide.
> Polysaccharides, oligosaccharides, and disaccharides must have the water removed from them (hydrolyzed) to form their component monosaccharides before being absorbed.
> Glyconutrients are nutrients composed of sugar (the Greek word "glyco" means "sweet").

Researchers have identified a small group of eight essential glyconutrients which are crucial to the proper structure and function of our 600 trillion cells. These glyconutrients combine with proteins and fats to create glycoproteins which coat the surface of virtually every cell in the body, thus forming a complex messaging system for "cell-to-cell" communication. If the cells do not have enough of the eight essential glyconutrients, then they cannot make the correct glycoproteins, and the cell-to-cell messages become disrupted. Subsequently, the immune system cannot effectively wage an offensive against bacterial and viral pathogens or rapidly dividing cancer cells. The result is the onset of disease.

Unfortunately, our modern diet is commonly providing only two of the eight essential glyconutrients (glucose and galactose). So, it is important to supplement your diet with a product that contains all eight (glucose, galactose, mannose, fucose, xylose, N-acetylglucosamine, N-acetylgalact-osamine, and N-acetylneuraminic acid). You guessed it! **Aloe vera contains all eight glyconutrients**. Without the essential glyconutrients, the immune system operates blindly and is very inefficient. Sort of like playing pin the tail on the donkey, if you're familiar with that game. Stripped of their ability to recognize pathogenic bacteria, viruses, and molds, your own cells will allow these foreign invaders to take over your body.

It is generally believed that aloe vera was introduced as a laxative by a Greek physician around 50 B.C. Aloe vera was also used during Biblical times. After Jesus was crucified, Joseph of Arimathea and Nicodemus took His body and prepared it for burial using 75 pounds of myrrh and aloes (*John 19:39*). The clinical use of aloe began in the 1930s with reports of successful treatment of x-ray and radium burns. In 1976, researchers isolated aloe emodin, a compound that showed significant antileukemic activity. One study published in the 1995 edition of *International Immunopharmacology* showed that aloe vera polysaccharides (called "polymannans") exhibited potent macrophage-activating activities. Remember, macrophages are leukocytes (white blood cells) that ingest foreign invaders and are an essential component of our immune system. Mannans are like the "mortar" that hold the building blocks of the immune system together, aiding macrophages and other components of immune response to "recognize" foreign invaders.

Aloe Immune is an excellent aloe product with all eight essential glyconutrients in a dehydrated powder rather than a freeze or spray dried powder, or diluted juice form. Aloe Immune is also less expensive than many other products on the market today. I have corresponded a few times with Scott Siegel, whose father (Dr. Robert Siegel) developed Aloe Immune. Interestingly, Dr. Siegel cured himself of three different cancers (prostate, colon, and kidney) using this product. You can purchase Aloe Immune at www.AloeImmune.com.

In summary, aloe vera is antibacterial, antiviral, and antifungal. This fact is well-known by herbalists around the world. Aloe vera also destroys cancerous tumors, boosts the immune system, and cures ulcers, IBS, Chron's disease, and Celiac disease. This is, in my opinion, the best single plant to have around your home.

APPLE CIDER VINEGAR

I am sure you've heard the old saying, *"An apple a day keeps the doctor away."* This could very well have a lot of merit. Apples are among the healthiest fruits available to us, and they are the central ingredient in apple cider vinegar (ACV). Hippocrates was said to have used ACV as a health tonic, and American soldiers are said to have used it to combat indigestion, pneumonia, and scurvy. ACV is a type of vinegar made by the fermentation of apple cider. During this process, sugar in the apple cider is broken down by bacteria and yeast into alcohol and then into vinegar. ACV is a powerful detoxifying and purifying agent. The amino acid in ACV is an effective antiseptic and antibiotic, whereas the acetic acid can aid in treatment of various fungal and bacterial infections.

ACV breaks down fatty, mucus, and phlegm deposits within the body. By breaking down these substances, ACV improves the health and function of the vital organs of the body (such as the kidneys, bladder, and liver) by preventing excessively alkaline urine. It also oxidizes and thins the blood, which is important in preventing high blood pressure.

A few years ago, Charlene had numbness and tingling in her foot, resulting in excruciating pain and making it difficult to walk. To remedy this, we combined ACV with blackstrap molasses, which contains many vitamins and minerals. She drank this concoction three times that day, and by the next morning, the pain had subsided and the numbness was nearly gone. She was back out walking and running with the children within two days, pain free and happy. She definitely is a "believer" in daily doses of ACV with blackstrap molasses. We're happy to say that it definitely works!

Top doctors have revealed that the combination of garlic, ACV and honey is a *"wonder potion."* In a study of arthritis victims, Dr. Angus Peters of the University of Edinburgh's Arthritis Research Institute found that a daily dose of ACV and honey reduced pains by 90%. Also, a daily dose of garlic and ACV has proved to be a powerful fat destroyer and weight reducer, according to Dr. Raymond Fish of London's famous Obesity Research Center. Dr. Hen Lee Tsno writes in China's respected *Journal of Natural Medicines*, *"Patients given this miracle drink before breakfast showed a remarkable reduction in high blood pressure and cholesterol in less than a week."*

Beware: Not all ACVs are created equal! Many commercial ACVs have been pasteurized, filtered, refined, or distilled in order to make the product look good. Unfortunately, this extra processing destroys much of the healthy goodness and thus many of the apple cider benefits that were in the product in the first place. The best type of ACV to use is one made from cold pressed, organically grown whole apples, in which no chemicals or preservatives have been added. We purchase Bragg ACV, which is raw and organic.

ASTRAGALUS

You've probably heard of natural cold remedies like echinacea, garlic, and goldenseal. But here is a remedy that may be even better!

So just what is this miracle remedy? It's an ancient Chinese herb called *"huang qi,"* which means *"yellow leader,"* but you probably know it by its more common name, *"astragalus."* Astragalus is a plant native to Asia, and the part of the plant used medicinally is the root, which is similar to a garlic bulb.

A myriad of studies show that astragalus is a powerful immune booster. However, a common misconception is that merely stimulating the immune system will be enough to "knock out cancer." Perhaps, in a few isolated cases, it will. However, the major problem with cancer is not only that the immune system has been compromised (which it has), but **also** that the immune response is not working. In other words, the cancer is "invisible" to the immune system and doesn't even appear on the "radar." As a result, when treating cancer, it is important to have a treatment that is both "immunomodulating" (*i.e.,* boosts the immune system) and "adaptogenic" (*i.e.,* corrects the immune response and "lights up the cancer radar").

Astragalus seems to be able to do both jobs. Firstly, it has phenomenal immune system modulating effects. In tests at the Hiroshima School of Medicine in Japan, it was shown to directly increase B-cell and T-cell levels, interleukin, and antibody production. But not only does astragalus increase the number of leukocytes, in particular the "hunter" T-cells; it also helps identify the viruses, bacteria, and other rogue cells. The University of Texas has shown astragalus to be an adaptogenic herb which enables viruses, bacteria, and even cancer cells to be "picked up" on the immune system's radar. In one study, astragalus was able to restore immune function in 90% of the cancer patients studied!

In a 1994 Italian study (*Morazzoni, Bombardelli*), breast cancer patients were given a combination of ligustrum and astragalus. Patients given this mix showed a decline in mortality from 50% to 10%. And in two other studies, cancer patients receiving astragalus had twice the survival rate of those who received the "Big 3" treatments. There is strong scientific evidence that it benefits liver function (often impaired in cancer patients). In China, astragalus is widely used in the treatment of hepatitis. It seems to reduce toxin levels significantly and boost interferon levels while having little or no effect on normal DNA. (*Zhang 1995, Fan 1996*)

In summary, this remarkable remedy boosts your immune system against colds and flu, bacteria, viruses, fungi, hepatitis, and even cancer. Unlike other immune-boosting herbs (like echinacea and goldenseal), you can take astragalus every day, with no adverse side effects.

BEE PRODUCTS

Bee Pollen

Bee pollen contains trace amounts of minerals and vitamins, is very high in protein and carbohydrates, and contains all the ingredients necessary for a balanced diet. Twenty-two nutrients required by the human body are found in this "perfect" food, including all of the B-complex vitamins, vitamin C, D, E, K, and Beta Carotene (vitamin A), plus numerous minerals, enzymes and coenzymes, plant-source fatty acids, carbohydrates, proteins, and 22 amino acids (including all eight "essential" amino acids that the body cannot manufacture for itself). Needless to say, bee pollen is one of the most complete foods available.

According to researchers at the Institute of Apiculture, Taranov, Russia, "*Honeybee pollen is the richest source of vitamins found in Nature in a single food. Even if bee pollen had none of its other vital ingredients,*

its content of rutin alone would justify taking at least a teaspoon daily, if for no other reason than strengthening the capillaries. Pollen is extremely rich in rutin and may have the highest content of any source, plus it provides a high content of the nucleics RNA and DNA."
www.shirleys-wellness-cafe.com/bee.htm

Doctors in Europe often prescribe it as a food supplement to increase energy and vitality. Another interesting fact about bee pollen is that it cannot be synthesized in a laboratory. When researchers take away a bee's pollen-filled comb and feed it "man-made" pollen, the bee dies even though all the known nutrients are present in the lab-produced "synthesized" food.

Thousands of chemical analyses of bee pollen have been made with the very latest diagnostic equipment, but there are still some elements present in bee pollen that man, with his finite wisdom, cannot identify. Evidently, the bees add some mysterious "extra" of their own. These unidentifiable elements may very well be the reason bee pollen works so marvelously against so many assorted health conditions.

NOTE: Do not give bee pollen to infants under 18 months old.

Raw Honey

Not only does this wonderfully rich golden liquid taste great, but it also contains all the essential minerals necessary for sustaining life. Raw Honey is virtually free of bacteria, which is why it rarely spoils, and it is also antiviral and antifungal. Raw honey supplies two stages of energy. The glucose in honey is absorbed by the body quickly and gives an immediate energy boost, then the fructose is absorbed more slowly providing sustained energy. Raw honey contains all the substances necessary to sustain life (including enzymes, vitamins, minerals, and water), and it's the only food that contains "pinocembrin" (an antioxidant associated with improved brain functioning).

It's best if you buy locally grown organic raw honey whenever you can, since it's produced by bees which are from the environment in which you live. It is always best to grow or consume foods from the area in which you live as they contain the immune stimulating properties needed for your body to adapt to its environment.

NOTE: Since raw honey contains a natural presence of botulinum endospores, do not give it to infants under one year old, as their intestinal track is not mature enough to inhibit the growth of clostridium botulinum.

Propolis

While propolis is just now enjoying a rediscovery, the usefulness of propolis can be traced back to the time of Hippocrates, who used it to heal sores and ulcers. One of the most powerful antibiotics found in nature, propolis is a highly complex mixture of waxes, resins, balsams, oils, and a small amount of pollen. Bees use this substance to seal their hives, protecting it from outside contaminants.

God created bees as some of the most sterile creatures on earth, with the bee hive being the most sterile place in nature. Propolis is the substance responsible for neutralizing any bacteria, fungi, or viruses which enter the hive. Interestingly, in World War II, it was used by the Soviet Union to treat battle wounds, since it is such a potent antibiotic (with no side effects) and immune system booster. Propolis is sometimes called "nature's penicillin" and has also been shown to fight bacterial strains that have become resistant to synthetic antibiotics.

Except for vitamin K, propolis has all the known vitamins. Of the minerals required by the body, propolis contains them all with the exception of sulfur. Today, propolis is used in the manufacture of chewing gum, cosmetics, creams, lozenges, and ointments.

Royal Jelly

Royal jelly is a thick, extremely nutritious, milky-white, creamy liquid secreted by the hypopharyngeal glands of the nurse bees. It transforms an ordinary female bee into a "Queen Bee," increases her life span of three months to over five years, and enables her to produce twice her own weight in eggs each day (over 3,000 eggs).

Although some of the elements found in royal jelly are in microgram quantities, they still can act supremely with co-enzymes as catalysts or can act synergistically. **Translation:** the elements' action combined is greater than the sum of their actions taken separately.

Royal jelly is rich in protein, the B-complex vitamins, vitamin C, vitamin E, and inositol. It's a great supplement to use for stress reduction. In fact, it contains 17 times as much pantothenic acid (vitamin B5), which reduces stress, as that found in dry pollen. Royal jelly contains gamma globulin, known to stimulate the immune system and fight off infections. It also supplies the minerals, calcium, copper, iron, phosphorous, potassium, silicon and sulfur.

Researchers at Valhalla, New York, have found that royal jelly contains a complex compound that stimulates glands and normalizes the reproductive systems of both men and women and acts as a natural hormone. Royal jelly is also rich in nucleic acids, RNA and DNA. Gelatin, another significant component, is one of the precursors of collagen, which is another component of royal jelly. Collagen is an anti-aging element that keeps the skin looking smooth and youthful.

According to Albert Einstein, *"If the bee disappears from the surface of the earth, man would have no more than four years to live."* In light of this quote by Albert Einstein, the fact that the bee population is rapidly diminishing is quite disturbing, isn't it?

BETA 1, 3-D GLUCAN

Beta glucans are polysaccharides (complex sugar molecules) present in a number of cereal grains such as barley, oats, rye, wheat, but also mushrooms, algae, baker's yeast, and even bacteria. Their very powerful immuno-modulating properties have been known for over 50 years. Beta glucans enhance the immune system by improving the immune response when the immune system is confronted with a foreign body it sees as "non-self" (i.e. viruses, bacteria, fungi, cancer, parasites, etc).

But not all beta glucan products are created equal. In May 2007, the *Journal of American Nutraceutical Association (JANA)* published the most comprehensive and complete, peer-reviewed, study ever published entitled *"An Evaluation of the Immunological Activities of Commercially Available B1, 3-Glucans,"* in which they ranked their immunological benefits. The study is groundbreaking, as it also includes prescription mushroom-based beta glucan known as PSK Krestin, which is used as the primary treatment for cancer in many Asian countries.

The *JANA* study showed that **Transfer Point Beta 1, 3-D Glucan** has the highest proven immunological benefits: Eight times more effective than any mushroom based beta glucan, including the prescription products (PSK Krestin) used thought out Asia, and 160x more effective than many of the popular internet products being sold. http://www.betterwayhealth.com/Beta-Glucan-Studies/JANA2008.pdf

Transfer Point Beta 1, 3-D Glucan is an intensely purified, biologically active complex of beta glucans. When absorbed and converted, it attaches to specific sites on all immune cells that have CR3 receptors (macrophages, neutrophils, eosinophils, monocytes, and NK cells). By attaching, or binding, to these specific sites, Beta 1, 3-D Glucan puts these immune cells on "high alert" to foreign bodies. This process is called "immune modulation."

Hundreds of scientific papers have been published by researchers from the University of Louisville, Tulane University, Brown University, Cornell University, Memorial Sloan Kettering Cancer Clinic, and Harvard University, to name a few. These research papers describe in detail how Beta 1, 3-D Glucan acts on the immune system.

Dr. Vaclav Vetvicka is one of the world's leading researchers on beta glucan, with over 20 years of research on beta glucan, 200 peer-reviewed publications, seven books, and five international patents. He also recommends Transfer Point Beta 1, 3-D Glucan. That's why the brand which my family takes each day is ... you got it ... Transfer Point Beta 1, 3-D Glucan from Better Way Health. Their website is BetterWayHealth.com or you can call them and order at 800-746-7640. Much of the information in this section came from A.J. Lanigan at http://aboutbetaglucan.com/faq and also Dr. Vaclav Vetvicka at http://glucan.us/glucanfaq.html.

CARNIVORA ®

Carnivora® is the 100% pure extract from the Venus Flytrap plant and was developed by Dr. Helmut G. Keller, an oncologist from Germany. As a young doctor, Keller was disenchanted with the dismal success of the "Big 3" treatments and considered dropping out of oncology. By a strange twist of fate, he discovered the Venus Flytrap as he was purchasing a bouquet of flowers for his wife. As Keller observed the Flytrap (a carnivorous plant), he deduced that it must possess an advanced immune system able to distinguish between harmful intruders and its own cells and was intrigued at its ability to recognize and digest animal protein from insects and spiders. Dr. Keller had a hunch that this insect-eating plant could become a medical breakthrough. Turns out he was correct!

In 1988, the active component of Carnivora®, "plumbagin," was isolated. It has proven itself to be, in vivo and in vitro (in live subjects and in the laboratory), a powerful immuno-stimulant, stimulating cytokines and also inhibiting protein kinases, thus stopping abnormal cell growth and proliferation of cancer cells. Carnivora® is reported to work therapeutically to shrink solid cancer tumors, and in fact works for any type of cancer except for blood abnormalities (like leukemia). Several celebrities have used Carnivora® successfully for cancer treatment including former president Ronald Reagan, who went to Germany for therapy. According to Dr. Morton Walker, *"He (Keller) now has more than three decades of lab analysis, clinical investigation, and treatment of about 15,000 cancer patients to back him up. This plant is packed with 17 different substances that boost your immune system."* www.naturalcancerremedies.net

Carnivora® has had a dramatic effect on patients infected with the HIV virus, since it increases the number and activity of the T-cells and other immune system components. In an article entitled, "The Carnivora Cure for Cancer, AIDS and Other Pathologies," Dr. Morton Walker stated that Carnivora® *"is highly effective for the total elimination of the HIV virus in vivo from human blood and may be considered a cure for the autoimmune deficiency syndrome AIDS."* (*Immune Perspectives*, Summer 1994)

In addition to cancer and HIV, Carnivora® has been successful in treating arthritis, Lyme disease, hepatitis C, Chrohn's disease, lupus, chronic fatique syndrome, ulcerative colitis, and multiple sclerosis. According to Dr. Dan Kenner, *"If I could only choose a single plant medication to use, the answer would be simple: Venus flytrap. Why Venus flytrap? In a word, its extract is the most versatile plant-based substance for the treatment of chronic infections and degenerative disease that I have ever experienced."* www.dankennerresearch.com

Warning: Do not take Carnivora® if you are pregnant. For more information on Carnivora®, please visit www.carnivora.com.

CAT'S CLAW (UÑA DE GATO)

Cat's claw is a plant of the Amazon rain forest which has two main species ("uncaria tomentosa" and "uncaria guianensis"). In the USA, you see mainly "uncaria tomentosa" and in Europe you will see mainly "uncaria guianensis." Commonly called *"uña de gato"* in Spanish and *"cat's claw"* in English, the name comes from the thorns on the plant's leaves that look like the claws of a cat. This wonder herb, according to Indian folklore, has been used to treat digestive problems, arthritis, inflammation, ulcers, and even to cure cancer. The part used medicinally is the root bark.

Although virtually unheard of in the USA until recently, the beneficial effects of cat's claw have been studied at research facilities in Peru, Austria, Germany, England, Hungary, and Italy since the 1970s. These studies have shown it to be an immuno-modulating herb which increases white blood cell levels and stimulates the production of NK ("natural killer") cells, T-cells, and macrophages. Four alkaloids in particular boost phagocytosis (literally "cell eating") where the white blood cells attack, wrap up, and carry off the rogue cells in the body.

Cat's claw possesses amazing healing abilities and benefits to the immune system with a plethora of therapeutic applications. Dr. Julian Whitaker reports using cat's claw for its immune-stimulating effects, for cancer, to help prevent strokes and heart attacks, to reduce blood clots, and for diverticulitis and irritable bowel syndrome (IBS). Due to its anti-inflammatory properties, cat's claw has been used for rheumatoid arthritis and osteoarthritis. Compounds in cat's claw bark and roots (called "quinovic acid glycosides") block the body's production of substances called "prostaglandins" and "tumor necrosis factor" (TNF) which cause inflammation.

Cat's claw also seems to have the ability to break through severe intestinal disorders that no other available products can touch. Dr. Brent Davis refers to cat's claw as the "opener of the way" for its ability to cleanse the entire intestinal tract and its effectiveness in treating stomach and bowel disorders such as Crohn's disease, leaky bowel syndrome, ulcers, gastritis, diverticulitis, and other inflammatory conditions of the bowel, stomach, and intestines. According to Dr. Mary D. Eades in her book <u>The Doctor's Complete Guide to Vitamins and Minerals</u>, *"Many of the single chemicals found in this powerful herb have been patented for use in treating AIDS, cancer, arthritis, and other diseases. However, using the whole plant can be more potent than any one isolated ingredient."*

CAYENNE

The hot fruit of the cayenne plant ("capsicum annuum") has been used as superb culinary spice for centuries. However, did you know that in addition to tickling your tongue, cayenne is perhaps the most valuable medicinal herb in the herb kingdom, not only for the entire digestive system, but also for the heart and circulatory system? Cayenne acts as a catalyst and increases the effectiveness of other herbs; the active ingredient in cayenne is called "capsaicin."

In 2004, Dr. Sanjay K. Srivastava and colleagues (University of Pittsburgh School of Medicine) treated pancreatic cells with capsaicin and found that it disrupted mitochondrial function and induced apoptosis (programmed cell death) in the cancerous cells without affecting normal pancreatic cells. The results of the study were published in the April 20, 2005, issue of *Innovations Report*, in which Dr. Srivastava stated: *"Our results demonstrate that capsaicin is a potent anticancer agent, induces apoptosis in cancer cells and produces no significant damage to normal pancreatic cells, indicating its potential use as a novel chemotherapeutic agent for pancreatic cancer."* www.innovations-report.com/html/reports/studies/report-43316.html

In an article published in *Reuters* on March 16, 2006, entitled, "Hot Pepper Kills Prostate Cancer Cells in Study," Dr. Soren Lehmann of the

Cedars-Sinai Medical Center and the UCLA School of Medicine asserted: *"Capsaicin had a profound anti-proliferative effect on human prostate cancer cells in culture. It caused 80% of the prostate cancer cells growing in mice to commit suicide in a process known as apoptosis."* Researchers in Japan have also shown that cayenne pepper can dramatically slow the development of prostate tumors.

And if cayenne's cancer-fighting capabilities weren't enough, its effects upon the venous structure and heart are nothing short of miraculous. Cayenne is incredibly nourishing to the heart and has been known to stop heart attacks within 30 seconds. If you want to carry something in your first aid kit for a heart attack, carry a cayenne tincture. Even a bottle of Tabasco Sauce® might be good enough. According to Dr. John R. Christopher, *"In 35 years of practice, and working with the people and teaching, I have never on house calls lost one heart attack patient and the reason is, whenever I go in (if they are still breathing) I pour down them a cup of cayenne tea (a teaspoon of cayenne in a cup of hot water) and within minutes they are up and around."* www.herballegacy.com/Cayenne.html

Cayenne has traditionally been used for overcoming fatigue and restoring energy. It is a natural stimulant without the threatening side effects (palpitations, hyper-activity or rise in blood pressure) of most other stimulating agents. Rubbed on the skin, cayenne is a potent remedy for rheumatic pains and arthritis due to what is termed a "counterirritant effect." A counterirritant is something which causes irritation to a tissue to which it is applied, thus distracting from the original irritation (such as joint pain in the case of arthritis). But that's not all.

Cayenne can also rebuild the tissue in the stomach and the peristaltic action in the intestines. It aids elimination and assimilation, and helps the body to create hydrochloric acid, which is so necessary for good digestion and assimilation, especially of proteins. There is also evidence to suggest that cayenne may be useful in the treatment of obesity. Results of one trial showed that consumption of 10 grams of cayenne pepper with meals helped to reduce appetite, while results of another revealed that cayenne increases the metabolism of dietary fats. Lastly, herbalists from centuries past would pour cayenne pepper directly on fresh wounds in order to sterilize and stop the bleeding.

Truth be told, the amazing curative powers of cayenne are almost mind-boggling. Clearly, it should be considered nothing less than a "wonder herb" that has scientifically proven its worth!

According to Dr. Richard Schulze, *"If you master only one herb in your life, master cayenne pepper. It is more powerful than any other."*

303

CocoChia™ Bars & CocoPure™ Chocolate Tea

I think it's only fitting for this chapter to include two delicious chocolate "snacks." To be honest, chocolate is one of life's most misunderstood foods. Too often it's considered an unhealthy indulgence, rightly so if you're talking about milk chocolate bars, chocolate candies, chocolate ice cream, or chocolate syrup. However, just the opposite is true when you eat or drink a pure cocoa extract. Believe it or not, pure cocoa froths with many cancer preventing compounds.

Do you know that many of the most popular "healthy" energy bars on the market are in all likelihood just as bad for your health as regular candy bars? Many energy bars contain pasteurized milk and soy protein, two foods that can cause significant damage to your tissues every single time you eat them. However, there is one snack bar which is just as good for you as it is yummy: **CocoChia™ bars.**

These bars deliver four powerful "superfoods" (raw cocoa, coconut, chia seeds, and almonds) in a great-tasting, convenient form. And the ingredients are **100% organic.** The unprocessed whole chia seeds provide a steady, slow-burning source of energy, while the organic coconut gives essential fats the body needs. Organic raw almond butter, micro-encapsulated probiotics, non-GMO brown rice protein, Therasweet™, and organic cocoa round out the healthy ingredient list, providing excellent nutrition and great flavor with no sugar added or alcohol.

CocoChia™ bars are high in fiber and gluten-free, making them a good choice for many people who have digestive disorders. They also are low in calories and have a low glycemic rating, making them a good choice for those who are looking to reach and maintain their ideal weight and those who have trouble regulating their blood sugar and insulin levels. My family absolutely loves to snack on CocoChia™ Raw Food Bars. You can purchase CocoChia™ bars at www.livingfuel.com.

A few years ago, I discovered a healthy hot chocolate drink which my entire family absolutely loves: **CocoPure™ Chocolate Tea**. Each cup of CocoPure™ has 4,000 milligrams of concentrated cocoa, but that's not all. In addition, the health benefits of cocoa have been further fortified by adding resveratrol, green tea, and soluble fiber. This unique combination of nutrients supports cardiovascular health, arterial health, increased blood flow, digestive health, and the immune system. This is a great "bedtime" drink which we enjoy almost every night.

Studies on the nutrients in CocoPure™ have been published in the *Journal of the American Medical Association, American Journal of Physiology*, and *Heart and Circulatory Physiology* to name a few. CocoPure™ is available at www.newvitality.com.

COENZYME Q10

Commonly know as coenzyme Q10 (CoQ10), "ubiquinone" is a vitamin-like substance found in every cell in the body which is converted into a potent antioxidant ("ubiquinol") and is vital to energy production. There's no question that if you're over 30 years old, you should be taking a good "ubiquinol" CoQ10 supplement each day, since the body's production of CoQ10 diminishes with age as does the ability to convert it into ubiquinol.

When you start taking the proper CoQ10 supplement in "ubiquinol" form, and in the right CoQ10 dosage, you'll feel the difference right away in your energy and stamina. A good CoQ10 supplement fuels energy production in every single cell in your body by facilitating production of adenosine triphosphate (ATP) in the mitochondria. This improved energy output from CoQ10 therapy has proven to be quite valuable in treating neurologic disorders such as Parkinson's disease, multiple sclerosis, amyotrophic lateral sclerosis (Lou Gehrig's disease), Alzheimer's disease, Huntington's disease, and strokes.

If you're taking statin drugs, a good CoQ10 supplement is even more important because statin drugs deplete your body's CoQ10 supplies. And without an adequate supply of CoQ10, your heart cannot function properly. University of Texas professor and biochemist, Dr. Karl Folkers, encouraged a cardiologist, Dr. Peter H. Langsjoen, to use CoQ10 to treat congestive heart failure, with great success. According to Dr. Langsjoen, *"The clinical experience with CoQ10 is nothing short of dramatic. It is reasonable to believe that the entire field of medicine should be reevaluated in light of this growing knowledge. We have only scratched the surface of the biomedical and clinical applications of CoQ10 and the associated fields of bioenergetics and free radical chemistry."* http://faculty.washington.edu/ely/coenzq10.html

In the 1970s, Dr. Folkers followed the course of six cancer patients who were taking CoQ10 for congestive heart failure. Four of them had lung cancer and two had breast cancer. All six experienced remissions of cancer due to CoQ10 therapy. Folkers persuaded one of his financial backers, who had developed "terminal" small cell carconoma of the lung with widespread metastasis, to try CoQ10. He was given less than a year to live by his oncologist. After one year of CoQ10 use, he had no sign of metastases, and he was still alive 15 years later! The only therapy he received was CoQ10. Dr. Folkers, who died in 1998, recommended the use of 500 milligrams of CoQ10 daily in patients with malignancies.

In a study at the University of Scranton in Pennsylvania, scientists found that daily treatment with a topical CoQ10 lotion provided antioxidant protection to the skin of both young and middle-aged subjects. Interestingly, end stage AIDS has been associated with a significant deficiency in CoQ10.

Dr. Mercola has an excellent CoQ10 supplement for sale on his website (www.mercola.com) and so does the Life Extension Foundation (www.lef.org). One excellent way to improve the absorption of CoQ10 is to put the capsules in a cup of hot tea. And since fat also improves absorption, add a teaspoon of coconut oil to the tea.

Thanks to the late Dr. Jim Howenstine for much of this information on CoQ10.

CURCUMIN (TURMERIC)

Turmeric (curry) is known as "the golden spice of life" and has been used in Indian cuisine for thousands of years. As a matter of fact, it is impossible to think of Indian food without turmeric. **Curcumin**, the active ingredient in turmeric, has several cancer-fighting properties. A recent study found that curcumin can actually repair DNA that has been damaged by radiation. This is very good news, because one cannot avoid all radiation sources. According to University of Chicago scientists, curcumin inhibits a cancer-provoking bacteria associated with gastric and colon cancer. (Magad GB, *Anticancer Research*, Nov-Dec 2002)

Yet another anti-cancer property of curcumin is that it is a powerful antioxidant. It can therefore protect our bodies from free radicals that damage DNA. This is also why turmeric (which contains curcumin) can be used for preserving foods. Tests in Germany, reported in the *Journal of Pharmacy & Pharmacology* in July 2003, found that "*all fractions of the turmeric extract preparation exhibited pronounced antioxidant activity.*" Turmeric extract tested more potent than garlic, devil's claw, and salmon oil.

In the January 27, 2007, issue of the *Journal of Clinical Immunology*, scientists at M. D. Anderson Cancer Center in Houston stated: "*Curcumin can suppress tumor initiation, promotion and metastasis. Pharmacologically, curcumin has been found to be safe. Human clinical trials indicated no dose-limiting toxicity when administered at doses up to 10 g/day. All of these studies suggest that curcumin has enormous potential in the prevention and therapy of cancer."* (Aggarwal, BB et al, *Anticancer Research*, Jan-Feb 2003) And in the June 1998 issue of *Molecular Medicine*, researchers at Harvard Medical School published their findings that curcumin inhibits angiogenesis (the formation of new blood vessels) which tumors use to nourish themselves as they spread.

Curcumin can also protect cells against xenoestrogens because it can fit to the same receptor as estrogen or estrogen-mimicking chemicals. In a study on human breast cancer cells, curcumin reversed growth caused by a certain form of estrogen by 98% and growth caused by DDT by 75%. Turmeric has been considered to be "skin food" in India and other cultures for thousands of years, due to the fact that it cleanses the skin, helps it maintain elasticity, nourishes the skin, and balances the effects of skin flora. Several animal studies have demonstrated that turmeric inhibits the growth of a variety of bacteria, parasites, and pathogenic fungi.

Since curcumin is found in the spice turmeric, and turmeric is the principal ingredient in curry, you can enjoy the protective benefits of curcumin by just adding curry spice to your foods. If you combine curcumin with black pepper, it multiplies the effectiveness of curcumin by **1,000 times**. It makes it the most powerful "natural chemotherapy" you can ever experience. In the words of Mike Adams, *"You eat curry and pepper, and add some broccoli, and for the next 48 hours, your body will be destroying cancer tumors better than any chemotherapy known to modern science!"*

ECHINACEA

Echinacea is one of herbs with the most beneficial effects upon human health. Also known as "American Coneflower," it has been used since ancient times by Native Americans in order to prevent or treat frequent health problems (such as cold or flu) and also as an antidote for snake bites and poisonous stings.

In the 1930s, Dr. Gerhard Madaus (a German scientist) carried out comprehensive studies on this "miracle herb" and discovered that its potency is derived from its impressive list of ingredients, including vitamins A, C, and E and a large number of nutritive minerals (copper, iron, potassium, and iodine). It is also rich in antioxidants and other beneficial elements (oils, alkylamides, polysaccharides, phenols, and flavonoids).

Echinacea stimulates and strengthens our immune system by activating white blood cells, specifically macrophages, lymphocytes, and T-cells. It also slows (and even prevents) the formation of an enzyme called "hyaluronidase," which is found in reptile venom and functions by dissolving the protective gel-like substance around human cells. Hyaluronidase is also used by other dangerous bacteria to dissolve the connective tissue in our body and to get more easily and deeper into our bodies, but echinacea prevents its formation.

Echinacea is a potent natural antibiotic; it fights off infections, prevents inflammation, and may also increase production of interferon (an important part of the body's response to viral infections). In 2007, Dr. Craig Coleman (University of Connecticut School of Pharmacy) reported that combining echinacea and vitamin C reduced cold incidence by 86%, while echinacea alone reduced colds by 65%. http://news.bbc.co.uk/2/hi/6231190.stm

ELLAGIC ACID

Ellagic acid is a naturally occurring substance found in almost 50 different fruits and nuts (like red raspberries, strawberries, blueberries, grapes, pomegranates, and walnuts). It belongs to the family of phytonutrients called "*tannins*" and is viewed as being responsible for a good portion of the antioxidant activity of these fruits and nuts. "*Ellagitannins*" are products that contain ellagic acid in its natural form. For this section, I will use the terms interchangeably.

The Hollings Cancer Institute at the University of South Carolina conducted a nine year (double blind) study on 500 cervical cancer patients. The study, published in 1999, showed that ellagic acid stops mitosis (cell division) within 48 hours and induces apoptosis (normal cell death) within 72 hours, for breast, pancreas, skin, colon, esophageal, and prostate cancer cells. http://hcc.musc.edu/

In addition to preventing mitosis and inducing apoptosis, ellagic acid also prevents the binding of carcinogens to DNA and strengthens connective tissue. Ellagic acid is also considered a potent antibacterial and antifungal, and it protects the liver. European medical studies also demonstrate that ellagic acid lowers the incidence of birth defects, promotes wound healing, and reduces heart disease. www.hopeforcancer.com/Ellagic.htm

Dr. Daniel Nixon of the Medical University of South Carolina studied ellagitannins (from raspberries) from 1993 through 1996 and published the following results and observations:

> ➤ Cervical cancer cells (HPV) exposed to ellagitannins from red raspberries experienced apoptosis.
> ➤ Ellagitannins lead to "G_1 arrest" of cancer cells, thus inhibiting and stopping mitosis (cancer cell division).
> ➤ Ellagitannins prevent destruction of the p53 gene by cancer cells.
> ➤ The tests reveal similar results for breast, pancreas, esophageal, skin, colon, and prostate cancer cells.

According to British scientific researchers, red raspberries also prevent heart disease, as they contain a natural form of aspirin called "salicylates." Herbalists also believe that ellagitannins are effective in treating diarrhea and nausea.

ESSENTIAL OILS & FATS

The two essential fatty acids (EFAs) are linoleic acid (LA), an omega-6 fat, and alpha-linolenic acid (ALA), an omega-3 fat. Vegetables and nuts (corn, safflower, cottonseed, peanuts, and soybeans) are the highest in omega-6 fats. Since approximately 90% of these oils (except peanut oil) produced in the USA are genetically modified (see chapter 14), I recommend you eat only organic, cold pressed oils made from these foods, or find other sources of omega-6. LA is the primary omega-6 fat, which a healthy human will convert into gamma linolenic acid (GLA). Other omega-6 fats include conjugated linoleic acid (CLA), dihomo-gamma-linolenic acid (DGLA), and arachidonic acid (AA). Ocean fish (such as salmon, tuna, and mackerel) and certain nuts/seeds (such as flax/linseed, and walnuts) are the highest in omega-3 fats. ALA is the principal omega-3 fat, which a healthy human will convert into eicosapentaenoic acid (EPA) and later into docosahexaenoic acid (DHA) and docosapentaenoic acid (DPA).

Good health requires the proper ratio of omega-6 and omega-3 fats; the ideal ratio is around 2:1. Both essential fats are bountiful in the leafy plants consumed by roaming animals, providing nearly equal ratios of these EFAs. For example, hemp seed oil has an optimum balance of omega-3 and omega-6 fats. Before the introduction of harvested grains as feed, cattle thrived on lush green grasses, which provide a complete and balanced diet and promote healthy growth without excessive fat production. In light of this fact, it is important to make sure that you only eat meat from animals that feed on grass, since their meat has the perfect ratio of omega-6 to omega-3 fats, and it is rich in CLA. A great many studies have shown that CLA fights cancer in lab animals. Animals that naturally graze have from 3-5 times more CLA than animals fattened on grain.

Superficially, CLA resembles linoleic acid, but they appear to have opposite effects. Whereas an overabundance of linoleic acid promotes tumor growth, CLA blocks it. In fact, CLA may be one of our most potent cancer fighters. In a recent study feeding rats small amounts of CLA shrank mammary tumors by 45%. Scientists added very small amounts of CLA to breast cancer cells growing in a culture. By the 8th day, the CLA had killed 93% of the cells.

A group of Finnish researchers found that women who consumed the most CLA had a 60% lower risk of breast cancer than other women. (www.drstallone.com/cancer_article19.htm) CLA also stimulates the immune system, improves insulin sensitivity, improves blood lipid levels, improves lean body mass to fat ratios, and has no known practical toxicity levels.

Modern farming practices have led to a steady decline in the amount of CLA supplied in the diet over the past half century. Today's dairy products have only around 25% of the CLA content they used to have around 1960. A good case could be made that the cancer, heart disease, diabetes, and obesity epidemics we are now experiencing are largely due to the decline of CLA in the diet. Unfortunately, if you go to the supermarket to purchase beef, you will get beef that has been **grain**-fed. As a result the omega-6 to omega-3 ratio will be completely out of whack and you will not be getting the CLA content that you would from **grass**-fed beef.

In my opinion, coconut oil is the healthiest oil; one of the most impressive features of coconut oil is that it is extremely rich in lauric acid (about 50% by volume). The only other abundant source of lauric acid found in nature is in human breast milk. A great deal of research has established the fact that lauric acid is used by humans to destroy viruses, and various pathogenic bacteria and microbes such as yeasts, fungi, bacteria, parasites, and molds.

According to Mary Enig, the USA's leading expert on fats: "*Coconut oil has a unique role in the diet as an important physiologically functional food. The health and nutritional benefits that can be derived from consuming coconut oil have been recognized in many parts of the world for centuries...coconut oil provides a source of antimicrobial lipids for individuals with compromised immune systems, and is a non-promoting fat with respect to chemical carcinogenesis.*" www.westonaprice.org/know-your-fats/541-new-look-at-coconut-oil.html

Coconut oil contains no trans-fats and about 2/3 of the saturated fat in coconut oil is made up of medium-chain fatty acids (MCFA's). By contrast, most common vegetable or seed oils are comprised of long-chain fatty acids (LCFA's), which put strain on the pancreas and the liver, are chiefly stored in the body as fat, and harden the arteries with cholesterol. The MCFA's in coconut oil have antimicrobial properties, are beneficial to the immune system, are easily digested for quick energy, and cause weight loss. That's right...eating coconut oil will help you **lose weight**!

Over 50% of Americans are overweight. One of the principal benefits of coconut oil lies in its ability to stimulate your metabolism. Back in the 1930s, Dr. Weston Price (a dentist) traveled throughout the South Pacific, examining traditional diets and their effect on dental and overall health. He found that those eating diets high in coconut products were healthy and trim, despite the high fat concentration in their diet. Then in the 1940s, farmers found out (by accident) that when they tried using inexpensive coconut oil to fatten their livestock, it didn't work! Instead, coconut oil made the animals lean! Since then, many animal and human research studies have demonstrated that replacing LCFA's with MCFA's results in both decreased body weight and reduced body fat percentage. So, by changing the fats in your diet from the unsaturated LCFA's found in vegetable or seed oils to the MCFA's in coconut oil, you will lose weight!

We've all heard the rhetoric about saturated fat being unhealthy, but this is complete nonsense. The saturated fat in coconut oil is actually health promoting. How did that rumor get started? Well, it was based on some flawed studies performed almost 50 years ago. The studies used hydrogenated coconut oil, and the myth was perpetuated by the vegetable oil industry (aided by the FDA) back in the 1980s. The fact of the matter is that **all** hydrogenated oils are bad, since they have been chemically altered. But virgin coconut oil is wonderful for the human body. That is the only coconut oil we consume. As a matter of fact, we use so much coconut oil that we purchase it a gallon at a time! According to Dr. Bruce Fife, "*coconut oil is the healthiest oil on earth.*"

Olive oil is the only vegetable oil that can be consumed fresh pressed, and it is the most prominent source of omega-9 fats, also known as oleic acids. The beneficial health effects of olive oil are due to both its high content of monounsaturated fatty acids and its high content of antioxidants. Studies have shown that olive oil offers protection against heart disease by controlling LDL ("bad") cholesterol levels while raising HDL ("good") levels. No other naturally produced oil has as large an amount of monounsaturated fatty acids as olive oil. We use olive oil all the time in salad dressings and vegetable medleys.

When buying olive oil you will want to obtain a high quality **extra virgin** olive oil. The oil that comes from the first "pressing" of the olive is cold pressed (extracted without using heat or chemicals) is awarded "extra virgin" status. This is the best oil because it is handled less, thus it is closer to its natural state and contains higher levels of antioxidants, vitamin E, and phenols. However, while you should include olive oil as a healthy part of your diet, you should **not** cook with olive oil, as heat can damage the fatty acids and create toxins called acrylamides. If you are going to cook with oil, use coconut oil, since it does not undergo toxic chemical changes when heated. We love making French fries with coconut oil, and Charlene also makes really great fried green tomatoes with this oil.

Avocados are a superb source of fats, specifically omega-3 and omega-9. According to the late Dr. Robert Atkins, *"avocados are not only nourishing they are a heart promoting, cancer-fighting fruit that offers unequaled health benefits."* Not only are avocados a rich source of omega-9 oleic acids, which have been shown to offer significant protection against breast cancer, but these fruits also contain the highest amount of the carotenoid lutein of all commonly eaten fruits, as well as measurable amounts of related carotenoids (zea-zxanthin, alpha-carotene, and beta-carotene) plus significant quantities of tocopherols (vitamin E).

In a laboratory study published in the January 2005 issue of the *Journal of Nutritional Biochemistry*, an extract of avocado containing carotenoids and tocopherols inhibited the growth of both androgen-dependent and androgen-independent prostate cancer cells. However, when researchers tried exposing the prostate cancer cells to lutein alone, the single carotenoid did not prevent cancer cell growth and replication.

Not only was the whole matrix of carotenoids and tocopherols in avocado necessary for its ability to kill prostate cancer cells, but the researchers also noted that the significant amount of monounsaturated fat in avocado plays an important role. Carotenoids are lipid (fat)-soluble, which means fat must be present to ensure that these bioactive carotenoids will be absorbed into the bloodstream.

GARLIC

There has been more written about the wonderful benefits of **garlic** than any other food source known. Its history dates back 3,500 years. Hippocrates, the father of medicine, was the first to write that garlic was an excellent medicine for eliminating tumors. Recent studies on garlic have shown that it kills insects, parasites, bad bacteria, and fungi. It also eliminates various tumors, lowers blood sugar levels, lowers harmful fats in the blood, and prevents clogging of the arteries.

Researchers have also shown that allicin (the organic compound which gives garlic its aroma and flavor) acts as a very potent antioxidant.

It has been discovered that the diallyl disulfide in garlic reduces the formation of carcinogens in the liver. (*Cancer Research*, 1988; 48:23) Dr. Sujatha Sundaram, a researcher at Pennsylvania State University, found that diallyl disulfide caused human bowel cancer tumor cells to shrink and die when transplanted into mice.

It is interesting to note the similarity between diallyl disulfide and dimethyl sulfoxide (DMSO). According to Dr. David Gregg, "*They both consist of one sulfur with two organic molecules attached. In the case of dimethylsulfide two methyl groups (CH_3) are attached, in the case of diallyl sulfide, to allyl groups (C_3H_5) are attached...There is an equilibrium established between dimethylsulfide (no oxygen attached), DMSO (one oxygen attached to the sulfur) and MSM (two oxygen's attached to the sulfur). Because of this equilibrium, this set of molecules can act as an effective oxygen transport system. Since diallyl sulfide is a very similar molecule and the same bonding sites are available on the sulfur, one would expect it to behave in a similar manner, and it seems to ... This would suggest that one of the major anticancer contributions of diallyl sulfide (and thus garlic) is to enhance oxygen transport to the cancer cells.*" www.krysalis.net.

The first scientific report to study garlic and cancer was performed in the 1950s. Scientists injected "allicin" (an active ingredient in garlic) into mice suffering from cancer. Mice receiving the injection survived three times longer than the other mice. Many studies have shown that "allyl sulfur" (another active ingredient in garlic) is effective in preventing cancer and tumor development. In addition, ajoene, another major compound of garlic, has been shown to induce apoptosis in human leukemic cells. (Dirsch VM et al, *Molecular Pharmacology*, March 1998)

Garlic also contains germanium, which is a powerful sulfur-containing antioxidant. Germanium not only boosts oxygenation but spares oxygen as it chelates toxic metals such as mercury, lead and cadmium from your body. It has been shown to restore normal function to lymphocytes (T-cells, B-cells, and NK cells) and stimulate the production of antibodies. We eat garlic in almost everything – dips, salad dressings, sauces, soups, wraps, you name it. But remember ... **cooking kills** garlic's cancer-fighting properties. There are cases on record where cancer was beaten with a good detox program and garlic alone. Here's a powerful anti-cancer concoction: blend up some ginger, onions, raw broccoli, and garlic juice. If you can stand the taste, it's one of the most potent cancer-fighting concoctions available.

GINGER

Aromatic, pungent and spicy, ginger adds a special flavor and zest to stir fries and many fruit and vegetable dishes. Ginger's benefits as a healing food are well-known in Asia where it is frequently called "the universal medicine." Ginger is regarded as an excellent "carminative" (a substance which promotes the elimination of intestinal gas) and "intestinal spasmolytic" (a substance which relaxes and soothes the intestinal tract).

Ginger's anti-vomiting action has been shown to be very useful in reducing the nausea and vomiting of pregnancy. Ginger's effectiveness as a digestive aid is due largely to its active phytonutrient ingredients: "gingerols" and "shogaols." These substances help to neutralize stomach acids, enhance the secretion of digestive juices (stimulating the appetite), and tone the muscles of the digestive tract. But that's not all. Both gingerols and shogaols have been shown to fight cancer as well.

Gingerols are phytonutrients responsible for ginger's distinctive flavor. Scientific research has been shown that gingerols have antibacterial properties to inhibit the growth of "helicobacter pylori," involved in the development of gastric and colon cancer and suppress the growth of human colorectal carcinomas. Lab experiments presented by Dr. Rebecca Lui (and colleagues from the University of Michigan) at the 97th Annual Meeting of the American Association for Cancer showed that gingerols kill ovarian cancer cells by inducing apoptosis (programmed cell death) and phagocytosis (self-digestion).

In a 2007 study published in the *Journal of Agricultural and Food Chemistry*, Dr. Chung-Yi Chen (and colleagues in the American Chemical Society) presented compelling evidence that ginger's shogaols effectively induce apoptosis in cancer cells. A 2007 Rutgers University study supported the cancer-fighting properties of both shogaols and gingerols. http://pubs.acs.org/doi/abs/10.1021/jf0624594

Ginger has been shown to reduce the stickiness of blood platelets and may thereby reduce the risk of atherosclerosis. It is an outstanding source of manganese, magnesium, potassium, copper, and vitamin B_6. Ginger is one of world's healthiest foods to be consumed freshly grated, dried ground, or as a tea. Remember that the phytonutrients in ginger are heat sensitive, so for maximum effectiveness, you should eat fresh ginger root and/or take a ginger supplement (such as ginger root powder or ginger extract).

In 2010, I corresponded with a man named Bill, a former Stage IV cancer patient who cured his cancer with ginger. For a 150 pound person, Bill recommends taking between four and six grams of ginger root powder per day. The ginger root should be taken for one to three days. His exact words are, *"I had previously been using ginger root powder in 500mg capsules for stomach upset. But then tried it successfully at a higher than label dosage instead of antibiotic. When prostate cancer spread to and blocked my colon, I tried ginger. I took up to six capsules, four times a day. I was very lucky. It worked!"*

GINSENG

Ginseng is perhaps the most well-known Chinese herb and the most widely recognized plant used in traditional medicine. The life-extending properties of ginseng were first described around 500 AD in a Chinese medical textbook by Shennong, and various forms of ginseng have been used in medicine for thousands of years. The two most common types of ginseng are *"panax ginseng"* (aka Asian, Korean or Chinese ginseng) and *"panax quinquefolius"* (aka American, Canadian, or North American ginseng). The word *"panax"* is derived from the Greek word *"panacea"* which means *"all healing,"* and the benefits of ginseng are recognized as such.

Ginseng is commonly used as an adaptogen, meaning it normalizes physical functioning depending on what the individual needs. For example, it will lower high blood pressure, but it will raise low blood pressure. Ginseng is also effective in combating cancer, diabetes, stress, and fatigue. These effects of ginseng are mainly attributed to a group of compounds called "ginsenosides."

In a study conducted by Dr. Taik-Koo Yun (and colleagues) published in the June 1998 *International Journal of Epidemiology*, consumption of ginseng resulted in a 67% decreased risk for stomach cancer and 70% for lung cancer. Animal studies have shown that ginseng stimulates the production of interferons and increases NK ("natural killer") cell activity. According to a report published in the *Chinese Medicine Journal*, the genisenosides in ginseng fight cancer by preventing angiogenesis (creation of new blood vessels), inducing apoptosis (normal cell death), and preventing metastasis (spreading) and proliferation of cancer. www.cmjournal.org/content/2/1/6

Other Chinese studies indicated that ginsenosides also increase protein synthesis and activity of neurotransmitters in the brain, thus ginseng is used to restore memory and enhance concentration and cognitive abilities. Additional research has shown specific effects that support the central nervous system, liver function, lung function, and circulatory system.

GLUTATHIONE

According to Dr. Mark Hyman, *"[Glutathione] is the most important molecule you need to stay healthy and prevent disease -- yet you've probably never heard of it. It's the secret to prevent aging, cancer, heart disease, dementia, and more, and necessary to treat everything from autism to Alzheimer's disease. There are more than 89,000 medical articles about it -- but your doctor doesn't know how to address the epidemic deficiency of this critical life-giving molecule ... What is it? I'm talking about the mother of all antioxidants, the master detoxifier and maestro of the immune system:* **glutathione**.*"* http://twitter.com/markhymanmd

Technically speaking, the "glutathione system" is comprised of glutathione, glutathione peroxidase (GPx) and glutathione reductase (GR). For purposes of this section of the book, I will use the term "glutathione" as a general term referring to either the entire glutathione system or its constituent parts, depending upon context. Glutathione is produced naturally in your body, specifically the liver and is composed of three amino acids: cysteine, glutamic acid, and glycine. N-Acetylcysteine (NAC) is a biologically active precursor for the amino acid cysteine, which, in turn, is a precursor for glutathione.

In the words of Dr. Hyman, *"Glutathione is critical for one simple reason: It recycles antioxidants. You see, dealing with free radicals is like handing off a hot potato. They get passed around from vitamin C to vitamin E to lipoic acid and then finally to glutathione which cools off the free radicals and recycles other antioxidants. After this happens, the body can 'reduce' or regenerate another protective glutathione molecule and we are back in business."* Glutathione is also essential for DNA synthesis and repair, protein and fat synthesis, the regulation of enzymes, and amino acid transport.

The **good** news is that our bodies produce glutathione. The **bad** news is that stress, aging, trauma, infections, radiation, pollution, toxins, drugs, and poor diet all significantly reduce your glutathione reservoir. Studies have shown that our body's supply of glutathione begins to decline by 10% to 15% per decade starting at the age of twenty. Individuals who have low levels of glutathione are susceptible to chronic illness. As we now know, a lowered immune system can bring about illness and disease. While you need glutathione for a productive immune system, a weakened immune system hampers the production of glutathione. This is a ferocious cycle.

The secret of glutathione's potency lies in the sulfur chemical groups it contains. Sulfur is a sticky, smelly molecule that acts like "fly paper." As a result, all the "bad guys" in your body (like heavy metals and free radicals) stick to glutathione which then carries them into the bile and the stool, then out of your body. Sulfur-rich foods (like garlic, onions, and cruciferous vegetables) support glutathione production.

Reduced (*i.e.*, "active") glutathione is also known as "GSH," while oxidized (*i.e.*, "inactive") glutathione is known as "GSSG." Studies have shown that when GSH falls below 70%, your body is in big trouble. This being so, it makes sense to feed the body GSH precursors, right? "Cysteine" is one of the three amino acids that generate GSH in the liver and is considered to be fundamental to this process, since cysteine is not as plentiful as glycine & glutamic acid, thus it is the availability of cysteine that controls the production of GSH.

Whey (a by product of cheese or yogurt processing) is a great source of cysteine and the amino acid building blocks for GSH synthesis. Please note that the whey protein must be bioactive and made from non-denatured (*i.e.*, natural and not broken down) proteins, such as raw milk which contains no pesticides, hormones, or antibiotics. "Immunocal®" is a bioactive non-denatured whey protein that is an excellent product to stimulate GSH production. *"Depletion of this small molecule is a common consequence of increased formation of reactive oxygen species during increased cellular activities. Bioactive whey protein concentrate has been shown to represent an effective and safe cysteine donor for GSH replenishment during GSH depletion in immune deficiency states."* (*Anticancer Research* 20: 4785-4792, 2000)

As you may have guessed, all meats are high in cysteine, but if the animal was injected with rBGH and fed on pesticide-laden grains and grass, the hormones and toxins will virtually neutralize GSH. However, asparagus, avocado, broccoli, watermelon, walnuts, and dark green leaf vegetables are good choices for GSH enhancement. In addition to bioactive whey protein and sulfur-rich foods, exercising also helps boost GSH levels. Other substances which assist the production of GSH are alpha lipoic acid ("ALA"), the B vitamins (specifically folic acid, B_6, and B_{12}), selenium, and milk thistle. As I've mentioned, Immunocal® is a super GSH supplement.

My family uses a product called "One World Whey" each day in our healthy "super green" shakes. It's also an excellent source of glutathione. You can find this product at www.cocoonnutrition.org.

Much of the information in this article was gleaned from an article by Dr. Mark Hyman entitled *"Glutathione: The Mother of All Antioxidants,"* posted here: www.huffingtonpost.com/dr-mark-hyman/glutathione-the-mother-of_b_530494.html.

GOLDENSEAL

Goldenseal (aka "orangeroot") is an herb native to the eastern North America. The use of goldenseal was taught to early American colonists by Cherokee medicine men and women. In 1798, Benjamin Smith Barton included it in his *Essays Towards a Materia Medica of the United States*, noting that American Indian groups used it for treating a wide range of conditions, including eye infections, diarrhea, liver disease, whooping cough, and pneumonia. It was even used in many cancer treatments by such successful physicians as John Pattison, who began his career using bloodroot and changed to goldenseal because he regarded it as clinically superior.

Goldenseal is a potent antimicrobial, antiparasitic, antiseptic, and antibiotic agent. Many people swear by goldenseal for common ailments (such as colds and wounds) as well as long-term (chronic) conditions. Conjunctivitis (aka "pink eye") can be effectively treated by using goldenseal eyewash. In addition to the above, goldenseal is a very popular treatment for infection of the gums or gingivitis. Gargling with goldenseal tincture is found to be extremely helpful in curing strep throat problems. Used externally, goldenseal it is very successful in treating cuts, wounds, and other bacterial skin infections and fungal infections.

Studies have shown that the combination of its three main alkaloids (berberine, hydrastine, and canadine) creates a synergy that is more potent than the sum of its parts. These alkaloids are known to increase blood circulation to the liver and spleen and also stimulate the secretion of bile. All these properties of goldenseal help in smooth and effective functioning of the pancreas, thyroid, and lymphatic system.

The goldenseal herb contains many important and useful vitamins, including vitamin A, various B vitamins, vitamin C, and vitamin E. It also contains zinc, potassium, calcium, iron, manganese, phosphorus, and selenium. Generally, the health benefits of goldenseal are enhanced when echinacea and goldenseal are combined. Since goldenseal has uterine-stimulating properties, it should not be used during pregnancy.

HYDROGEN PEROXIDE (H_2O_2)

Although hydrogen peroxide has already been mentioned in the section on bio-oxidative therapies, it is important enough to mention again. Did you know that you probably had your first sip of hydrogen peroxide (H_2O_2) shortly after you took your first breath? That's right! Mother's milk, sprecifically colostrum, contains tremendously high concentrations of H_2O_2. In light of the fact that we know that one of the main functions of mother's milk is to activate and stimulate the immune system in the infant, the fact that it contains abnormally large amounts of H_2O_2 makes sense.

When ozone mixes with moisture in the air, it forms H_2O_2, which comes down in rain and snow. H_2O_2 occurs naturally in fresh fruits and vegetables, some coming from rain and some manufactured during photosynthesis. Most people are familiar with the common drugstore variety of 3% hydrogen peroxide, used for everything from sterilizing a cut to cleaning kitchen tables. The sterilizing power comes from its extra oxygen atom. H_2O_2 has a similar cleansing power in the body. But please remember that the drugstore variety of H_2O_2 should **never** be used internally, because of the chemicals it contains as stabilizers. For internal consumption, you will need **food grade** H_2O_2.

Dr. Charles Farr has shown that H_2O_2 stimulates oxidative enzyme systems throughout the body, which triggers an increase in the metabolic rate, causes small arteries to dilate and increase blood flow, clears out toxins, raises body temperature, and enhances the body's distribution and consumption of oxygen. H_2O_2 stimulates NK ("natural killer") cells, which attack cancer cells as they attempt to spread throughout the body. In the body's immune response, H_2O_2 is released by T-cells to destroy invading bacteria, viruses and fungi. Blood platelets release H_2O_2 on encountering particulates in blood. In the large intestine, acidophilus lactobacillus produces H_2O_2 which keeps the ubiquitous candida yeast from multiplying out of control. When candida spreads out of the intestine, it escapes the natural control system and can gain a foothold in the organs of the body, causing what is called chronic fatigue syndrome.

Any cancer patients who use hydrogen peroxide internally should also use a quality proteolytic enzyme (such as Vitälzym) which will cut through the protein coating on the cancer cells and will enable the H_2O_2 to penetrate the cell wall. If you are on the Budwig Diet, you should avoid ingesting food grade H_2O_2 since the interaction of the fats with the H_2O_2 may cause stomach damage. Bathing in hydrogen peroxide is the best way to get it into the body and is an inexpensive treatment. The recommended rate is 8 ounces of 35% food grade hydrogen peroxide in a tub of non-chlorinated water, soaking 30 minutes. For an excellent **free** ebook on food grade H$_2$O$_2$, please visit www.foodgrade-hydrogenperoxide.com.

If you feel like you're getting sick, try dropping a few drops of H$_2$O$_2$ into each ear. The H$_2$O$_2$ begins working in minutes killing the cold or flu. It will probably bubble, which is a sign that it's killing the "bad guys." Wait until the bubbling subsides, drain from the ear, and repeat with the other ear. Hydrogen peroxide is one of the few "miracle substances" still available to the general public. And best of all, it is safe and dirt cheap!

IODINE

Iodine is responsible for the production of every hormone in your body. It is antibacterial, antiparasitic, antiviral, and a potent cancer fighter. Most Americans (over 95%) are iodine deficient. Why are we all iodine deficient? For many years iodine was added to bread in generous quantities which prevented iodine deficiency. Each slice of bread contained 150 micrograms of iodine, which was the recommended daily allowance. Fifty year ago, the average American consumed about one milligram of iodine daily with bakery products accounting for about 75 % of the total.

However, in the 1970s, the food industry decided to remove iodine from baked goods and replace the iodine with bromine. According to the late Dr. Jim Howenstine, *"Iodine and bromine appear similar to the thyroid gland and bromine easily binds to the thyroid gland's receptors for iodine. Bromine, however, is of no value to the thyroid gland unlike iodine, and it inhibits the activity of iodine in the thyroid gland. Bromine also can cause impaired thinking and memory, drowsiness, dizziness and irritability. This substitution of bromine for iodine has resulted in nearly universal deficiency of iodine in the American populace."* www.newswithviews.com/Howenstine/james37.htm

Iodine assists the body in eliminating heavy metals and toxins (like lead, arsenic, aluminum, mercury, and fluoride). Interestingly, fluoridated drinking water actually depletes iodine absorption. Iodine deficiency leads to cancers of the breast, prostate, ovaries, uterus, and thyroid. Iodine deficiency can also lead to mental retardation and infertility. So, how can we correct an iodine deficiency? To correct an iodine deficiency by taking iodized salt is not feasible, since you would need 20 teaspoons of iodized salt daily to get adequate quantities of iodine.

Dr. Jay Abrahams developed an iodine preparation (named "Iodoral®") to treat iodine deficiency. My family takes this supplement almost daily. Dr. Abrahams believes that the correct quantity of iodine needed to maintain sufficient amounts of iodine in the body is 13 milligrams daily (1 tablet of Iodoral®). Amazingly, this is 100 times more than the USRDA for iodine. Japanese women (who eat lots of seaweed) have the highest average iodine intake (13.8 milligrams daily) of women anywhere in the world. They also have the lowest incidence of breast cancer in the world. In addition Japan has one of the lowest incidences of iodine deficiency, goiter (enlarged thyroid gland), and hypothyroidism. Iceland, another high iodine intake country, has low rates of goiter and breast cancer.

Fish contains iodine, but you may want to limit your intake due to high levels of mercury. However, sardines have such a short life span they do not get contaminated with mercury. My suggestion would be to buy cans of sardines packed in tomato sauce so you can avoid the trans-fats used in oil packed sardines. Also, remember that selenium, vitamin C, and magnesium enhance the effectiveness of iodine. In the end, you may still need an iodine supplement like Iodoral®. If so, then check out this website: www.iodoral.org.

IP6 / INOSITOL

IP6, also known as "inositol hexophosphate" or "phytic acid," is composed of inositol (one of the B vitamins) bound with six molecules of phos-phorous and is found naturally in seeds, bran, whole grains, and legumes. IP6 is one of nature's most effective cancer fighters. IP6 selectively removes iron from cancer cells, which effectively deprives them of their primary growth factor. However, IP6 does not remove iron from red blood cells which are tightly bound to hemoglobin. Unlike cancer drugs, healthy cells are not affected with IP6, so IP6 has very low toxicity. (Deliliers GL, *British Journal of Haematology*, 117: 577–87, 2002)

Why is the iron-chelation so important? Because iron is needed by cancer cells to produce new DNA. Also, excess iron stored in tissues promotes insulin resistance, leading to high levels of both glucose and insulin, neither of which is beneficial for cancer control. IP6 removes excessive copper, needed to produce new blood supplies for the cancer.

IP6 also removes heavy metals such as mercury, cadmium, and lead, while not removing beneficial minerals such as potassium and magnesium. It activates NK cells, promotes cell differentiation (turning cancer cells into more normal cells), reduces tumor sizes, and helps the tumor suppressor gene p53 that is often defective in cancers. There have been numerous studies that conclusively prove IP6 is an effective and non-toxic cancer-fighting molecule.

Since the late 1980s, Dr. Abulkalam Shamsuddin, a scientist at the Maryland University School of Medicine, has been the pioneer researcher of IP6. He discovered that when properly combined with inositol, IP6 forms two molecules of IP3 in the body. Inositol, the backbone structure of IP6, has six carbon atoms that are capable of binding phosphate molecules; when all six carbons are occupied by six phosphate groups IP6 is formed. However, when only three of the carbon groups are bound by phosphate, it is called IP3.

This chemistry is important because although IP6 is gaining all the attention, it is really IP3 that is doing all the work. IP3 plays an important role inside the cells of our bodies. It basically functions as an "on/off" switch for human cancers according to in vitro studies. When IP3 levels are low (as in cancer cells), the cells replicate out of control. That basically is what occurs in cancer. When cancer cells are bathed in a broth of IP3, they literally "turn themselves off." This action reflects the central role that IP3 plays in controlling key cell functions, including replication and communication.

Dr. Shamsuddin recommends taking a daily dose of 800 to 1,200 milligrams of IP6 along with 200 to 300 milligrams of inositol as a general preventative measure. In patients with cancer or at high risk for cancer, he recommends a dose in the range of 4,800 to 7,200 milligrams of IP6 along with 1,200 to 1,800 milligrams of inositol. This should be taken on an empty stomach. Dr. Shamsuddin's remarkable product is called "IP6 Gold."

LIVING FUEL ™

Living Fuel's "Super Greens" contains concentrated sources of vitamins, minerals, proteins, essential fats, enzymes, co-enzymes, herbs, botanical extracts, and soluble and insoluble plant fibers from fresh, high-quality, mostly organic, non-GMO, nutrient-rich foods and supplements. Super Greens is a whole, raw, wild-crafted, complete, foundational "super food." It is a blend of organic, all natural foods that have been optimized with the most bio-available and usable nutrients. This product combines the nutrients of more vegetables and fruits than you could possibly eat. It even includes chlorella, spirulina, and probiotics.

Living Fuel's "Super Berry" will also provide you total nutrition and great taste, but rather than getting the greens in the "Super Greens," the

"Super Berry" contains whole organic strawberries, raspberries, blueberries, and cranberries. Living Fuel provides you with high quality nutrition and has more potassium than bananas, more calcium than milk, more fiber than oatmeal, more friendly bacteria than yogurt, more protein that six eggs, and more vitamins, minerals, and antioxidants than a whole day's supply of fruits and vegetables.

Those concerned about their health and those with allergies and other conditions can confidently consume either of these products because they have no GMO, no pesticides, no sugar, no wheat, no dairy, no eggs, no maltodextrin, no fillers, no artificial colorings, no irradiation, no herbicides, no soy, no yeast, no whey, no nuts, no preservatives, no artificial colors, and no hydrogenated oils.

In my opinion, Living Fuel's "Super Greens" and "Super Berries" are in **a league of their own.** My family drinks these shakes every day as an important part of our healthy lifestyle. I'm good friend with the owners of Living Fuel, KC and Monica Craichy. They are both Christians and have impeccable character, integrity, and honesty. You need to be taking Living Fuel every day. Period. No questions asked. No, I don't make any money for endorsing Living Fuel. It's just the best. ☺ The website is www.livingfuel.com.

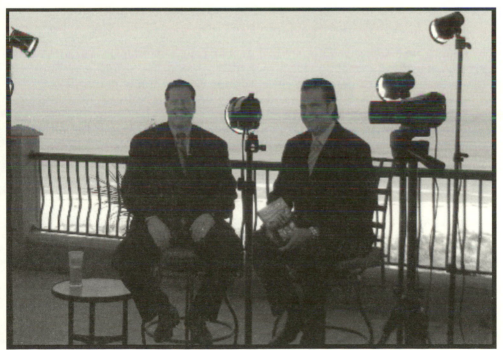

On the set of Living Fuel TV with my good friend, KC Craichy

MELATONIN

Did you know that if you sleep with a nightlight, you are increasing your risk of cancer? It has been shown that light exposure at night suppresses your production of melatonin. This, in turn, can lead to increased risk of cancer.

So, what exactly is melatonin? Melatonin is a hormone which modulates our neurotransmitters. It is produced from the amino acid tryptophan by the pineal gland (a pea-sized gland in the brain) when the lights go out at night. It's the reason you get sleepy when it's dark. Melatonin also is produced by the retina and, in vastly greater amounts, by the gastrointestinal system. Melatonin levels peak during the night but also increase after eating, which explains why you get sleepy after a meal. Melatonin is highly fat soluble and also water soluble, thus enabling it to easily penetrate the cell membrane, cytoplasm, and nucleus.

According to Dr. Eileen Lynch, "*Melatonin's amphiphilicity, or ability to both absorb and repel water - in conjunction with its ability to act as a weak preventive antioxidant, a weak metal ion chelator, and in certain circumstances, a direct free radical scavenger – enables it to counteract oxidative stress within the chaotic tumor microenvironment.*" www.lef.org/magazine/mag2004/jan2004_report_melatonin_01.htm

Due to the fact that over 75% of cancer cells exhibit oxidated DNA damage, the statement by Dr. Lynch above is very important. As a free radical scavenger, melatonin rivals vitamin C in its ability to counteract the oxidating effects of toxins. Not only does melatonin act as a free radical scavenger; it also is a hormone that **kills** cancer cells! According to Dr. Lynch, "*Melatonin plays a critical role in the host defense system against cancer's progression by activating the cytokine system, which exerts growth-inhibiting properties, and by stimulating the cytotoxic activity of macrophages and monocytes.*"

Multiple studies have indicated the cytotoxic effects of melatonin, including a 2002 article in *Tumor Biology* published by Dr. K. Winczyk and colleagues entitled "Possible involvement of the nuclear RZR/ROR-alpha receptor in the antitumor action of melatonin on murine Colon 38 cancer." In another article by Dr. P. Lissoni and colleagues in the 1989 *European Journal of Cancer & Clinical Oncology*, melatonin has also been shown to boost the immune system. In his 2004 report to the American Association for Cancer Research, Dr. David E. Blask reported that melatonin puts breast cancer cells to sleep, and it also slows breast cancer growth by 70%. Breast cancers get "turned on" by linoleic acids (omega-6 fats); however, melatonin interacts with linoleic acid. At a news conference, Dr. Blast stated, *"This breast cancer rev-up mechanism gets revved down by melatonin. Nighttime melatonin is a relevant anticancer signal to human breast cancers. Ninety percent of human breast cancers have specific receptors for this signal."*

Blask's team exposed lab mice with human breast cancers to constant light. Guess what happened: tumor growth **skyrocketed**. Dr. Blask asserts, *"With constant light, tumors grow seven times faster and soak up incredible amounts of linoleic acid. During the day, the cancer cells are awake and linoleic acid stimulates their growth. At night cancer cells go to sleep. When we turn on lights at night for a long time, we suppress melatonin and revert back to the daytime condition."*
www.webmd.com/content/article/71/81159.htm

Additional research corroborates the fact that melatonin can kill many different types of human tumor cells, including a groundbreaking 2000 study performed by three Russian physicians, Riabykh, Nikolaeva, and Bodrova. A report by Dr. R.M. Sainz et al in the 2003 issue of *Cellular Molecular Life Science* indicates that melatonin is a naturally produced cytotoxin which can induce tumor cell death (apoptosis). Interestingly, Dr. Lissoni also discovered that melatonin inhibits angiogenesis, which is the development of new tumor blood vessels. (Dr. P. Lissoni, et al, *Neuroendocrinology Letter*, 2001)

A growing body of evidence linking increased light at night (LAN) to certain types of cancer has led researchers to suspect it could be connected to the steady increase in cases of childhood leukemia. Scientists presenting research at the First International Scientific Conference on Childhood Leukemia said that light at night and working night shifts (which disrupts the body's circadian rhythm, or internal clock) have both been associated with an increased risk of breast and colorectal cancer.

You have to wonder if the rapid growth of television and video games over the last 30 years has contributed to the growth in childhood leukemia. Children are staying up later and later, and this LAN may be suppressing the natural production of melatonin that would otherwise fight the free radicals that damage DNA and lead to cancer. Is it just a coincidence that childhood leukemia has literally exploded at the same time as the escalation of television and video games?

"Compared with other working women, female night-shift workers have about a 50% greater risk of developing breast cancer," says William Hrushesky of Dorn Veterans Affairs Medical Center in Columbia, S.C. That presumably explains why the original Harvard study of nurses, which was led by Eva S. Schernhammer, found that shift workers had an elevated risk of breast cancer. (*Science News*, 1/17/01, p. 317) More recently, Schernhammer and her Harvard

colleague Susan E. Hankinson found that women who happen to have above-average melatonin concentrations are relatively unlikely to develop breast cancer. *"Those with higher levels seem to have lower breast cancer risk,"* said Schernhammer. She and Hankinson reported the data in the 7/20/2005 *Journal of the National Cancer Institute*.

One would hypothesize that if melatonin production is triggered by darkness, then those who would have the greatest production would be blind people, correct? In a 1998 study by Doctors Feychting and Osterlund, higher melatonin levels were found in blind and visually impaired people, along with correspondingly lower incidences of cancer compared to those with normal vision, thus suggesting a role for melatonin in the reduction of cancer. ("Reduced cancer incidence among the blind," *Epidemiology*, 1998)

Several studies have shown that the circadian rhythm is involved in tumor suppression at various levels and also regulates the immune response. This being so, it only makes sense that the disruption of the circadian rhythm could lead to a weakened immune system and the growth of cancerous tumors. However, melatonin has been shown to act as a "circadian referee" and is able to regulate the body's internal clock, thus keeping the immune system at its highest level of surveillance. *"Sleep per se is not important for melatonin,"* says Dr. Russel J. Reiter, a neuroendocrinologist at the University of Texas Health Science Center in San Antonio, quoted in the January 7, 2006, issue of *Science News*, "...***but darkness is***."

Recent studies have found reduced levels of melatonin in the cerebrospinal fluid of patients with Alzheimer's disease compared to age-matched control subjects. (H. Tohgi, 1992; D.J. Skene, 1990) Due to the fact that circadian rhythms are disrupted in Alzheimer's disease, it is interesting to speculate whether restoration of melatonin to normal levels in these patients would alleviate other symptoms as well. Melatonin should probably be taken 30-45 minutes before sleeping. You can find melatonin in any health food store. Cherries are a good natural source of melatonin, thus they are a great bedtime snack.

Medicinal Mushrooms

Mushrooms have been treasured as both medicine and food for thousands of years. Across the globe, many people take pleasure in hunting for wild mushrooms, appreciating the variety of colors, shapes, and sizes. In Japan, street vendors sell many species of medicinal mushrooms to health conscious citizens who utilize them to maintain health and promote long life. Some Japanese people travel hundreds of miles in order to collect wild mushrooms that only grow on very old plum trees. Likewise, for thousands of years, the Chinese have valued many mushrooms for their healing properties, particularly tonics for the immune system.

Most medicinal mushrooms contain polysaccharides (complex sugar molecules) called "beta-glucans" that increase DNA and RNA in the bone marrow where immune cells (like macrophages and T-cells) are made. In Japan, extracts containing various types of beta-glucans have been used to successfully assist in treating cancer patients for the last 20 years. Beta-glucans enhance immunity through a variety of mechanisms, many similar to those of echinacea and astragalus. Researchers at Alpha-Beta Technology in Massachusetts examined the effects of beta-glucans on human blood. When the two were incubated together, beta-glucans enhanced the growth of myeloid and megakaryocyte progenitor cells (which develop into immune cells) and triggered a burst of free radicals in white blood cells, enhancing the cells' antibacterial activity. Interestingly, the white blood cells' bacterial killing capacity was proportional to the beta-glucan dose.

In the July 1984 issue of *Immunopharmacology*, Dr. R. Seljelid (and colleagues) reported that beta-glucans stimulate the production of small protein compounds called cytokines within the phagocytic cells. This cytokine stimulation increases the capacity of macrophages to stop tumor cell growth and kill the tumor in its entirety. In 1975, the *Journal of the National Cancer Institute* published the results of a study conducted by Dr. P.W. Mansell which reviewed the cancer-fighting effects of beta-glucans on nine cancer patients. The patients (who had skin, breast, or lung cancer) had beta-glucans injected into their tumors. In all nine cases, the beta-glucans initiated an immediate immune response, and the tumors were reduced within five days.

Reishi mushrooms have been used as a medicine in Asia for over 4,000 years. In Chinese, they are called *"Ling Zhi"* (translated as *"mushroom of immortality"*). Reishi is known to promote respiratory and cardiovascular health as well as blood sugar levels. One substance in reishi (called canthaxanthin) slows down the growth of tumors, according to author Phyllis A. Balch and other experts. As a result of these amazing anti-cancer abilities, the Japanese government officially recognizes reishi as a cancer treatment. In the USA, this hard red mushroom can be found at the base of living deciduous trees (especially maple) from May through November.

Maitake mushrooms are commonly known as *"hen of the woods"* due to their interesting shape. In Japanese, *"maitake"* actually means *"dancing mushroom"* since people are said to dance for joy when they find one. These mushrooms are specifically recommended for the stomach and intestines and are known to regulate blood sugar and pressure. Maitake also contains "grifolan" (a beta-glucan) which has been shown to activate macrophages in the immune system. In China, a maitake extract was shown to have an anti-cancer effect in patients with stomach cancer, lung cancer, and leukemia.

Shiitake mushrooms are used to treat nutritional deficiencies, to lower blood pressure, and alleviate liver ailments. Recently, shiitake was found to contain tremendously high levels of vitamin D when dried in the sun. In Japan, clinical studies have also been conducted with "lentinan" (a beta-glucan) found in shiitake. These studies have shown that treatment of advanced cancer patients with intravenous lentinan results in increased number and activity of immune killer cells and in prolonged survival (sometimes five or more years). Shiitake is a cultivated mushroom in the USA and is not found in the wild.

Turkey tail mushrooms are known for their strong antiviral, antimicrobial, and antitumor properties. These properties have been attributed to polysaccharide-K (PSK Krestin) and polysaccharide-P (PSP). The Japanese government approved the use of PSK in the 1980s for treating several types of cancers, and it is currently used along with the "Big 3" treatments. Accoding to Julie Diaz, a writer for Natural News, *"PSK was shown to significantly extend survival at five years or beyond in cancers of the stomach, colon/rectum, esophagus, nasopharynx and lung (non-small cell types) in Japanese trials since 1970. Polysaccharide-P (PSP) was discovered more recently and has been studied mainly in China. In double-blind trials, PSP significantly extended five-year survival in esophageal cancer patients. PSP significantly improved quality of life, provided substantial pain relief and enhanced immune status in 70-97 percent of patients with cancers of the stomach, esophagus, lung, ovaries and cervix. Both PSK and PSP boosted immune cell production and alleviated chemotherapy symptoms. Research indicates that PSP may slow the growth of certain tumors and help protect the immune system, particularly from the effects of cancer treatment. Additionally, a 7-year study funded by the National Institutes of Health and reported in November 2010 found that the use of turkey tail mushroom significantly boosted immunity in women who had been treated for breast cancer."*
www.naturalnews.com/042965_turkey_tail_mushroom_cancer_treatment_scientific_study.html

A 2009 UCLA study showed that breast cancer patients who ate medicinal mushrooms two times per day prevented their cancers from returning. This was concluded to be due to the mushrooms' anti-estrogen activity. So eat your mushrooms, and add a little olive oil and chopped garlic ... very tasty! And remember that all mushrooms must be cooked to get the nutritional value. The cell walls cannot be digested unless they are tenderized by heat.

MISTLETOE

Mistletoe is actually a powerful medicinal plant used since ancient times. References to mistletoe's "cure-all" properties date back as far as the ancient Greeks and the Druids. It has been used for centuries to treat epilepsy, arthritis, and hypertension. And though it's potent for many uses, it's especially deadly on cancer tumors.

There are two types of mistletoe:

1. American mistletoe (*Phoradendron* species) is poisonous and should not be ingested. Death has been shown to occur within 10 hours of ingestion.
2. European mistletoe (*Viscum album*) has been used to treat some diseases over the past few decades. The plant is also known as Golden Bough or Herb de la Croix (French for "herb of the cross").

Based on the information above, I think it's patently obvious that we're going to be discussing medicinal uses for European mistletoe in this section of the book. The modern focus on mistletoe as a treatment for cancer began around the 1920s, and it has steadily become more widespread. In certain European countries, products made from European mistletoe are among the most prescribed therapies for cancer patients. In fact, doctors in Germany treat over 50% of their cancer patients with mistletoe in one form or another. Many of these therapies are detailed in the special report, <u>German Cancer Breatkthrough</u>, which is a guide to the best German alternative cancer clinics. My friend and colleague, Andy Scholberg, calls mistletoe *"the laetrile of Germany."*

Mistletoe extracts are marketed under several trade names in Europe, the most well-known of which is Iscador®. One of the primary functions of Iscador® is that it stimulates parts of the immune system (NK cells) that can slow the growth of cancer cells and does so with very limited side effects. As a result, another reported benefit is a dramatic increase in quality of life while battling cancer. So if you are undergoing the "Big 3" treatments, mistletoe reduces the adverse effects of chemo and radiation.

In the May 1, 2001, edition of *Alternative Therapies*, Dr. R.G. Maticek (and colleagues) published a the results of a 30 year long study (with more than 35,000 participants) which concluded that extract of mistletoe (Iscador®) greatly improves survival rate for a wide variety of cancers (including breast cancer) through enhancing the immune system, halting tumor growth, and preventing metastatic growth of cancer.

The most common treatment is to inject the mistletoe extract under the skin. Of course, the FDA doesn't allow injectable mistletoe to be sold or used in the USA except for research. So if you live in the USA, your only options are oral formulas or traveling to another country for injections. So, the next time you hang a bough of mistletoe in your doorway, you'll have more to appreciate than its power to get you a holiday kiss.

MORINGA OLEIFERA

Moringa oleifera is a tree brought from the mind of God to the hands of man. It was recognized by the National Institutes of Health as the Botanical of the Year for 2007, and praised again in 2011 and 2012. It is valued worldwide for its ability to treat over 300 diseases. It has the ability to retain high concentrations of electrolyte minerals, allowing it to stay internally hydrated in the driest of conditions. Africans have honored it with names that translate to: "Never Die," and "The Only Thing that Grows in the Dry Season," and "Mother's Milk." This plant has saved more lives in Third World countries than any other.

It's an unfortunate fact that our own "civilized" food supply no longer feeds us well nutritionally. Our food is comforting, and tastes good, but as far as our cells are concerned, too much of what we eat is over-processed, denatured and acidic, and ends up depleting our bodies — robbing us rather than feeding us. We all need to supplement our diets in the most efficient and economical means possible. The Moringa tree is working in remote areas to solve hunger and malnutrition.

With its **90 nutrients**, **46 antioxidants**, **36 anti-inflammatories**, and more, Moringa oleifera has proven to be the most nutrient-dense and enzymatically active botanical known to man. It contains all 9 essential amino acids (the building blocks of protein), properly sequenced and in the optimal ratios. Moringa oleifera also contains the vitamins, minerals, fatty acids, phytonutrients, and antioxidants necessary to sustain life. It also contains plant hormones (cytokinins such as zeatin) with anti-aging properties in humans.

Today's western diet has double the caloric intake of a consumer in 1965 and we are receiving 75% less nutrient value for current calories consumed. Seeking daily, quality nutrient supplementation is no longer an option but a **requirement** for health. If your desire is to get healthy and stay healthy, I highly recommend moringa oleifera, which I personally take each and every day. It has become the backbone of my daily nutritional regimen. You can learn more about some exceptional moringa oleifera products at www.MoringaMagicTeam.com.

OIL OF OREGANO

Oil of oregano, an herbal product that has been used since Biblical times, is extracted from wild oregano plants. Oil of oregano has been shown to kill parasites and viruses, bacteria, and some types of fungi, as well as being an antihistamine. Oil of oregano has been used for centuries to treat infections and it might be a savior for sufferers of colitis, an inflammation in the gastrointestinal system. It is derived from the wild oregano plant (member of the mint family) that grows naturally in the mountains of the Mediterranean region and is usually bottled and mixed with olive oil or coconut oil because of its potency.

The lead ingredient in oregano oil is carvacrol, a strong antimicrobial used to preserve food and protect against mold and other common bacteria, making it the largest healing agent of the oil. Thymol is the second most active ingredient important as a fungicide and is the leading anti-halitosis (*i.e.,* bad-breath fighting) agent in Listerine. The rest of the ingredients provide more antibacterial support, prevent the damage caused by free radicals, act as allergen-blockers, and inhibit the growth of cancer cells.

Oil of oregano also contains copper, calcium, niacin, zinc, boron, beta-carotene, vitamins A, C, and E, potassium and iron among others. Jean Valnet, in his book The Practice of Aromatherapy, describes how oil of oregano has superseded anti-inflammatory drugs in reversing pain and inflammation and is nearly as powerful as morphine as a painkiller. It possesses significant antioxidant power and also stimulates the flow of bile in the liver, which greatly aids digestion.

Dr. Cass Ingram wrote a book called The Cure is in the Cupboard: How to Use Oregano for Better Health about his life-saving encounter with oil of oregano. This "super oil," he claims, is helpful in calming or healing over 170 different bodily conditions – everything from athlete's foot to worms, diarrhea to diaper rash, a bee sting to shortness of breath. Makes you want to go buy some oil of oregano right now, doesn't it?

However, before you go online or to your local herb store, make sure you do your research. Whichever brand you decide to purchase, make sure that the oil is at least 70% carvacrol. It is important to note that oil of oregano is not recommended for anyone allergic to oregano, thyme, basil, mint, or sage. Oil of oregano can also reduce iron intake within the body, so you should consider taking a good iron supplement. Due to this fact, pregnant women shouldn't take oil of oregano. The body of positive evidence for oregano oil as a major antibiotic is growing. Among 52 plant oils tested, oregano was considered to have "pharmacologic" action against common bugs such as Candida albicans (yeast), E. coli, Salmonella enterica, and Pseudomonas aeruginosa. (*Journal Applied Microbiology*, Volume 86, June 1999)

Also, oil of oregano is not to be confused with common oregano in the kitchen spice cupboard, which is usually marjoram rather than true oregano. My favorite source of oil of oregano (undiluted and 85% carvacrol) is from Kurt Wilson, the "Armchair Survivalist." His website is www.se1.us. Kurt's oil of oregano is 100% pure essential oil. This being so, do **not** put directly on your skin or in your mouth. It will burn! If this happens, flush with a dairy product such as milk, yogurt, or ice cream immediately. But don't worry, it won't cause permanent damage.

PAU D'ARCO

Lapacho is a huge evergreen canopy tree found in the rainforests of South America, specifically Paraguay, Brazil, and Argentina. The medicinal part of the tree is the inner lining of the bark (called the "*phloem*") which contains compounds known as "*naphtha-quinones*" (aka N-Factors). Lapacho is more commonly known by its Portuguese name of "*pau d'arco.*" It is also known by tribal names such as "*taheebo*" and "*ipe roxo.*"

Throughout South America, tribes living thousands of miles apart have used pau d'arco for the same medicinal purposes for thousands of years, including the treatment of malaria, influenza, lupus, respiratory problems, syphilis, colitis, and fungal infections. It has also been used to relieve pain (arthritis and rheumatism), kill germs, increase the flow of urine, and even as an antidote to poisons and snakebites. However, it was the reported cures for various types of cancers which fueled much of the early research in the early 1960s. The chemical constituents and active ingredients of pau d'arco have been well documented, and researchers have concluded that one of its most important chemicals is the N-Factor "lapachol." Quercitin, xloidone, and other flavonoids are also present and contribute to its effectiveness in the treatment of tumors and infections. In a 1968 study, lapachol demonstrated highly significant activity against cancerous tumors in rats.

According to Dr. Daniel B. Mowry, "*Part of the effectiveness of lapacho (pau d'arco) may stem from its observed ability to stimulate the production of red blood cells in bone marrow. Increased red blood cell production would improve the oxygen-carrying capacity of the blood. This, in turn, could have important implications for the health of tissues throughout the body. Also needed for oxygen transport by red cells is iron. This might explain the augmentation in lapacho's therapeutic properties when it is combined with iron-rich yerbamate, another South American plant; in fact, it is native practice to almost always combine these two plant species ... While there can be no doubt that lapacho is very toxic to many kinds of cancer cells, viruses, bacteria, fungi, parasites and other kinds of microorganisms, the substance appears to be without any kind of significant toxicity to healthy human cells."* www.pau-d-arco.com/Dr.Mowry.html

Pau d'arco has become a standard form of treatment for some kinds of cancer and for all kinds of infections in hospitals throughout Brazil, Argentina, and other countries in South America. Not surprisingly, using pau d'arco is still considered "tribal quackery" in the USA. However, it's interesting to note that Big Pharma regularly screens pau d'arco for the presence of substances (like lapachol) that could be the basis for new drugs. Of course, once Big Pharma tries to isolate, copy, and patent a natural substance, it **never** works as well as the natural substance. Also, no isolated component of pau d'arco comes anywhere close to being equal to the combined activity of all constituents (*i.e.*, the whole herb).

Pau d'arco is available in health food stores as capsules, tablets, alcohol solutions, dried bark, and tea. In many ways, pau d'arco parallels the immune stimulating properties found in echinacea and ginseng. Much of the information in this section was gleaned from an article entitled "Into the Light" written by Dr. Daniel B. Mowry, and available at www.pau-d-arco.com/Dr.Mowry.html.

PROBIOTICS / SBOs

It is commonly believed that all bacteria are bad. But this is not so. Optimal gastrointestinal health depends on the balance of beneficial bacteria and pathogenic bacteria. When illness strikes, it is usually because the beneficial bacteria have diminished (oftentimes due to antibiotics, a diet high in sugar, steroids, chemotherapy, or other medications). It is well established that infection and toxins from pathogenic bacteria, fungi, and viruses are one of the causes of cancer.

As long as the beneficial bacteria flourish, they prevent pathogenic bacteria and fungi from colonizing. In this way, beneficial bacteria help keep you healthy through naturally boosting the immune system. They produce natural antibiotics that inhibit the growth and activity of pathogenic bacteria, while increasing the body's production of gamma interferon (an important antiviral molecule made by T-cells) and increasing enzyme production such as proteases and lipases. However, if our intestinal environment is disrupted, pathogenic bacteria, fungi, and parasites move in, multiply, and attack the beneficial bacteria.

Anyone who has ever taken a round of antibiotics should read this. According to Dr. Joseph Mercola, *"Antibiotics destroy the normal, protective gut bacteria, allowing intestinal yeast and fungi to grow unchecked. These internal, gut yeasts make toxins, too. This can lead to immune suppression, symptoms of any autoimmune disease, or even cancer."* www.mercola.com

That's right. Antibiotics not only kill off your enemies (the bad bacteria), but they also kill off your bodyguards (the good bacteria). When your bodyguards are lying dead you have no defense, then your digestion will suffer and so will your overall health. You see, we should have a balance of about 85% good to 15% harmful bacteria in the intestinal tract. But most of us today have the opposite ratio, creating a chronically unhealthy condition. But antibiotics aren't the only culprit. Did you know that chlorinated water not only kills harmful bacteria in drinking water, but also kills the good bacteria in your digestive tract as it passes through? It's no wonder that we are sick all the time! So, how do you replenish the healthy, protective bacteria in your gut? Probiotics and soil based organisms (SBO's) are a good start.

Probiotics are health promoting bacteria that, when introduced effectively into the intestinal tract, replenish the good bacteria and help the body to digest and absorb food as well as fight off many different illnesses and disease. Most friendly bacteria come from the Lactobacillus or Bifidobacterium groups. In 1908, Professor Elie Metchnikoff won a Nobel Prize for his work on the immune system. He later discovered lactobacillus (one of the bacterium in yogurt) and stated, *"Death begins in the colon."*

SBOs are beneficial bacteria that live in the dirt. Until the 19th century, when food processing replaced ingestion of raw fruit and vegetables, SBOs formed a regular part of our diet. By around 1900, their presence in the food chain had seriously dwindled. Both modern agricultural methods with their over-reliance on powerful pesticides, fungicides, and germicidal chemicals and heat-based food processing are toxic to SBOs. The gut of every healthy person contains about 3½ pounds of beneficial bacteria that produce essential vitamins and hormones. These bacteria, of which SBOs are a vital source, help your digestive system break down proteins, fats, and carbohydrates, as well as digest waste. Most importantly they compete with undesirable microorganisms, like yeasts, fungi, bacteria and parasites, to keep their numbers under control.

Some of the benefits of probiotics and SBOs:

> They stimulate activity in the thymus and spleen, which keeps our immune system at an optimal level by prompting the body to manufacture natural antibodies.
> Certain probiotic strains protect against the formation of tumors and promote production of interferon (a hormone that protects against cancer) by both the lymphocytes and the thymus gland. (Journal of Immunotherapy, 1991; 7:4)
> SBO's secrete specialized proteins which stimulate your immune system to produce more white blood cells and antibodies that dramatically boost your immunity.
> They both help reduce the amount of toxic chemicals in the body, *i.e.*, pathogenic bacteria and fungi that produce their own toxins.
> Both probiotics and SBOs result in an abundance of healthy flora in the digestive tract and enhance the breakdown of food, which results in a more alkaline environment.

Regular supplementation with probiotics and SBOs repopulates your intestinal tract with good bacteria, thus optimizing your immune system and fighting off disease. Any anti-cancer diet should include supplementation with both of these. By far, the best probiotic available on the market today is Natren's "Healthy Trinity." You can purchase it here: www.natren.com. The best SBOs I have found are called Primal Defense® (www.gardenoflife.com).

PROTANDIM®

As we age, our bodies become overwhelmed by free radicals, and it is typical for oxidative stress (cell damage caused by free radicals) to occur. Most folks believe that the best way to rid the body of free radicals and reduce oxidative stress is to consume more antioxidants. After all, that's what we have all been taught, right? Well, our bodies actually possess a far superior mechanism for getting rid of oxidative stress: triggering the production of free radical fighting enzymes known as superoxide dismutase (SOD), catalase, and glutathione. These enzymes have the power to eliminate free radicals much faster than antioxidants can. Protandim® is a unique blend of phytonutrients (ashwagandha, bacopa, curcumin, green tea, and milk thistle) that increases the body's natural antioxidant protection by inducing the production of these three important protective enzymes. According to

Dr. Joe McCord, *"Common antioxidants are very limited in their abilities-and in truth, they only offer benefits outside the antioxidant realm. The body's enzymes, however, can each eliminate approximately one million free radicals per second without being used up. The advantage of enzymes over antioxidants vitamins is almost mind blowing."* http://matthewneer.com/2010/05/protandimreview

From fading colors in clothes to paint that begins to chip, we can actually see the signs of something getting older. However, our bodies also have internal methods of chronicling age: thiobarbituric acid-reactive substances ("TBARS"). TBARS are the toxins in your blood produced by the free-radicals in your cells and are basically the laboratory "markers" for oxidative stress in the body. The sum of these TBARS has a direct correlation to the rate at which you age; as we get older, the amount of TBARS increases. Dr. McCord conducted the clinical trials of Protandim® by measuring the TBARS in men and women of a variety of ages. The amount of TBARS in their blood was consistent with their age (*i.e.*, the older the subject, the higher number of TBARS in their blood). The test subjects took one Protandim® pill each day for thirty days. The results were remarkable. The study revealed that after only 30 days, TBARS levels decreased an average of 40%, which was equivalent to the aging rate of a 20 year old! www.raysahelian.com/protandim.html

Oxidative stress is an important contributor to cancer development, and the association between chronic inflammation and cancer is well established. The protective antioxidant enzymes (especially SOD) have been demonstrated to reduce formation of tumors, suppress cell proliferation, and also reduce inflammation. The cancer fighting properties of Protandim® were published in an April 2009 study by Louisiana State University researchers (Dr. Jianfeng Liu and colleagues) in *PLoS ONE* (www.plosone.org). Protandim® is marketed via multilevel marketing, but don't let that scare you off. It's a very good product, in my opinion.

PROTEOLYTIC ENZYMES

The chemistry of digestion is really simple; with all the three major types of food being protein, carbohydrates, and fats. But remember, the important thing is not how much food we eat, but rather how much food we **digest.** And enzymes are the main component in food digestion. As I mentioned previously, there are also three main categories of digestive enzymes: proteases (for protein digestion), amylases (for carbohydrate digestion), and lipases (for fat digestion). We digest proteins into amino acids, carbohydrates into glucose, and fats into fatty acids.

Each day, the pancreas secretes about 1.7 liters of pancreatic juice in the small intestine. In this juice are enzymes (including lipases, proteases and amylases) required for the digestion and absorption of food. Lipases, along with bile, help digest fats. Amylases break down starch molecules into more absorbable sugars and are secreted by the salivary glands as well as the pancreas. The proteases secreted by the pancreas (trypsin, chymotrypsin, and carboxypeptidase) break protein molecules into single amino acids. There are also two plant-based proteases – bromelain (from the stems of pineapples) and papain (from unripe papayas). Let's take a close look at the proteases produced by our pancreas, oftentimes referred to as "proteolytic" (protein digesting) enzymes. When a "foreign invader" enters our system, it is our leukocytes that lead the charge of our immune response. However, cancer cells have a protein coating which renders them "unrecognizable" to the leukocytes and keeps them from destroying the cancer cells. In this scenario, would it not make sense to have something strip away the outer protein coating of the cancer cells? Of course it would. That idea has made sense in Europe and Asia for almost half a century where they have been throwing highly proteolytic and fibrinolytic (scar tissue eating) enzymes at cancer with great success. Earlier in the book, we learned about Dr. William Kelly who had an enzyme-based cancer treatment he effectively used on tens of thousands of cancer patients.

Proteolytic enzymes destroy cancer cells by breaking down the protein coating around the cell, and then the leukocytes attack the remaining cancer cell and destroy it. However, when we eat a diet high in overcooked proteins, which lack food enzymes, our own proteolytic enzymes are called upon to digest the proteins. We only have a limited supply of these proteolytic enzymes, and if this supply is being exhausted to digest protein in foods, then little or none is left to break down the protein coating on cancer cells. Thus, the cells begin to flourish and multiply because our leukocytes cannot kill them. The truth is that cancer is oftentimes a disease of protein metabolism because the proteolytic enzyme "cancer-fighting mechanism" can be overwhelmed by consuming protein-rich foods at inappropriate times or in excessive amounts. The body needs about 12 hours each day without protein consumption for its enzyme cancer-fighting mechanism to work optimally.

Around the age of 30, your body's production of enzymes drastically diminishes, so it's essential to begin supplementing immediately if you are older than 30. What is the best enzyme? My wife and I take Vitälzym every day. Vitälzym contains serrapeptase, which is an enzyme produced in the intestines of silk worms to break down cocoon walls. This enzyme is proving to be a superior alternative to the non-steroidal anti-inflammatory agents (NSAIDs) traditionally used to treat arthritis. However, if you are a cancer patient, Wobenzym contains more trypsin and chymotrypsin than any other enzyme, so this might be the best choice for you. In my opinion, you can't go wrong with either Vitälzym or Wobenzym, both of which you can purchase at www.iherb.com.

RESVERATROL

Resveratrol is a bioflavonoid found in the skin of dark grapes that is produced naturally when the plant is under attack by pathogens such as bacteria or fungi. Since resveratrol's prime function in nature is to protect the fruit against pathogens, it only makes sense that it would exhibit potent antifungal activity in the human body, which it does. It also destroys candida albicans. It has been suggested that resveratrol underlies the phenomenon known as the "French paradox" (the unexplained fact that the French, who have the same cholesterol levels as the rest of us, have only one-third the rate of heart disease).

Why? Because the French drink wine with meals, and red wine contains a high concentration of resveratrol. The WHO has suggested that resveratrol can reduce cardiovascular risks by up to 40%, since it blocks platelet "stickiness," prevents oxidation of LDL's, reduces triglyceride levels, and (most importantly) reduces tension levels, thus relaxing and dilating the arteries. Reseveratrol is virtually non-toxic since, after oral ingestion, it is quickly metabolized by the liver, attached to a detoxification molecule called "glucuronate," which renders it harmless. However, at the tumor site, the resveratrol is unzipped by an enzyme called "glucuronidase" that uncouples it from the glucuronate and makes it available to "go to work" on the cancer cells. In the April 2004 *Journal of Alternative and Complementary Medicine*, researchers at Cornell University's Weill Medical College published the results of tests on breast cancer and brain cancer cells. In these tests, resveratrol was shown to induce apoptosis (normal cell death) via the p53 gene, which repairs DNA. In studies published in the March 2004 *Anticancer Research*, resveratrol and curcumin impeded tumor cell growth and induced apoptosis in neuroblastomas (brain cancer) by activating the p53 gene pathway. In studies on neuroblastomas in mice, resveratrol halted cellular proliferation and altered the cellular structure of the tumor cells, leading to apoptosis. (*Surgery*, July 2004)

In addition to inducing apoptosis, resveratrol appears to kill off cancer cells by depolarizing (*demagnetizing*) mitochondrial membranes (*the energy source*) within tumor cells, which results in a decrease in the cell's potential to function. Resveratrol is a **dozen cancer-fighting substances** all wrapped up into one. It is another of God's natural cancer killers and fights cancer in so many ways that researchers can't find a cancer-promotion pathway it doesn't inhibit. In November 2008, researchers at the Weill Medical College of Cornell University reported that dietary supplementation with resveratrol significantly reduced plaque formation in animal brains, a component of Alzheimer's and other neurodegenerative diseases. According to the University of Basel, resveratrol increases cell viability through offering "neuro-protective" and antioxidative benefits by enhancing the body's production and assimilation of glutathione, the "master antioxidant."

One of the most interesting developments concerning resveratrol has come in the area of calorie restriction. Research studies with rats show that calorie deprivation results in increased longevity; a 10% to 30% calorie reduction can almost double their life span. In 2007, Harvard Medical School researchers reported that large daily doses of resveratrol could offset an unhealthy, high-calorie diet, thus having the same effect as calorie reduction: an increased life span.

Not surprisingly, resveratrol has also caught the eye of several Big Pharma companies who are already trying to capture its benefits in a synthetic, patentable, and expensive drug. My prediction: it will **not** work. Any time man tries to modify what God made and "improve" on His creation, it never works! Also remember, it is likely that pesticide-laden or genetically modified fruits will not produce significant quantities of resveratrol, as they have little need to naturally protect themselves from pathogenic attack.

In summary, resveratrol not only protects against bacteria, fungi, yeasts, and viruses, but it also fights cancer, heart disease, diabetes, and Alzheimer's. And if that's not enough, it also promotes longevity. Biotics Research Corporation sells a terrific product called ResveraSirt-HP® which contains 250 mg of resveratrol along with quercetin and IP6. It's the best resveratrol product I've found in my research. You can purchase it at www.bioticsresearch.com.

SEA CUCUMBER

Despite the name, sea cucumber is **not** a vegetable. It's a marine creature (related to the sea urchin and starfish) that lives all over the world on the ocean floor and has been used in traditional Chinese medicine for hundreds of years. In 2011, researchers at the Robert H. Lurie Cancer Center (in Chicago) studied the effects of sea cucumber extract on human **pancreatic cancer** cells and quickly discovered that this amazing extract is able to stop cancer cells from spreading and even activates apoptosis (*programmed cell death*). Amazingly, pancreatic cancer cells were actually dying **within five minutes** of exposure to the extract! Since then, in vitro (test tube) studies have shown that the fatty acids and saponins found in sea cucumber prohibit cancer from metastasizing and creating new blood vessels, while inducing apoptosis. http://www.ncbi.nlm.nih.gov/pubmed/12712407

Additionally sea cucumber has the ability to activate the immune system's killer cells to attack **breast cancer** cells. As reported by Ethan Evers, author of The Eden Prescription, previous research shows that sea cucumber is effective at killing lung, skin, colon, prostate and liver cancer cells. Frondoside A (a component of the sea cucumber) is believed to be a key component in the battle against cancer. A recent study, published in *PLoS One*, has confirmed just how powerful frondoside A truly is. According to the study, frondoside A *"can kill 95% of ER+ breast cancer cells, 95% of liver cancer cells, 90% of melanoma cells, and 85-88% of three different types of lung cancer."* When given to mice with non-small cell lung cancer, frondoside A was found to shrink tumors by 40% in only 10 days. Studies have shown frondoside A to be as effective as chemo at killing cancer cells ... but without **any** side effects. www.ncbi.nlm.nih.gov/pubmed/23308143

While your doctor won't likely be recommending sea cucumber extract to treat cancer, you can find dried and powdered sea cucumber in health stores and on www.iherb.com either as a single ingredient supplement or mixed with other ingredients in a formulation. The liquid extract is often a part of a formula (for inflammation and/or joint pain), but tablets consisting of pressed ground, dried sea cucumber are normally available.

WARNING: Do not take sea cucumber in any form if you have an allergy to seafood, or if you are taking anticoagulants as it may act as a blood thinner.

SELENIUM

From my research, I have begun to realize that selenium is possibly the most powerful anticancer nutrient there is. I am certainly not alone in singing the praises of selenium. Dr. E. J. Crary states, *"Selenium is the most potent broad-spectrum anticarcinogenic agent that has yet been discovered."* **That's right.** The trace mineral, selenium, has been shown in multiple studies to be an effective tool in warding off various types of cancer, including breast, esophageal, stomach, prostate, liver, and bladder cancers. The scientific and medical literature is filled with studies that demonstrate selenium's anticancer effects in humans. For example, in an epidemiological study, Dr. Raymond Shamberger categorized the states and cities in the USA according to whether there was high, medium, or low selenium availability in the diet. He demonstrated an inverse association between selenium availability and age-adjusted mortality for all types of cancer. To put it simply, **the more selenium available, the lower the levels of cancer.**

In a worldwide study Dr. Gerhard Schrauzer, M.D., Ph.D. (professor of medical chemistry at the University of California at San Diego) analyzed the blood-bank data from 27 countries around the world. He compiled a list in order of their blood selenium levels disclosing an inverse proportional relationship to cancer incidence, reporting specifically that areas with low levels of selenium in the diet had higher levels of leukemia and cancers of the breast, colon, rectum, prostate, ovary, and lung. In other words, the number one nation in blood selenium level (Japan) had the lowest cancer level (and consistently has rated highest in longevity) while the number two selenium level nation had the second lowest cancer rate, etc. etc.

Selenium was initially used in conventional medicine as a treatment for dandruff, but our comprehension of the mineral has dramatically increased over the past 20 years. It is an essential component of a powerful antioxidant manufactured by the body. This antioxidant, called glutathione peroxidase, defends specifically against peroxides, a type of free radical that attacks fats. Like other antioxidants, glutathione peroxidase also reduces the risk of developing cancer and heart diseases and stimulates the immune system's response to infections. This important enzyme is selenium dependent, with each molecule of the enzyme containing four atoms of selenium. Research shows selenium (especially when used in conjunction with vitamins C, E, and beta-carotene) works to block many chemical reactions that create free radicals in the body. Remember, free radicals can damage our cellular DNA, which eventually can lead to degenerative diseases like cancer. Selenium also helps to prevent damaged DNA molecules from reproducing and proliferating, a process called mitosis. In other words, selenium acts to prevent tumors from developing.

"It contributes towards the death of cancerous and pre-cancer cells. Their death appears to occur before they replicate, thus helping stop cancer before it gets started," according to the late Dr. James Howenstine in <u>A Physician's Guide to Natural Health Products That Work</u>. Selenium research over the past 20 years has focused heavily on a novel form of selenium: methylselenocysteine (MSC). A relatively simple organic selenium compound, MSC is formed naturally in various plants, including garlic, broccoli, wild leeks, and onions grown on high selenium soil. MSC is easily converted to methylselenol by an enzyme called beta-lyase, which is widely distributed in the body.

According to Dr. Daniel Medina (Baylor College of Medicine Department of Molecular and Cellular Biology), methylselenol has been shown to be an effective anti-cancer form of selenium that kills cancer cells through apoptosis, which is programmed cell death. ("Se-methylselenocysteine: A new compound for chemoprevention of breast cancer," *Nutrition & Cancer* 2001, 40:12-17) Methylselenol is also known to inhibit angiogenesis (creation of new blood vessels) in beginning cancer tumors and represents the safest and most effective anti-cancer form of selenium available today. One of the most important blind studies on selenium and cancer was a double-blind intervention trial conducted by Dr. L.C. Clark (and colleagues) at the University of Arizona Cancer Center. When all the results were tabulated, it became clear that the selenium-treated group developed almost 66% fewer prostate cancers, 50% fewer colorectal cancers, and about 40% fewer lung cancers as compared with the placebo group.

The old expression is *"an ounce of prevention is worth a pound of cure."* It would take almost 100 years at almost 800 mcg daily of selenium to consume a pound. Only 200 mcg daily supplementation of selenium has been documented to dramatically reduce cancer incidence, when in a grown, food-formed variety. A daily intake of 400 mcg was recommended by Dr. Schrauzer, mentioned earlier in this article. A daily intake of 600 mcg has been documented for residents of Japan on a traditional Japanese diet where cancer incidence is lowest and longevity is the greatest in the world. If every man, woman, and child supplemented with 200 mcg of selenium, we could almost wipe out the cancer epidemic over night! There is no downside to selenium supplementation, except perhaps to Big Pharma and the Medical Mafia, as this would definitely cut into their revenue stream!

Some of the best natural sources of selenium are Brazil nuts, garlic, broccoli sprouts, and brussel sprouts. All of these foods contain selenium in the form of MSC. Although garlic has the greatest concentration of MSC, you are not likely to eat enough of it to produce the desired results, so Brazil nuts, broccoli sprouts, and brussel sprouts are your best choices. My family takes "Innate Response" selenium at www.choosetobehealthy.com, recommended by my friend, Chris Barr.

SILVER

Colloidal silver is a suspension of extremely fine (submicroscopic) particles of pure silver suspended in water by a positive electric charge on each particle. The particles remain suspended throughout the water because these positive-charged particles repel each other with a greater force than gravity. Colloidal silver is an "umbrella term" that often includes forms of silver that contains salts, proteins, or other stabilizers that allow manufacturers to put more silver into the water. But more silver is not necessarily better.

A powerful germicidal, silver is an exceptional metal in that is non-toxic to healthy mammalian cells but lethal to over 650 disease-causing bacteria, viruses, fungi, parasites, and molds. The daily ingestion of small quantities of colloidal silver is like having a "second immune system." I remember Granddad telling me that they used to put silver dollars into milk to keep it fresh longer, before they had refrigerators. It is well-known that the ancient Greeks knew the medical value of silver. They realized that families who used silver utensils were rarely sick and had few infections.

This knowledge passed on to kings, emperors, sultans, and their families and members of their royal courts. They ate from silver plates, drank from silver cups, used silver utensils, and stored their food in silver containers. As a result of this use, the silver particles were released and mixed with their foods and drinks. As a general rule, they were much healthier than the peasants who ate with dishes made of earthenware and utensils made of iron. This is why royalty became known as "blue bloods," since their skin had a blue-grey tint from the accumulation of minute traces of pure silver. This is also where the phrase *"born with a silver spoon in your mouth"* arose.

While studying regeneration of limbs, spinal cords and organs in the late 1970s, Dr. Robert O. Becker, author of <u>The Body Electric</u>, discovered that silver ions promote bone growth and kill surrounding bacteria. The March 1978 issue of *Science Digest,* in an article, "Our Mightiest Germ Fighter," reported: *"Thanks to eye-opening research, silver is emerging as a wonder of modern medicine. An antibiotic kills perhaps a half-dozen different disease organisms, but silver kills some 650. Resistant strains fail to develop. Moreover, silver is virtually non-toxic."* The article ended with a quote by Dr. Harry Margraf, a biochemist and pioneering silver researcher: *"Silver is the best all-around germ fighter we have."*

How does it work? The presence of colloidal silver near a virus, fungus, bacterium or any other single celled pathogen disables its oxygen metabolism enzyme. In other words, it disables the pathogen's "chemical lung" so that it cannot breathe. Within a few minutes, the pathogen suffocates and dies and is cleared out of the body by the immune, lymphatic, and elimination systems. Unlike pharmaceutical antibiotics (which destroy beneficial bacteria and enzymes), positively charged silver ions first target microbes having a negative charge (most commonly pathogenic). This is why under normal use there is little healthy gut ecology disruption. It is difficult to know whether the colloidal silver made by home generation units are producing pure particles small enough to interact successfully with the microbial world, much less carry that all-important positive charge. In order for the body to use and excrete it successfully, you should seek photographic proof of particle size as is only possible with electron microscopy.

Taken orally, colloidal silver, particularly bioactive silver hydrosol (particles smaller than 10 nanometers), is absorbed from the mouth into the lymph and bloodstream then transported quickly to the cells. Swishing the liquid under the tongue briefly before swallowing may result in more efficient absorption across the mucosa. Active silver works very rapidly with a short half-life in the lymph and even shorter in the blood, so repetitive dosing is essential in acute situations. Prolonged administration may be needed for chronic immune disorders with doses spaced further apart than in acute situations.

The hydrosol form of colloidal silver is excreted via the liver (Phase II glutathione conjugation) and out through the colon as solid waste. Lesser forms of colloidal silver (which include compounds of salts or combinations of protein) are more difficult for the body to bind and excrete. Although the kidneys will attempt to eliminate the compounds unable to be excreted by the liver, their lack of complete elimination results in accumulation within the organs and skin (argyria – benign cosmetic discoloration of the skin). Additionally, silver has a tremendous affinity for oxygen. The warmer the silver is, the greater its oxygen carrying capacity, up to 10 times its atomic weight! Why is this important? Cancer cells abhor oxygen and silver floods your body's cells with copious amount of oxygen.

Prior to 1938, colloidal silver was used by physicians as a mainstream antibiotic treatment and was deemed to be a "cutting edge" treatment for a variety of ailments. Not surprisingly, however, Big Pharma moved in and caused colloidal research to be set aside in favor of financially lucrative drugs, particularly patented antibiotics. The best silver available for purchase, in my humble opinion, is "Sovereign Silver," which is manufactured by Natural Immunogenics Corporation. At only 10 parts-per-million, it outperforms colloidal silvers of much higher concentration, which makes it safe for long term use. Their website is http://www.sovereignsilver.com/. They manufacture a brand for health professionals as well, known as Argentyn 23.

VITAMIN D

Ultraviolet light from the sun comes in two main wavelengths – ultraviolet A ("UVA") and ultraviolet B ("UVB"). Think of UVA as the "bad guy" and UVB as "the good guy," since UVA penetrates the skin more deeply and causes more free radical damage, whereas UVB helps your skin produce vitamin D. Technically speaking, vitamin D is not really a vitamin, per se, but is more appropriately classified as a "pro-hormone." Regardless, vitamin D has been shown to be crucial in preventing cancer. The mechanisms by which vitamin D reduces the risk of cancer are fairly well understood. They include enhancing calcium absorption, inducing cell differentiation, increasing apoptosis (programmed cell death), reducing metastasis and proliferation, and reducing angiogenesis (formation of new blood vessels).

So, where do I buy the best vitamin D supplement? The truth be told, most vitamin D supplements are virtually worthless. Here's why: The vitamin D in milk and in most vitamin supplements is vitamin D2 and is synthetic. Vitamin D2 is also called "ergocalciferol." It is **not** the form of vitamin D that you need to prevent cancer and degenerative diseases. In actuality, the form of vitamin D which you need is vitamin D3 (aka "cholecalciferol") and is produced from the UVB rays in sunlight. That's why I frequently refer to sunshine as the *"most affordable cancer-fighting nutrient in the world."* Think about it, you can get a lifetime supply for **free**!

Don't fall for the "sunscreen myth." Despite what we hear from the Medical Mafia, sunlight is actually good for you (especially the UVB rays), and sunscreens filter out UVB! The main chemical used in sunscreens to filter out UVB is octyl methoxycinnamate (aka "OMC") which has been shown to kill mouse cells even at low doses. Plus, it was also shown to be particularly toxic when exposed to sunshine. And guess what? OMC is present in **90%** of sunscreen brands!

The most popular brands of sunscreens also contain other toxic chemicals (such as dioxybenzone and oxybenzone) that are absorbed through the skin where they enter the bloodstream, generate free radicals, wreak havoc on the immune system, damage the liver and the heart, and even promote systemic cancer. The time required in the sun is probably 15 to 30 minutes per day. The optimal time for UVB production of vitamin D is around the middle of the day when the ratio of UVB to UVA is highest and the required exposure times are shortest. However, this works only when the sun is elevated high enough. During winter months, it is oftentimes impossible to produce any vitamin D from sunlight, depending upon how far north you live.

But you do **not** want to burn! If you are going to be out in the sunlight for prolonged periods of time, you need to protect your skin from burning. Aloe vera gel is a natural sunscreen (if you have sensitive skin), and it also helps to heal sunburn. We use Dr. Mercola's *"Natural Sunscreen with Green Tea"* if we are going to be out in the sun for prolonged periods of time. However, when sunlight (specifically UVB) is not available, an excellent source of vitamin D that will also provide beneficial omega-3 fatty acids DHA and EPA (which are pivotal in preventing heart disease, cancer, and many other diseases) is cod liver oil. The highest quality and best tasting cod liver oil (with the lowest price) is Carlson's Cod Liver Oil found at www.iherb.com.

You must be cautious when using cod liver oil, as it is possible to overdose on vitamin D. For this reason, cod liver oil should be consumed only in cool weather months unless you can test your vitamin D levels to make sure that they are not too high. In warm weather, most people get enough vitamin D from sunshine, so don't take cod liver oil during summer months. Researchers in Belgium appear to be the first to show that vitamin D lowers C-reactive protein (CRP), a measure of inflammation in the body, in critically ill patients. CRP is elevated when there is inflammation in the body, and chronic inflammation is a risk factor for a number of conditions including coronary heart disease, diabetes, and cancer.

WATER

Water is probably the most important topic. Without food, most humans will die in a month. Without water, we're dead in less than ten days. Water makes up over 70% of the body, around 90% of the blood, and about 85% of the brain.   The problem with most of us is that we have been sold a bill of goods – when you're thirsty, drink a soda, or the latest "sports drink" (chock full of sugar, by the way). Americans drink coffee and sodas and beer and anything else we've been conditioned to buy, but most of us forget to drink enough **water**.

Many people drink distilled or osmotic water, but in my opinion, this is dead water. Yes most of the toxic chemicals have been removed, but also missing are the alkaline minerals and oxygen...especially in the case of distilled water, since it is "acidic." My family drinks tap water that has been filtered with our Big Berkey water filter, which filters out lead, arsenic, chlorine, fluoride, etc. All that remains is pure water. We used to drink bottled water, but the plastic leaching was a concern to us, so we switched to filtered water.

If you are thirsty, it means your cells are already dehydrated. A dry mouth should be regarded as the last outward sign of dehydration. That's because thirst does not develop until body fluids are depleted well below levels required for optimal functioning. Some statistics show that as much as 90% of us are walking around in a chronic state of dehydration. One way to tell if you're dehydrated is to check the color of the urine. If it's dark all the time, you're probably dehydrated.

Physicians rarely promote the curative properties of water, but the late Dr. Fereydoon Batmanghelidj (aka "Dr. Batman") studied water's effect on the human body and found it to be one of the best pain relievers and preventative therapies. His pioneering work shows that Unintentional Chronic Dehydration (UCD) contributes and even produces pain and many degenerative diseases which can be prevented and treated by increasing water intake.

Dr. Batman was born in Iran in 1931, and he practiced medicine in the UK before returning to Iran where he played a key role in the development of hospitals and medical centers. When the Iranian Revolution broke out in 1979, Dr. Batman was placed in the infamous Evin Prison as a political prisoner for thirty-one months. It was there he discovered the healing powers of water. One night, Dr. Batman had to treat a fellow prisoner with crippling peptic ulcer pain. With no medications at his disposal, Dr. Batman gave him two glasses of water. Within several minutes, his pain completely disappeared. He was instructed to drink two glasses of water every three hours and became absolutely pain free for his four remaining months in the prison. While in prison, Dr. Batman successfully treated over 3,000 fellow prisoners suffering from stress-induced peptic ulcer disease with **water alone**.

While in prison he conducted extensive research into the medicinal effects of water in preventing and relieving many painful degenerative diseases. Evin Prison proved an ideal "*stress laboratory,*" and despite his being offered an earlier release, Dr. Batman chose to stay an extra four months in prison to complete his research into the relationship of dehydration and bleeding peptic ulcer disease. The report of his findings was published as the editorial of the *Journal of Clinical Gastroenterology* in June 1983.

On his release from prison in 1982, Dr. Batman escaped from Iran and came to America. He wrote his ground-breaking book <u>Your Body's Many Cries for Water</u> in 1992, which has been translated into 15 languages and continues to inspire readers worldwide. In his book, he stated that a dry mouth is not a reliable indicator of dehydration. The body signals its water shortage by producing pain. Dehydration actually produces pain and numerous degenerative diseases, including asthma, arthritis, hypertension, angina, adult-onset diabetes, lupus, and multiple sclerosis. Dr. Batman's message to the world was, "*You are not sick, you are thirsty. Don't treat thirst with medication.*" Learn more at <u>www.watercure.com</u>.

ZEOLITES

Zeolites are natural volcanic minerals with a unique, complex crystalline structure. Zeolites, in general, have been used for almost 1,000 years as a traditional remedy throughout Asia to promote overall health. One amazing property of zeolites is that their honeycomb framework of cavities and channels (like cages) work at the cellular level trapping heavy metals and toxins. As you know, toxins poison our air, our water, our food, and our bodies. According to the EPA, 80,000 chemicals are used commercially in the United States, and 75,000 of them are potentially hazardous to our health. The Environmental Defense Council reports that more than four billion pounds of toxic chemicals are released into the environment each year, including 72 million pounds of known carcinogens.

Zeolites are one of the few negatively charged minerals in nature. Basically, they act as magnets, attracting positively charged heavy metals and toxins, capturing them, and removing them from the body. They are an extremely effective chelating agent. Here's how: within the structure of the zeolites, there are certain "cages," inside of which are positive ions. The positive ions switch places with the heavy metals, pesticides, or herbicides, which are also positive ions, and then the cage structure of zeolites tightly binds them. One amazing quality of this "caged binding" effect is that the toxins and heavy metals are 100% excreted. In other words, they don't get "relocated" to another spot in the body, they actually get evicted!

Zeolites are effective against harsh microorganisms such as bacillus, fungi, mildew, staphylococcus, and streptococcus. They function as a broad spectrum antiviral agent, help balance pH levels in the body, reduce allergic reactions, chelate heavy metals, neutralize acids, increase oxygen levels, fend off microorganisms, and support immune system function. The main problem with zeolites is that they all "push" aluminum and lead into gastric acid, so there are other "complementary" products that **must** be used along side of zeolites, in order to minimize their "heavy metal footprint." To learn more about these products, please visit http://www.ToxinsAway.com.

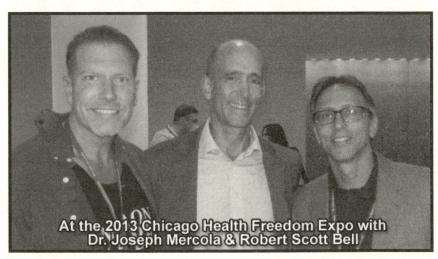

At the 2013 Chicago Health Freedom Expo with Dr. Joseph Mercola & Robert Scott Bell

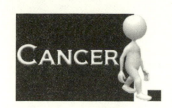

CHAPTER 13
THE "DIRTY DOZEN"

> "WHEN YOU SEE THE GOLDEN ARCHES, YOU ARE
> PROBABLY ON YOUR WAY TO THE PEARLY GATES."
> -DR. WILLIAM CASTELLI

The last couple of chapters have dealt with which herbs, foods, and supplements you should consume. Now for the items you should **avoid.** I have labeled this chapter "*The Dirty Dozen*" because it details twelve foods/toxins which can pose serious health problems if consumed or ingested regularly. Actually, a few of them can cause serious problems if only consumed/ingested even occasionally.

Is it possible to eliminate these substances completely? Probably not, but at least you will be aware of which ones are the worst, since food and toxins are integral components of the cancer equation. As a matter of fact, a report by the Columbia University School of Public Health estimated that **95%** of cancers are caused by diet and environmental toxicity. The journal of *Pharmaceutical Research* summarized in 2008 that the development of cancer is 90-95% dependant upon the everyday battle between environmental carcinogens and the natural cancer-fighting agents which lessen the impact of carcinogens in your body.

Here are a few more startling statistics:

> ➢ There are over 80,000 chemicals produced in North America.
> ➢ There are over 3,000 chemicals added to our food supply.
> ➢ There are over 10,000 chemical solvents, emulsifiers, and preservatives used in food processing.
> ➢ There are over 1,000 new chemicals introduced each year.

This chapter is a veritable "buffet" of foods, toxins, and poisons to avoid like the plague if you have cancer! The first section is entitled *"Franken-Foods"* and the last section is entitled *"Terrible Toxins."*

"FRANKEN-FOODS"

This section is entitled "Franken-Foods" because, if you will notice, all of the foods have been altered from their natural state or they contain ingredients which have been altered. The 5 foods/food ingredients in this section not only have little nutritional value, but they also give your body a healthy (or is it "unhealthy") dose of carcinogenic toxins, which should make the idea of eating them really *"hard to swallow."*

1. "Fake-Fats" (Trans-fats & Hydrogenated Oils)

"Trans-fats" are manufactured fats, produced by pushing hydrogen into vegetable oils to produce a solid fat, hence they are also called "hydrogenated" or "partially hydrogenated" oils. Trans-fats are in fried foods, margarines, and baked goods, packaged snacks, cookies, pie crusts, and donuts. Even "healthy" low-fat muffins and cereals may contain trans-fats. The trouble is that trans-fats are bad for us even in tiny quantities. Research has shown that they are implicated in increased cardiac disease, cholesterol levels, and yes, **cancer**.

According to Dr. Brian Olshansky, Professor of Internal Medicine at Iowa University, *"The problem with trans fatty acids is that your body doesn't know what to do with them. Trans fatty acids may help preserve food so that it tastes good, but your body can't break them down and use them correctly. Normal fats are very supple and pliable, but the trans fatty acid is a stiff fat that can build up in the body and create havoc. The chemical recipe for a trans fatty acid involves putting hydrogen atoms in the wrong place. It's like making a plastic."* www.psa-rising.com/eatingwell/transfats092003.htm

In order to mass produce and distribute foods high in oils, food manufacturers deliberately alter the chemical composition of the oils, which gives them longer "shelf lives." Another problem with many processed foods is that they are not only irradiated, but they are made with genetically modified foods. If we look at corn chips, we see a product that is likely made with genetically modified corn, then processed in trans-fats, and then irradiated. After all of this, the chips are packaged in a bag which says *"All Natural."* But don't be deceived...there is nothing "natural" about fried corn chips.

In the 1950s, Dr. Johanna Budwig proved that these chemically-altered, hydrogenated fats (which she called "pseudo" fats) destroy cell membranes. She demonstrated that these hydrogenated, processed fats and oils shut down the electrical field of the cells and make us susceptible to chronic and terminal diseases.

CounterThink

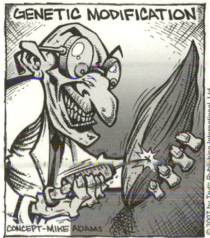

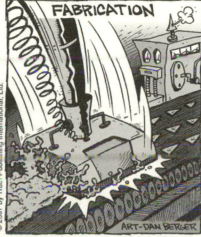

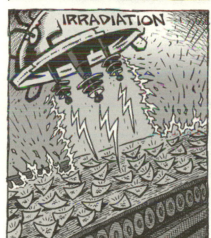

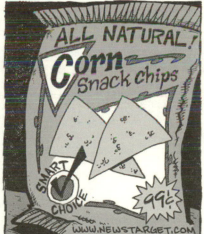

FACT: THE "ALL NATURAL" CLAIM ON FOOD PRODUCTS IS MEANINGLESS. GET THE FACTS: www.HonestFoodGuide.org

Thanks to Mike Adams and *www.NaturalNews.com* for the cartoon above.

In healthy fats there is a vital electron cloud which enables the fat to bind with oxygen. Healthy, oxygenated fats are capable of binding with protein and in the process become water-soluble. This water solubility is vital to all growth processes, cell damage restoration, cell renewal, brain and nerve functions, sensory nerve functions, and energy development. In fact, the entire basis of our energy production is based on lipid metabolism. Hydrogenation destroys the vital electron cloud, and as a result, these "pseudo" fats can no longer bind with oxygen or with protein. These fats end up blocking circulation, damaging the heart, inhibiting cell renewal, and impeding the free flow of blood and lymph.

Three of the most popular foods which contain trans-fats are donuts, French fries, and chips. Donuts are nothing but big balls of sugar, trans-fats, and white flour. They have no nutritional value. Most French fries and chips have been soaked in trans-fats to such extent that there is virtually no nutrition left in them. Some companies have tried to make them more "healthy" by eliminating the trans-fats, but all donuts and chips and fries that are cooked in oil (regardless of what type oil) contain cancer-causing acrylamides.

The chemical, acrylamide, which is used industrially in the manufacture of some plastics, is also formed by the heating of starches. And guess what...three foods with especially high levels of **acrylamides** are donuts, French fries, and potato chips. Acrylamides are only allowed in your drinking water at a level of 0.12 micrograms per serving by the EPA. Alarmingly, a six ounce helping of French fries at your local fast food joint will contain anywhere from 50 to 70 micrograms of acrylamides. That's between **400 and 600 times** the EPA limit! I have heard it said by numerous doctors that a French fry is worse for your health than a cigarette. I agree.

In light of the fact that they have been shown to cause so many health problems, why do food manufacturers continue to use trans-fats? The answer is plain and simple: **money.** Trans-fats greatly prolong the shelf life of processed foods.

2. Sugar, Syrup, & Sodas

I decided to combine these three items since they typically go "hand in hand" in our "Big Gulp" society, despite what you hear from the sugar industry and its efforts to prevent the distribution of information that accurately links refined sugars to chronic disease. Sugar, high-fructose corn syrup (HFCS), and sodas are all on the "no no" list if you want to obtain optimal health.

Remember, cancer cells grow by anaerobic respiration. In other words, they ferment sugar. If you've ever made wine, you'll know that fermentation requires sugar. There are many nutritional cancer therapies, but not a single one allows foods high in carbohydrates and not a single one allows sugar, because **sugar feeds cancer cells**.

During my lifetime, HFCS has taken our food shelves by storm. It is present in almost everything we eat today, including breads, sweets, sodas, oatmeal, barbeque sauce, ketchup, jelly, jam, yogurt, chocolate milk, pop tarts, and cereal, to name a few. But isn't HFCS a healthy alternative to sugar? Well, in a word, "**no**." A few months ago, I remember seeing commercials about HFCS, the core message of which was that HFCS is made from corn, has no artificial ingredients, has the same calories as sugar, and is OK to eat. The ads are priceless in their total misrepresentation of facts and in their complete lack of respect for the IQ of the viewing public.

The truth is that HFCS doesn't actually exist anywhere in nature. It is a manufactured product created by using enzymes (two natural, one synthetic) to increase the fructose content of corn syrup to about 90%. This super HFCS is then blended "down" with a 100% glucose corn syrup to be added to our foods. When HFCS is ingested, it travels straight to the liver which turns the sugary liquid into fat. According to the USDA, HFCS depletes the body of chromium, which is important in helping glucose pass from the bloodstream into the cells. This depletion of chromium in combination with an overworked pancreas frequently results in diabetes.

But isn't HFCS made from corn? Yes, it's absolutely true that HFCS is made from corn, but that means nothing. Biodiesel is also made from corn, but you don't want to eat biodiesel! The bottom line is that just because you start with a natural, safe substance doesn't automatically make derivatives of that substance safe. Let's think about this for a moment. What do farmers feed cows when they want to fatten them up for market? Corn, of course! So, if you want to look like a cow, all you have to do is eat lots of corn and corn by-products, including HFCS.

And to make matters worse, two separate studies – one published in the *Journal of Environmental Health* and the other conducted by the Institute for Agriculture and Trade Policy (IATP) – recently revealed the fact that HFCS may also contain mercury. And if that's not enough, **over 86% of corn in the USA is now genetically modified** (see the next chapter on GMO)!

"*But why didn't my doctor warn me about HFCS?*" Remember, it wasn't too long ago when doctors were being paid by cigarette companies to actually endorse cigarettes. So it's really no surprise that there are some doctors who are clueless on the dangers of HFCS, despite the fact that it's basically common sense to anyone who has half a brain and has spent more than a few minutes studying the issue.

One can of soda has almost 13 teaspoons of sugar, most of which is fructose from HFCS. Another reason to avoid carbonated sodas is that they have a pH of around 2.0, which will contribute to a highly acidic terrain. According to Dr. James Howenstine, in his book A Physician's Guide to Natural Health Products That Work: "*In an interesting experiment the sugar from one soft drink was able to damage the white blood cells' ability to ingest and kill gonococcal bacteria for seven hours...Soft drinks also contain large quantities of phosphorus, which when excreted pulls calcium out of the bones. Heavy users of soft drinks will have osteoporosis along with their damaged arteries.*"

In 1951, Dr. Clive McCay, a Navy nutritionist at the Naval Medical Research Institute, found that human teeth softened and started to dissolve in a short period of time after sitting in a cup of Coca Cola. He stated the acidity of cola beverages is about the same as vinegar, only it is masked by the sugar content. Maybe this is why sodas are also referred to as "**soft** drinks" – because they soften your teeth and bones!!

And if you think diet sodas are better, think again. Diet sodas typically have a lower pH than normal soda, and they also contain harmful artificial sweeteners like aspartame. If you want to sweeten foods, I recommend **stevia**, which is an herb 300 times sweeter than sugar. Its medicinal uses include regulating blood sugar, preventing hypertension, treatment of skin disorders, and prevention of tooth decay. Other studies show that it is a natural antibacterial and antiviral agent as well. So, while it will make your food tasty, stevia is also actually good for you! For the cancer patient, sugar is a definite "no no." If you hate your cancer, then starve it. If you regularly drink sodas, try drinking water instead. Eliminating sugar, HFCS, and sodas from your diet is one of the easiest ways to immediately improve your health.

3. Excitotoxins (MSG & Aspartame)

What is an excitotoxin? These are substances, usually amino acids, which react with specialized receptors (neurons) in the brain in such a way as to lead to the destruction of certain types of brain cells. Humans lack a blood-brain barrier in the hypothalamus, which allows excitotoxins to enter the brain and cause damage. Simply put, as described in Dr. Russell Blaylock's book, Excitotoxins: The Taste That Kills, they are exactly what they sound like: **toxins that excite your brain cells to death**!

No strain of rat or mice is naturally obese, so the scientists have to create them. They make these morbidly obese creatures by injecting them with monosodium glutamate (MSG) when they are first born. The MSG triples the amount of insulin the pancreas creates, causing rats to become obese. MSG creates a lesion in the hypothalamus that correlates with abnormal development, including obesity, short stature and sexual reproduction problems. MSG has also been shown to kill brain cells as well as to cause nausea, vomiting, migraine headaches, depression, and heart problems. Unfortunately, MSG is often disguised under other names; thus, you may not be able to detect it in a list of ingredients.

Some synonyms for MSG are *"Glutamate Textured Protein"* or *"Glutamic Acid Yeast Extract"* or *"Gelatin Yeast Nutrient"* or *"Hydrolyzed Vegetable Protein."* They hide MSG under many different names in order to fool those who catch on. Food companies learned that MSG could increase the flavor and aroma and enhance acceptability of commercial food products, so it is doubtful that they will ever quit using this brain killing additive to our food supply. Take a quick trip to your kitchen and check the pantry and the fridge. You will realize that MSG is in everything: soups, the chips, the ramen, the hamburger helper, the gravy, the salad dressings, the corn oil, the broth, and so on.

Aspartame is also an excitotoxin, and it has been shown to erode intelligence and affect short-term memory. Believe it or not, aspartame was once on a Pentagon list of biowarfare chemicals submitted to Congress! It is made from two amino acids and methanol (wood alcohol). Although test studies showed that it is extremely toxic to the brain, the government suppressed this fact, and it was officially approved as a food additive for use in soft drinks in 1983. The FDA ignored complaints of headaches, dizziness, nausea, vomiting, seizures, convulsions, blurred vision, and a multitude of other negative reactions to aspartame.

A few years ago, we watched a documentary on aspartame called "Sweet Misery." It was amazing...and disturbing. You can see the trailer and also see the first five minutes here: http://aspartamekills.com. Later in the book, there is an entire chapter dedicated to exposing the frauds surrounding aspartame.

4. rBGH / Sodium Nitrate

In 1994, Monsanto and the FDA introduced rBGH (recombinant bovine growth hormone) into the market. This is a powerful genetically engineered drug which, when injected into dairy cows, will force them to produce up to 25% more milk. However, when a cow is injected with rBGH, its milk production is stimulated, but not directly. The presence of rBGH in the cow's blood stimulates production of another hormone, called Insulin-Like Growth Factor (IGF). It is IGF that stimulates milk production.

IGF is a naturally occurring hormone-protein in both cows and humans. Numerous studies have shown that the IGF in cows is chemically identical to the IGF in humans. The use of rBGH increases the levels of IGF in the cow's milk, and the IGF is **not** destroyed by pasteurization. Since IGF is active in humans and causes cells to divide, an increase in IGF in milk raises obvious questions as to whether it will cause inappropriate cell division and growth, leading to growth of tumors.

Since the emergence of rBGH on the market in 1994, every industrialized country in the world (except for the USA) has **banned** it. The fact of the matter is that rBGH was never adequately tested before the FDA allowed it on the market. A standard test of new biochemically produced products and animal drugs requires 24 months of testing with several hundred rats. But rBGH was tested for only 90 days on 30 rats. This short term rat study was submitted to the FDA but never published. The FDA refused to allow anyone outside that agency to review the raw data from this truncated study, saying it would "*irreparably harm*" Monsanto.

In February of 1997, two veteran news reporters for Fox TV in Tampa, Florida, were fired for refusing to water down an investigation reporting that rBGH may promote cancer in humans who drink milk from rBGH treated cows. Monsanto pressured Fox TV to water down the series, offering to pay the two reporters if they would leave the station and keep silent about their report, but they refused and were fired. On April 2, 1998, they filed their own lawsuit against the TV station. After a five week trial and six hours of deliberation which ended August 18, 2000, a Florida state court jury unanimously determined that Fox "*acted intentionally and deliberately to falsify or distort the plaintiffs' news reporting on rBGH.*" The jury awarded $425,000 in damages. Why was Monsanto so determined to keep the reporters quiet?

Here's why. In 1998, Canadian scientists managed to acquire the full Monsanto studies for the first time. They were stunned to find out that the FDA never even looked at Monsanto's original data on which the agency's approval had been based. In reviewing the data, the scientists learned that Monsanto's "secret" studies showed that rBGH caused prostate cancer and thyroid cancer in laboratory rats!

In August 2008, Eli Lilly agreed to buy rBGH from Monsanto. This seemed to be a peculiar choice at the time. Why on earth would Eli Lilly's veterinary division (Elanco) pay $300 million for a drug that other companies wouldn't touch with a ten foot pole? Then I began to connect the dots. Back in college, I read a story about an owner of an auto body shop who was arrested for "keying" hundreds of cars. What a way to increase business! Eli Lilly was doing the "drug equivalent" of keying cars and then getting paid to fix them!

You see, Eli Lilly also sells cancer drugs. So, while Eli Lilly is pushing a milk drug (rBGH) that causes cancer, they are also planning on "coming to the rescue" with other drugs to "treat" the cancer that the rBGH just created. Just call it the perfect business "double play." But that's not all ... it gets even better for Eli Lilly. Cows treated with rBGH have much higher incidence of mastitis (udder infection). You guessed it. Eli Lilly is more than happy to sell antibiotics to treat the infection. Meanwhile, Eli Lilly is laughing all the way to the bank.

Sodium nitrate ($NaNO_3$) and its close relative **sodium nitrite** ($NaNO_2$) are preservatives that you find in lots of processed meats. Stuff like salami, pepperoni, hot dogs, bologna, ham, bacon (even turkey bacon), livestock feed (yet another reason to only eat grass-fed beef), and SPAM all normally contain sodium nitrate as one of the ingredients. It's the ingredient that gives these meats that pretty "reddish-pink" color rather than their natural rotten grey. It makes meats appear "fresh" even if they've been on the shelves for months.

Almost all processed meats are made with sodium nitrite, despite the fact that it is a precursor to cancer causing chemicals called **nitrosamines**. An enormous amount of evidence indicates that nitrosamines are human carcinogens. For instance, tobacco-specific nitrosamines are one of the major groups of chemical carcinogens in tobacco products. Just remember, when you eat bologna or pepperoni or bacon, you are also eating sodium nitrite, which forms nitrosamines, which promotes the growth of cancer cells. Back in the 1970s, the USDA attempted to ban sodium nitrite but failed due to lobbying efforts of the meat processing industry.

Do you want statistics? The University of Hawaii conducted a study that lasted seven years on almost 200,000 people. The results of the research indicated that people who consumed processed meats (such as hot dogs and sausage) had a **67%** increased risk of pancreatic cancer over those who consumed little or no meat. (www.naturalnews.com/007024.html) Now, I'm not saying that meat products are bad, as I have already discussed grass-fed beef. But almost all processed meats and meats from rBGH cows...**they're terrible!** One of the reasons is sodium nitrite. And this is just the tip of the iceberg.

5. Soy

According to most health professionals, soy beans are the most versatile, natural, heart-friendly, health-improving foods on earth. Soy is the largest cash crop in the USA, and it is being touted as having a myriad of health benefits. But according to Dr. William Wong, *"Soy is poison, period!"* In his article entitled "Soy: The Poison Seed," Dr. Wong describes several reasons why soy is poison. Soy contains two isoflavones (estrogen-like substances) which are basically built in insecticides for the soybean. He asks, *"If they kill bugs, are they good for humans?"* Good point.

According to nutritionist Mary Enig, PhD, *"The reason there's so much soy in America is because they (the soy industry) started to plant soy to extract the oil from it and soy oil became a very large industry. Once they had as much oil as they did in the food supply they had a lot of soy protein residue left over, and since they can't feed it to animals, except in small amounts, they had to find another market."* And another market was exactly what they found: **the unsuspecting American public**. After tens of millions of dollars spent on advertising, a propaganda campaign that makes Hitler look like a rank amateur and intense lobbying to the FDA, approximately 75% of American consumers now believe soy products are healthy.

If you're thinking the health claims surrounding soy sound too good to be true you just may be right. Soy contains **phytin**, which removes essential minerals such as iron, zinc, and magnesium before they can be absorbed. Soy also contains **trypsin inhibitors** – remember trypsin is essential in the recognition and digestion of both proteins and cancer cells. Beyond these, soybeans also contain **hemagglutinin**, a clot promoting substance that causes red blood cells to clump together. These clustered blood cells are unable to properly absorb oxygen for distribution to the body's tissues.

According to Dr. Tim O'Shea, *"Yet another toxin found in some processed soy products is aluminum, which is said to be 10 times higher in infant soy formulas than in milk-based formulas--and 100 times higher than in unprocessed milk. Levels are even higher when soy products are hydrogenated. Aluminum, a cause of Alzheimer's, can also damage the newly forming kidneys of an infant who drinks soy formula. Worse yet, aluminum can directly damage the infant brain because the blood-brain barrier has not formed yet. Processed soy can also contain a known carcinogen called lysinoalanine. It is a by-product of a processing step called alkaline soaking, which is done to attempt to eliminate enzyme inhibitors. Even though the beans are thoroughly rinsed, the lysinoalanine by-product can remain from the*

interaction of the soybeans with the alkaline solution."
www.camaweb.org/library/nutrition/soy_con.php

The bottom line on soy is this: ***soybeans are not a complete protein, are not a natural food, contain several harmful and even carcinogenic substances, and most soybeans in the United States are genetically modified.*** According to Dr. Wong, *"Any opinions to contradict the facts noted above have been paid for by the agribusiness giants Monsanto and Archer Daniels Midland. Once public knowledge of their manipulation of public opinion and of the FDA becomes widely known, expect monster class action lawsuits against these folks. They'll deserve it in spades!"* See chapter 20 for more information about the dangers of soy.

"TERRIBLE TOXINS"

The toxins listed in this section are everywhere, so watch out! In all actuality, an entire book could be devoted to environmental and food toxins, but I have chosen just to mention a few of the most common toxins.

6. Asbestos

More than thirty million tons of asbestos in its various forms have been mined in the past century. Asbestos is one of the most pervasive environmental hazards in the world, present in more than 3,000 manufactured products. It was widely used from the 1950s to 1970s. Asbestos is actually a family of minerals that can be spun into fibers and then woven into cloth. Due to this fact, it will not burn; thus, it has been used heavily in the insulation industry as a fire retardant. Problems arise when the material becomes old and crumbly, releasing fibers into the air and then inhaled into our lungs. Asbestos won't burn; neither will it dissolve once inside the body. The fibers get caught in the lungs and other organs then irritate the tissues and cause lesions and eventually scarring.

There are three diseases that are triggered by inhaling asbestos fibers: asbestosis, mesothelioma, and lung cancer.

Asbestosis is caused when asbestos fibers are inhaled and become trapped in the lungs. In response, the body tries to dissolve the fibers by producing an acid. While not destroying the fibers, the acid serves to scar the lung tissue. Eventually the scarring can become so severe that the lungs become unable to function. **Mesothelioma** is a cancer of the outside tissue of the lungs. This cancer is solely linked to asbestos. The time from exposure to manifestation of these diseases is from 15 to 40 years.

The major sources of asbestos are insulation on floors, ceilings, heating ducts, and water pipes from the 1950s to the 1970s. Even though the use of asbestos in office buildings ceased over 30 years ago, millions of office workers are still working in older buildings which contain asbestos insulation. It's estimated that over 50% of the skyscrapers in America still contain asbestos. Both of the *"Twin Towers"* that were brought down (in classic "controlled demolition"style) on 9/11/01 were full of asbestos.

There have been concerns about a possible asbestos cover up by the EPA and the federal government during the cleanup of the World Trade Centers. In fact, the United States is one of the few nations that have not yet placed a ban on asbestos – it is still an ingredient in thousands of products. That's right, amazingly, despite the known health risks, asbestos has **not** been banned in the USA. The Consumer Product Safety Commission (CPSC) abandoned its attempts to ban asbestos products in 1979, passing the responsibility to the EPA. In 1989, the EPA attempted a ban of its own, but in 1991, the U.S. 5th Circuit Court of Appeals overturned it. Insidious and deadly, asbestos has worked its way through the "cracks" of the consumer protection system for almost 30 years.

As a result, asbestos is still lodged deep in the tissue of American commerce, and almost no one is paying attention. Despite the fact that health experts expect asbestos to claim another 250,000 lives in the USA during the next several decades, asbestos is still being used as an ingredient in a multitude of everyday products ranging from brake pads to ceiling tiles. Imports of products containing asbestos are also on the rise. The bottom line is that virtually every man, woman, and child has been exposed to asbestos, due to its pervasiveness. Only time will tell the deleterious health effects which result from this dangerous carcinogen.

7. Fluoride

In early 2010, there was a huge volcanic eruption in Iceland. Currently, animals in southern Iceland are at risk of fluoride poisoning if they inhale or ingest the ash from the eruption. Fluoride poisoning can lead to internal bleeding, long-term bone damage, and tooth loss. According to BBC News (April 19, 2010): *"The fluoride in the ash creates acid in the animals' stomachs, corroding the intestines and causing hemorrhages. It also binds with calcium in the bloodstream and after heavy exposure over a period of days makes bones frail, even causing teeth to crumble."*

Most folks never "connect the dots" between the tragic poisoning of these animals due to a natural event, and the **intentional** poisoning of human beings through excessive fluoride exposure each and every day. The practice of adding fluoride to your tap water began in the 1940s, but contrary to popular opinion, fluoride doesn't stop tooth decay at all. Scientific studies actually prove that fluoride is neurotoxic and causes birth defects, cancer, and osteoporosis. Fluoride also damages the immune, digestive, and respiratory systems as well as the kidneys, liver, brain, and thyroid.

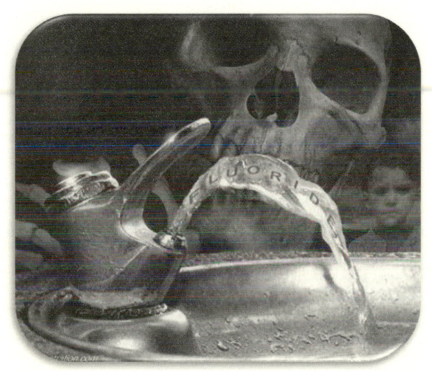

Thanks to David Dees for the picture above.

A 1936 issue of the *Journal of the American Dental Association* stated that fluoride at the 1 ppm (part per million) concentration is as toxic as arsenic and lead. There are more than 500 peer reviewed studies documenting adverse effects of fluoride ranging from cancer to brain damage. And yet, municipalities throughout the USA actually purchase this product and then drip it into the public water supply. Dr. Charles G. Heyd, former President of the AMA, declares, *"I am appalled at the prospect of using water as a vehicle for drugs. Fluoride is a corrosive poison that will produce serious effects on a long range basis. Any attempt to use water this way is deplorable."* www.apfn.org/apfn/poison.htm

There is **no scientific evidence** that fluoride is a beneficial additive to water, and in fact there is overwhelming scientific evidence that proves, without a doubt, that fluoride is harmful. It actually causes teeth to rot and crumble! The bottom line is that all federal health agencies have known these facts for years, but have been controlled by the political interests of the nuclear arms, aluminum, and phosphate manufacturers to keep it a secret. See chapter 16 for more information about the dangers of fluoride.

8. Mercury

Did you know that most of the fish we eat contains mercury? Why? Thousands of tons of mercury are released into the air each year through pollution and waste. Eventually, it accumulates in steams, oceans, water and soil. It also accumulates in the food chain, so each fish absorbs the mercury in other fish and organisms it eats. The bigger the fish, the more mercury it absorbs. Shark, swordfish, tilefish, mackerel, sea bass, marlin, halibut, oysters, salmon, and tuna contain the highest levels of methylmercury.

According to Dr. Joseph Mercola, *"Methylmercury toxicity can result in paraesthesia, depression, & blurred vision. In fetuses and developing infants it can also have negative effects on attention span, language, visual-spatial skills, memory and coordination. It is estimated that nearly 60,000 children each year are born at risk for neurological problems due to methylmercury exposure in the womb."* www.mercola.com/2003/jun/28/mercury_fish.htm

The Environmental Protection Agency (EPA) has issued health advisories about consuming fish due to mercury contamination. The *"Got Mercury? Calculator"* at www.gotmercury.org can help you decide how much and what type of seafood is safe for you and your family. Just enter your weight, the seafood type and quantity, and hit the calculator button. The online calculator will tell you whether your consumption exceeds the EPA's safe limit for mercury.

What about those mercury fillings in your mouth? Mercury amalgam dental fillings contain approximately 50% mercury. Initially, the American Dental Association (ADA) denied that mercury from these fillings leaked vapor, which is then absorbed into our bodies. But, in recent years, facing numerous studies to the contrary, the ADA has conceded that mercury fillings do leak mercury vapor, which is extremely toxic.

Did you know that the metallic mercury used by dentists to manufacture dental amalgam is shipped as a **hazardous material** to the dental office? Did you know that when mercury fillings are removed, they are treated as hazardous waste and are required to be disposed of in accordance with federal OSHA regulations? Over the past few years, Charlene and I have had all of our mercury fillings removed. I recommend that you do the same. Like mercury, other heavy metals (like arsenic, lead, aluminum, and cadmium) which are prevalent in many areas of our environment, can accumulate in soft tissues of the body and can cause a multitude of degenerative diseases, including cancer. These heavy metals are found in our drinking water, in fish, vaccinations, pesticides, antiperspirants, building materials, and dental amalgams, just to name a few sources. See chapter 18 for more information about the dangers of mercury.

9. Mycotoxins (fungal toxins)

Mycotoxins are poisonous substances produced by certain molds found primarily in grain and nut crops. They are basically "fungal poisons" which cause a wide range of health problems in humans. Corn is commonly contaminated with fumonisin and aflatoxin (both known for their cancer-causing effects). A 1993 study demonstrated 24 different types of fungi found in peanuts, including aflatoxin. (Costantini, A. "Etiology and Prevention of Atheroscler-osis," *Fungalbionics Series* 1998/99) Mushrooms also contain mycotoxins.

Now, I'm not recommending that you totally eliminate peanuts, since they are a very good source of fiber, vitamin E, potassium, folic acid, zinc, and magnesium. Peanuts also contain resveratrol (the substance found in dark grapes), flavonoids, and antioxidants, all of whose health benefits are increasingly being proven to help you prevent a wide variety of diseases. The key to consuming healthy peanuts is to make sure they are organic and grown in a region where the soil is dry and aflatoxin has therefore not been reported as a problem, such as New Mexico. My family loves peanut butter, so we buy Maranatha Peanut Butter, which is organic and uses Valencia peanuts from the arid soil of New Mexico; thus, they are free from aflatoxin, pesticides, and chemicals.

Reishi, shiitake, and maitake mushrooms have been shown to possess cancer-fighting properties, so I'm not against mushrooms either. The active anti-cancer constituent in these mushrooms is a polysaccharide called beta-glucan, a huge sugar molecule made up of many little sugar molecules chained together bound to amino acids. These intricate sugars stimulate or modulate the immune system by activating immune cells such as macrophage and helper T-cells, as well as increase the immunoglobin levels (immunoglobins are specific types of antibodies) to produce a heightened response to foreign cells, whether bacteria, viruses, or tumor cells.

To be honest, everything that's animal or vegetable can get moldy. Grains, nuts, fruits, tea and coffee plants, herbs, and vegetables all mold. While living things are alive, the mold attackers can be held at bay, but as soon as they are dead, molding begins. First it molds and then the bacterial action sets in; this is what makes things biodegradable. Without mold and decay, the streets of Fort Worth would still be full of horse manure from the days of the horse and buggy and our lakes too full of dead fish to swim in. There is absolutely no way that you can completely eliminate mycotoxins from your diet. However, in light of Dr. Tullio Simoncini's pioneering work relating to the potential fungal link to cancer, I highly recommend that you **minimize** the amount of mycotoxins which you ingest. That's definitely a good idea. And here is some good news for cooks: if you bake your own bread, you can extend the period your bread will be mold-free by adding a bit of vitamin C to the dough. It will also make the bread rise higher. You can do the same when cooking rice.

10. Organochlorines (Chlorine Byproducts)

Chlorine gas was a weapon used in both world wars and is a neurotoxin so poisonous that it was outlawed by international war codes. It cannot be screened out by our lungs, goes in faster than oxygen, is immediately absorbed into the bloodstream when it is inhaled, and if the concentration is adequate, death is instantaneous. As molecular biologist Joe Thornton explains, *"There are no uses of chlorine which we regard as safe."* Yet chlorination, considered one of the greatest advances ever in public health and hygiene, is almost universally accepted as the method of choice for purifying water supplies.

Most drinking water in the USA comes from a surface water source, that is, a lake or river. These lakes and rivers are typically rich in invisible organic matter produced by decaying leaves and algae. During disinfection, chlorine randomly attaches to this organic matter to form thousands of newly created chemicals called "organochlorines." Organochlorine compounds are not found naturally anywhere in the world, but once they are formed by combining chlorine with organic materials, they are extremely toxic and very stable. Most of them don't break down for hundreds of years.

Organochlorines are easily absorbed into our bodies and are lipophilic (stored in our fat cells) where they accumulate. According to molecular biologist Joe Thornton, *"Chlorination virtually always increases toxicity."* A growing number of studies have linked chlorinated drinking water to cancer in humans. The most esteemed cancer study is a compilation of 10 separate epidemiological studies on chlorinated drinking water and cancer known as the Morris study. It found disinfection by-products in chlorinated water to be responsible for 9% of all bladder cancers and 15% of rectal cancers in the USA. This translates into 10,000 additional deaths per year for just these two organs.

According to the U.S. Council of Environmental Quality, *"Cancer risk among people drinking chlorinated water is **93% higher** than among those whose water does not contain chlorine."* Prolonged exposure has also been shown to produce birth defects, immune system problems, and reproductive disorders.

Although water disinfection accounts for only a small percentage of total global organochlorine production, the effect on human health is proportionately greater because exposure to chlorinated drinking water is large and continuous. It is piped right into our homes. But organochlorines in our drinking water are just the tip of the iceberg! The most toxic organochlorine is **dioxin**, which is the most caustic man-made chemical known. "Dioxin" is a general term for hundreds of chemicals that are produced in industrial processes that use chlorine and burning. Disturbingly, it has a half-life of over **one hundred years** when it is leached into soil or embedded in water systems. Dioxin was the most harmful component in Agent Orange, which contributed to over half a million birth defects in Vietnam!

A draft report released for public comment in September 1994 by the U.S. EPA clearly describes dioxin as a serious public health threat. In 1997, the International Agency for Research on Cancer (part of the World Health Organization) announced that the most potent dioxin is now considered a Group 1 carcinogen, meaning a *"known human carcinogen."* Of course, the EPA maintains that low levels of dioxin are "safe."

Let me ask a question. If dioxin is so safe, why does the Veterans Administration make automatic payments for a wide range of claims that include several types of cancers and leukemia, liver disease, heart disease, Parkinson's disease and diabetes? American taxpayers are footing the bill for veterans' Agent Orange dioxin injuries that are estimated to cost over **$40 BILLION** over the next decade! I submit that Dow and Monsanto (*the top 2 producers of Agent Orange*) should pay for all damages... **NOT** the American taxpayer.

In addition to cancer, dioxin can cause reproductive and developmental disorders, liver damage, chloracne, skin rashes, skin discoloration, etc.

A typical American will receive 93% of his/her dioxin exposure from meat and dairy products. In fish, these toxins bioaccumulate up the food chain so that dioxin levels in fish are 100,000 times that of the surrounding environment. The main sources of dioxin are the paper production industry, the plastic production industry, and incinerators than burn chlorinated waste.

Recent scientific research has clearly demonstrated an association between organochlorines and breast cancer. Analyses of the breast fat of women with breast cancer found that DDT, its derivative DDE, PCBs, and other organochlorine pollutants actually concentrate in the cancer tissue itself, in contrast with surrounding non-cancerous tissue. Organochlorines are not only often overtly toxic, but they also possess estrogenic activity. In other words, they mimic estrogen. Chemicals that function like estrogen are called xenoestrogens (literally "foreign estrogens") and wreak havoc in a number of ways. A woman's earliest and most dangerous contact with them may be in the womb. Xenoestrogens have been linked to breast cancer as well as an increase in reproductive abnormalities in males, including prostate cancer and testicular cancer.

11. Plastic Pollutants

When you eat or drink things that are stored in plastic, taste it, smell it, wear it, sit on it, and so on, plastic is incorporated into you. In fact, the plastic gets into the food and food gets into the plastic and you. So, quite literally, you are what you eat, drink, and breathe. We are becoming "**plastic people**."

Water bottles are be made from various types of plastic, such as polycarbonate (PC), polyethylene terephthalate (PET), polypropy-lene (PP), high-density polyethylene (HDPE), low-density polyethy-lene (LDPE), polyvinyl chloride (PVC or vinyl), and others. Bisphenol-A (BPA) is a monomer used in the synthesis of PC plastics, epoxy resins, and composites, as well as a heat stabilizer in PVC.

The list of products containing BPA is long, as it is deeply imbedded in the products of modern society. BPA-based PC plastic is used as a coating for children's teeth to prevent cavities, as a coating in metal cans to prevent the metal from contact with food contents, as the plastic in food containers, refrigerator shelving, baby bottles, water bottles, returnable containers for juice, milk and water, microwave ovenware, and eating utensils.

As the plastic ages, then the BPA leeches. Experiments with rats demonstrate that low level exposure to BPA during fetal growth causes breast cancer in adults as well as insulin resistance. In a small prospective study, researchers in Japan report that BPA levels are higher in women with a history of repeated spontaneous miscarriages.

BPA is only one of a long list of plastic pollutants, a list that is so long that it would require its own book in order to have an exhaustive study. The bottom line is that BPA (and other plastic pollutants) are extremely toxic and are everywhere! What this all means is that most of your life, you will be within arm's length to BPA or another form of toxic plastic. www.ourstolenfuture.org

Phthalates are plasticizers used to make plastic products more flexible and also to lengthen the life of fragrances. About four million tons of phthalates are produced worldwide each year. Phthalates are recognized as toxic substances under environmental law, but companies are free to use unlimited amounts in cosmetics.

Some common phthalates and the products which contain them:

> **Di-ethyl phthalate** (DEP): Toothbrushes, auto parts, tools, toys, food packaging, insecticides, mosquito repellents, aspirin, nail polish, perfumes, hair sprays
> **Di-n-butyl phthalate** (DBP): Cellulose plastics, solvents for dyes, solvents for cosmetics, nail polish, food wrap, perfumes, skin emollients, hair spray, insect repellents
> **Benzyl butyl phthalate** (BBP): Plasticizers in adhesives, PVC flooring, wood finishes, biodegradable tampon ejectors

That new car smell, which is especially strong after the car has been sitting in the sun for a few hours, is the odor of phthalates precipitating from a hot plastic dashboard. Then, when it cools down in the evening, the phthalates condense to form an oily coating on the inside of the windshield. An environmental release of just 10 pounds of DBP must be reported to environmental authorities under the Superfund Law. However, the cosmetics industry puts thousands of tons of DBP into nail polish each year, with no requirements for safety testing or reporting to anyone.

But "why?" you may ask. Many pivotal court decisions implementing the 1976 Toxic Substances Control Act (TSCA) have basically hamstrung the EPA. You see, the EPA must prove an "*unreasonable risk of injury*" to human health before it can remove a chemical from the market. However, they cannot prove unreasonable risk of injury without first conducting safety studies, which are expressly prohibited until "substantial" or "significant" exposure is proved to be occurring. So, it's an endless loop, since the FDA can almost never prove that substantial or significant exposures are occurring because exposure data is extremely difficult to obtain. To put it simply, the EPA cannot regulate a chemical until it makes a finding of risk based on data which the law virtually prohibits it from collecting. This is absurd, isn't it?

Women who are pregnant, nursing or thinking about getting pregnant should look for and avoid all personal care products with the word phthalate on the label. The major sources of phthalates are plastic wrap, plastic bottles, plastic food storage containers, nail polish, and cosmetics. Phthalates have been shown to have estrogenic qualities, have toxic effects on the testicles, and to cause birth defects. They can also cause cancer, damage the endocrine system, and are particularly dangerous to children.

Have you heard about benzene? Almost 300,000 people per year are exposed to benzene in the workplace. Benzene is an aromatic hydrocarbon and a volatile organic compound (VOC) which is produced by the burning of natural products. It is a component of products derived from coal and petroleum and found in gasoline and other fuels. Most benzene is produced for use as a building block in the manufacture of a number of products, such as medicinal and industrial chemicals, plastics, rubber, resins, synthetic fabrics, and dyes.

Research has shown benzene to be **extremely carcinogenic;** it is a known carcinogen and one of the primary causes of leukemia in the USA. Generally, benzene exposure comes from tobacco smoke, gasoline and automobile exhaust. Benzene is also used as a solvent in waxes, paints, resins, and inks.

However, there is another source of benzene which is very disturbing: **sodas**. Two preservatives commonly added to sodas (ascorbic acid and sodium benzoate) react to produce, yes, you guessed it: **benzene**. The warmer the soda gets, the more benzene will be produced. The FDA and soda manufacturers have known about this "dirty little secret" since 1990 but failed to warn the public. So for almost two decades, people have unwittingly been drinking sodas which contain a known human carcinogen. In 2007, there was a class action lawsuit and several soda manufacturers (including Coca Cola, PepsiCo, and Sunny Delight Beverages) settled and agreed to reduce the amount of benzene in their drinks. However, numerous drink manufacturers are still using ascorbic acid (vitamin C) and benzoate salts in many drinks that are being sold worldwide. The exposed population is huge, probably in the billions.

On a related note, many brands of plastic dinnerware is made of melamine plastic, since it is hard and smooth and keeps its shape well. Did you know that up to 90% of the infant formula sold in the USA may be contaminated with trace amounts of melamine? According to recent tests (the results of which the FDA hid from the public), Nestle, Mead Johnson and Enfamil infant formula products were all contaminated with melamine.

The truth about the melamine only became public after the Associated Press filed a Freedom of Information Act (FOIA) request, demanding the test results from the FDA. Of course, the FDA claims that low levels of melamine are perfectly safe for babies to consume in unlimited quantity. Sure they are! I suppose BPA is safe, too? What about aspartame, MSG, fluoride, sodium nitrite, and every other poison? If you believe the FDA, all these toxic poisons are safe to consume. However, by this point in the book, I hope you now realize that the FDA (and the Medical Mafia) is nothing more than a legalized gang of unindicted criminals engaged in the tactics of intimidation, censorship, and oppression that can appropriately be described as health *"terrorism."*

12. The "Cides" (Pesticides, Herbicides, Fungicides, Insecticides)

Do you still think that the fruit you are eating is safe? Think again. A recent study from the UK indicates that pesticide residues on some common fruits are unusually high. Some apples, pears, raspberries, and grapes contained pesticide residues that exceeded the legal limits. Cherries, lettuce, and pumpkins all contained potentially dangerous levels of toxic pesticide residues as well. And the produce wasn't just from one area – it originated from all over the world from Brazil to Spain to Canada.

So remember that when you reach for that luscious fruit at the grocery you may be inadvertently feeding your children pesticides as well. Fruits and vegetables that are heavily sprayed include strawberries, cantaloupe, bell peppers, peaches, nectarines, celery, potatoes, carrots, and imported grapes. I recommend that you buy organic when it comes to these fruits and vegetables. If you can't find organic produce, try mixing twenty drops of grapefruit seed extract, one tablespoon of baking soda, one cup of vinegar, and one cup of water together in a spray bottle. Spray the produce, let it sit for about ten minutes, and then rinse thoroughly. This process should eliminate a good amount of pesticide residue. Blueberries, grapefruit, bananas, broccoli, mangos, cauliflower, avocados, asparagus, onions, California grapes, citrus, pineapple, and melons typically don't contain a large amount of pesticides.

According to the EPA, 60% of herbicides, 90% of fungicides and 30% of insecticides are known to be carcinogenic. Alarmingly, pesticide residues have been detected in over half of American foods. Most pesticides contain multiple toxins, and there is no class of pesticide which is free of cancer causing potential. The most convincing evidence that pesticides cause cancer is from epidemiological studies. The common lawn pesticide 2,4-D (aka "Weed-B-Gone") has been shown to increase the risk of lymphatic cancer in farmers six times the normal rate, according to a National Cancer Institute report. (Sinclair, W. *18* "Studies Show Why Pesticides Are More Dangerous than Previously Realized"). Most folks don't realize that 2,4-D is half of the recipe for Agent Orange, and is one of the top souces of dioxin in the USA. Dow Chemical is the biggest 2,4-D manufacturer.

Scientists believe that the use of lawn chemicals (like Weed-B-Gone) have been a significant factor in the 50% rise in non-Hodgkin's lymphoma over the past 20 years in the American population. (World Health Organization, 2,4-D *Environmental Aspects*. Geneva, Switzerland, 1989). 2,4-D has also been linked to malignant lymphoma in dogs. Pets are exposed to higher doses of pesticides because they are closer to the ground where concentrations are the highest. Studies show that the risk of lymphomas doubled in dogs whose owners treated lawns four times per year.

In light of the fact that 2,4-D is a known carcinogen and toxin, one would think that the EPA would want to prohib its sale. **Nay nay!** In November of 2013, the EPA rejected a petition that sought to prohibit the domestic sale of 2,4-D. And Dow Chemical believes that sales will skyrocket in the coming months, since they are awaiting federal approval of a genetically engineered crop they've created that will be resistant to 2,4-D. If approved, farmers will be able to plant the "franken-corn" and douse their fields with the pesticide to eliminate unwanted weeds with greater success. Although 2,4-D isn't currently used to a large degree on corn fields, all that could soon change for the USA's most successful crop if their new "franken-corn" is approved.

The Natural Resources Defense Council, an environmental watch group, has argued that expose to 2,4-D has caused in some cases cancer, hormone disruption, genetic mutations and neurotoxicity, reports the New York Times. In voting not to hear the petition against the pesticide, however, the EPA says that they believe there to be a lack of evidence that would be significant enough to raise suspicion.

In 1983 the National Cancer Institute studied 3,827 Florida pesticide applicators that had been spraying for more than 20 years. They found that these pesticide applicators had nearly three times the risk of developing lung cancer and two times the risk of developing brain cancer. There was no increased risk for pesticide applicators that had been spraying for only five years. (*Journal of the NCI*, July 1983)

Speaking of pesticides, DEET is a chemical that was patented by the US Army in 1946 and is still widely recognized as an effective mosquito repellent. In fact, most commercial insect repellents are made of varying concentrations of DEET. Currently, DEET is used in up to 230 different products. However, all is not well with DEET. When combined with other chemicals or medications, DEET can have toxic effects on the brain and body. DEET has been shown to cause seizures, neurological damage, memory loss, headaches, weakness, fatigue, muscle and joint pain, tremors, and shortness of breath. Children are even more susceptible to subtle brain changes caused by toxic chemicals in their environment because their skin more readily absorbs them. So you should **never** use any DEET-containing product on infants!

Since the late 1970s, there have been multiple reports linking pesticides to leukemia in children. A 1987 study by the NCI showed that children living in pesticide-treated homes had nearly a four times greater risk of developing leukemia. If the children lived in homes where pesticide was sprayed on lawns and gardens, the risk of developing leukemia was 6.5 times greater. (Dr. John Peters, USC, *Journal of the NCI*, July 1987)

Have you ever heard of Atrazine? Atrazine is a powerful herbicide applied to over 70% of America's cornfields. Traces of the chemical routinely turn up in American streams and wells and even in the rain, and residues of Atrazine are frequently found in our food supply. So what? Well, this toxic chemical, which was recently banned by the European Union, is a suspected carcinogen and endocrine disruptor that has been linked to low sperm counts among farmers. As a matter of fact, Tyrone Hayes, a herpetologist at UC Berkeley, while doing research on behalf of Syngenta (*the manufacturer of Atrazine*), found that even at concentrations as low as 0.1 part per billion, Atrazine will chemically emasculate a male frog, causing its gonads to produce eggs, in effect, turning males into hermaphro-dites. I don't know about you, but there is no way that I want my son to be exposed to Atrazine!

In a June 2006 article in the *New York Times* entitled "The Way We Live Now," author Michael Pollen comments, "*Atrazine is often present in American waterways at much higher concentrations than 0.1 part per billion. But American regulators generally won't ban a pesticide until the bodies, or cancer cases, begin to pile up - until, that is, scientists can prove the link between the suspect molecule and illness in humans or ecological catastrophe. So Atrazine is, at least in the American food system, deemed innocent until proved guilty – a standard of proof extremely difficult to achieve, since it awaits the results of chemical testing on humans that we, rightly, don't perform. I don't know about you, but as the father of an adolescent boy, I sort of like the idea of keeping such a molecule out of my son's diet..."*

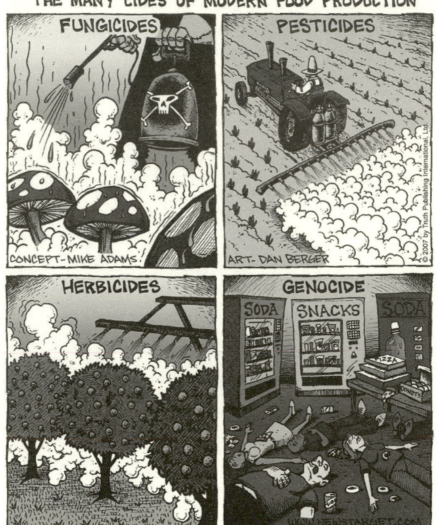

Thanks to Mike Adams and *www.NaturalNews.com* for the cartoon above.

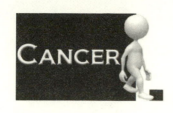

CHAPTER 14
SAY "NO" TO GMO!

> "CONTROL THE OIL AND YOU CAN CONTROL
> ENTIRE CONTINENTS. CONTROL THE FOOD AND
> YOU CONTROL THE PEOPLE." ~ HENRY KISSINGER

A FALSE SENSE OF SECURITY

The majority of American consumers erroneously believe that the FDA approves genetically modified foods through rigorous, in-depth, long-term studies. Nothing could be further from the truth. It is imperative to fully understand the severe ramifications of ingesting this laboratory created, if you will pardon the expression, "food." Genetic engineering/modification of food involves the laboratory process of artificially inserting genes into the DNA of food crops or animals. The result is called a genetically modified organisms ("GMO"). GMO can be engineered with genes from bacteria, viruses, insects, animals, or even humans. The primary reason the plants are engineered is to allow them to basically *drink poison*. They're inserted with foreign genes that allow them to survive otherwise deadly doses of poisonous herbicides, fungicides, and insecticides.

The only "testing" for safety that is required is for the GMO producer to submit a self-authored report on the new GMO safety. This scam was devised by Michael Taylor, a former FDA lawyer who established the "no testing" policy by reasoning that GMO are "substantially equivalent" to food, and food has already been determined to be safe. Taylor (second cousin to Tipper Gore) is notorious for his "revolving door" employment within the US government and Monsanto and was chosen by Obama as the FDA Deputy Commissioner for foods (aka the "food safety czar") in July 2009. While at Monsanto, Taylor's main responsibility was gaining regulatory approval of the GMO cancer-causing bovine growth hormone (rBGH). Effectively, in the area of American food safety, we now have the "fox" guarding the "henhouse."

You see, we have been given a false sense of security about the safety of our food supply. Ignorance is the key in this campaign of deception, as only about 25% of Americans even know if they've ever eaten GMO food in their lifetime! The five main GMO foods are soy, corn, cotton, canola, and sugar beets. Their derivatives are found in more than 75% of the foods in the grocery store. The fact of the matter is that GMO have been linked to toxic and allergic reactions, sick, sterile, and dead livestock, and damage to virtually every organ studied in lab animals. GMO food has been banned by food manufacturers in Europe and almost every other country in the world, yet GMO are present in the vast majority of processed foods in the USA and Canada.

According to Jeffrey M. Smith, bestselling author and filmmaker, "*GM foods are particularly dangerous for pregnant moms and children. After GM soy was fed to female rats, most of their babies died—compared to 10% deaths among controls fed natural soy. GM-fed babies were smaller, and possibly infertile. Testicles of rats fed GM soy changed from the normal pink to dark blue. Mice fed GM soy also had altered young sperm. Embryos of GM soy-fed parent mice had changed DNA. And mice fed GM corn had fewer, and smaller, babies. In Haryana, India, most buffalo that ate GM cottonseed had reproductive complications such as premature deliveries, abortions, and infertility; many calves died. About two dozen US farmers said thousands of pigs became sterile from certain GM corn varieties. Some had false pregnancies; others gave birth to bags of water. Cows and bulls also became infertile. In the US, incidence of low birth weight babies, infertility, and infant mortality are all escalating.*" www.ResponsibleTechnology.org

Dr. Joseph Mercola asserts, "*I strongly believe that one of the most obvious clues about the danger of GMO foods are that just about EVERY species of animal that is offered a GMO food versus a non-GMO food will avoid the GMO one. Many times they will do this to the point of starvation, as they have an intuitive sense of the danger of this food.*" http://articles.mercola.com

Monsanto is the corporation largely responsible for the introduction of poisonous GMO to our food supply. Yes, for the past 15 years, the same Monsanto that gave us Agent Orange, dioxin, and rBGH has been "pushing" GMO crops on the unwitting American public. Currently, Monsanto's mutated seeds comprise over 93% of the USA's soy crops, 86% of the corn crops, and wheat is next on their agenda.

Before we get rolling on this issue, I want to clarify the difference between GMO and hybrid plants. Farmers and gardeners have been cultivating new plant varieties for thousands of years through selective breeding. They did this by cross-pollinating two different (but related) plants over multiple generations, eventually creating a new plant variety. Hybrid seeds are just as natural as their historic counterparts, since they are merely cross-pollinated from two different (but related) plants.

Genetic modification, on the other hand, involves the laboratory process of artificially inserting genes into the DNA of food crops or animals. The result is called a genetically modified organism. GMO can be engineered with genes from bacteria, viruses, insects, animals, or even humans. The primary reason the plants are engineered is to allow them to basically *drink poison*. They're inserted with foreign genes that allow them to survive otherwise deadly doses of poisonous herbicides, fungicides, and insecticides. Genetic engineering creates combinations of plant, animal, bacteria, and viral genes that do not occur in nature. Scientists are putting fish genes into tomatoes and strawberries, human genes into corn and rice and sugarcane, jellyfish genes into corn, and even spider genes into goats!

Except for the "spider-goat" mentioned above, these techniques create different characteristics in the "franken plant," such as resistance to chemicals like Roundup® (glyphosate). When glyphosate is sprayed on GMO crops, they resist the herbicide. It kills the weeds, but not the crops. Farmers love it because they may get a higher yield from their farms. But how to these crops affect the people that eat them? This is the $64,000 question.

CONTAMINATED CORN

Imagine that you spray an insecticide on a plant, but you are unable to wash it off prior to eating it, because it has become part of the plant! Guess what happens when you eat the plant. You ingest that insecticide. **Case in point**: Monsanto has crossed genetic material from bacteria known as *Baccilus thuringiensis* ("Bt") with corn. This is one of the most common GMO traits, and crops that contain the Bt toxin are designed to kill insects and pests by breaking open their stomachs.

The resultant GMO plant (known as *"Bt Corn")*, is itself registered as a pesticide with the EPA, since the Bt toxin actually becomes part of every cell of the plant. In other words, if you feed this corn to your cattle, your chickens, or yourself, you'll be feeding them an actual pesticide, not just a smidgeon of pesticide residue. Bt corn has been implicated in the deaths of cows in Germany, and horses, water buffaloes, and chickens in the Philippines.

Speaking of intestines, the proliferation of GMO has corresponded with upticks in bowel diseases such as diverticulitis, colitis, and irritable bowel syndrome (IBS), Crohn's disease, leaky gut, and, especially in children, allergies. Coincidence? I don't think so. It's a massive human experiment, and we **all** are the guinea pigs. Leaky gut syndrome takes place when fissures open between cells lining the gastrointestinal tract. Partially digested food particles ooze through those fissures into the body and appear to be foreign invaders. The immune system activated to do what it does best: seek and destroy. This is one of the main problems with GMO – they introduce gene sequences that the body has never seen before. Our immune systems then attack the GMO as if it were a harmful pathogen (which it actually is).

Monsanto is in the process of unleashing its latest "frankenfood" experiment, a new version of GMO corn with eight abnormal gene traits called "Genuity SmartStax" corn. That's right, Smartstax has no less than **eight** "transgenes" (*i.e.,* mutated genes) combined or "stacked" together - six for insect resistance and two for herbicide tolerance. To give you a proper perspective, current stacked GMO crops only have up to three traits each. Smarstax corn contains a potpourri of transgenes claimed to control pests both above and below ground. Genuity, a subsidiary of Monsanto, uses a combination of fungicides along with clothianidin (an insecticide) in their GMO seeds. Clothianidin is a systemic insecticide that may be carried to all parts of the corn plant including the pollen-producing tassel and pollen visited by bees. The selection of clothianidin for seed treatment is rather "cavalier" because it has been implicated in the reduction of the bee population. (*Chemical & Engineering News,* 5/26/08) If GMO are wiping out the earth's pollinators (like bees), they are far more disastrous than merely the threat they pose to humans and other mammals.

The Committee of Research and Information on Genetic Engineering (CRIIGEN) and Universities of Caen and Rouen (France) studied three different types of Monsanto's GMO corn. The data *"clearly underlines adverse impacts on kidneys and liver, the dietary detoxifying organs, as well as different levels of damages to heart, adrenal glands, spleen and haematopoietic system,"* reported Gilles-Eric Séralini, a molecular biologist at the University of Caen. www.biolsci.org/v05p0706.htm#headingA11

Speaking of Séralini, a 2009 study by Benachour and Séralini published in *Chemical Research in Toxicology* examined the toxicity of four popular glyphosate based herbicide formulations on human placental cells, kidney cells, embryonic cells, and neonate umbilical cord cells. What they found was shocking: **Total cell death** of each of these cells within 24 hours. In an interview at the European Parliament, Professor Andrés Carrasco (Argentine government scientist) reported that childhood cancer increased by 300% and babies with birth defects by 400% during the past decade in parts of Argentina, where GMO soy is grown to supply European farmers with cheap GM animal feed. He also noted that Argentinian children were consuming so much GMO soy that they began developing breasts from the estrogenic effects. His studies show glyphosate exposure can cause defects in the brain, intestines, and hearts of fetuses. Moreover, the amount of Roundup® used on GMO soy fields was as much as 1,500 times greater than that which created the defects!

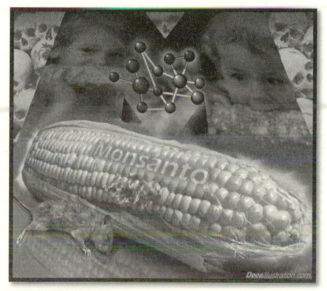

Thanks to David Dees for the picture above.

But now Monsanto is pushing GMO corn with eight transgenes! This is no laughing matter. If you live in America, your health and the health of your children and grandchildren are at stake. It seems more like a scene from a horror flick than something happening in modern day America.

STERILIZING SOY

In a recent Russian study (jointly conducted by the Institute of Ecology and Evolution of the Russian Academy of Sciences and the National Association for Gene Security), researchers found that GMO soy caused sterility in 3rd generation hamsters! The hamsters were fed the GMO soy for a period of two years, during which time the researchers evaluated three generations of hamsters. During the study, the 2nd generation GMO soy-fed hamsters had an infant mortality rate **five times** higher than "non-GMO-soy-fed hamsters." But then an even bigger problem became apparent, because nearly all of the 3rd generation hamsters (over 90%) were **sterile**! Disturbingly, this Russian study used the same GMO soy that is produced on over 90% of the soy acreage in the USA.

Back in 2005, Dr. Irina Ermakova (also with the Russian National Academy of Sciences) reported that over 50% of the babies from mother rats that were fed GMO soy died within three weeks. She wanted to perform further studies to analyze the organs she'd collected from the study, but she never got the chance. According to Jeffrey Smith (author of the bestselling book, Seeds of Deception *and* Genetic Roulette*): "She told me as we were sitting at the EU Parliament after giving a presentation there, that her boss had been pressured by his boss. So, she was told to do no more GMO food study on animals, her documents were burned on her desk, samples were stolen from her laboratory, and one of her colleagues tried to comfort her by saying, 'Well maybe the GM soy will solve the overpopulation problem on earth.' She wasn't impressed."* http://articles.mercola.com

In the only human "feeding" study ever published on GMO, seven volunteers ate so-called "Roundup-ready" soybeans (*i.e.*, soybeans that have herbicide-resistant genes inserted into them in order to survive being sprayed with otherwise deadly doses of Roundup herbicide). In three of the seven volunteers, the gene inserted into the soy transferred into the DNA of their intestinal bacteria, and continued to function long after they stopped eating the GMO soy! Imagine your digestive tract turned into a "Roundup factory" and other distorted genetic signals gradually and progressively rotting away your health. One of the primary functions of the liver is detoxification. Mice and rats fed GMO soy had profound changes in their livers. In some cases, livers were smaller and partially atrophied. Some were significantly heavier and inflamed.

"TERMINATOR TECHNOLOGY"

Since the early 1980s, the US government and companies like Monsanto have quietly been working to perfect a GMO technique whereby farmers would be forced to turn to their seed supplier each harvest to get new seeds. The seeds would only produce one harvest. After that the seeds from that harvest would "commit suicide" and be unusable.

This is referred to as "terminator technology" (aka Genetic Use Restriction Technology or "GURT"). This is a major violation of the rights of farmers to save and reuse their own seeds. And through pollen movement, in the first generation, terminator genes could "cross contaminate" farmers' crops. Escaped genes from GMO plants are causing cross contamination and pose threats to agricultural biodiversity and the livelihoods of farmers. Not surprisingly, Monsanto acquired Delta & Pine Land (DPL), the world's largest cotton seed company, which jointly holds three US patents on "terminator technology" with the USDA.

GURTs are a threat to the food security as well of North America, Western Europe, Japan and anywhere Monsanto and its elite cartel of GMO agribusiness partners enters a market.Rafael Alegría of Via Campesina (an organization representing over 10 million peasant farmers worldwide) asserts: *"Terminator is a direct assault on farmers and indigenous cultures and on food sovereignty. It threatens the well-being of all rural people, primarily the very poorest."*

GURTs are the answer to Big Agra's dream of controlling world food production. No longer would they need to hire expensive detectives to spy on whether farmers were reusing Monsanto or other GMO patented seed. Terminator corn or soybeans or cotton seeds could be genetically modified to "commit suicide" after one harvest season. In the words of Henry Kissinger, *"Control the food and you control the people."*

This technology could potentially wipe out food on the planet in one season. Food can be used as a weapon. Supreme Court Justice Scalia has made remarks that cross-contamination isn't *"the end of the world."* Well, he may be right, but it may be the end of America.

FEEDING THE WORLD?

In the past two decades, GMO have completely infiltrated our farm fields, grocery stores, and kitchens to such an extent that most folks have no idea how many GMO they actually consume daily. If you ingest processed foods, bread, pasta, crackers, cake mixes, canola oil, mayonnaise, soymilk, veggie burgers, corn tortillas, corn chips, corn oil, corn syrup, or anything else made from corn, soy, or cotton, you are usually consuming GMO. The first GMO food hit the market in 1994 (the "Flavr Savr" tomato). Since then, sugar beets, potatoes, corn, squash, rice, soybeans, vegetable oils and animal feed have all been manipulated. Each year, American farmers plant over 200 million acres of GMO crops. It is estimated that each person in the USA eats about 200 pounds of GMO foods per year!

But, hey, at least the GMO crops produce higher yields so we can "feed the world" right? **Think again.** In a 2013 study funded by the USDA, University of Wisconsin researchers refuted the "higher yield" argument for GMO. The researchers looked at data from that compared crop yields from various varieties of GMO corn between 1990 and 2010. While some GMO varieties delivered small yield gains, others did not. With the exception of one commonly used trait, the authors concluded, "*we were surprised **not** to find strongly positive transgenic yield effects.*" Please allow me to translate: Both the glyphosate-tolerant (Roundup® Ready) and the Bt toxin (for corn rootworm) caused yields to drop. That's right. They found that GMO crops produce **less** rather than more food!

In an article from the Cornucopia website, Maria Rodale cites a number of independent studies that point to the dangers of GMO. One study she cites, taken from a journal entitled *Nature Biotechnology*, states "*after we eat GMO soy, some of the GMO genes are transferred to the microflora of our intestines and those GMO genes are still active.*" She goes on to state that a study found in the journal *Reproductive Toxicology*, "*found Bt-toxin (used in genetically modified Bt corn) in the blood of 93% of the pregnant women studied and their babies.*"

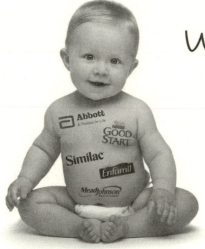

Who's making your baby a lab rat?

Our babies deserve better than GMOs

GMO INSIDE

C'MON ... BE FAIR

Am I being fair? Only giving one side of the story? God forbid! So let's check out Monsanto's own website and see what they say about GMO. After all, they are one of the largest producers of GMO. On their website (www.Monsanto.com), they refer to "*a large body of documented scientific testing showing currently authorized GM crops safe"* through a body called the Center for Environmental Risk Assessment (CERA). They were even kind enough to give a link to CERA's website. Thanks Monsanto!

So, when I visited the CERA website (www.CERA-gmc.org), I found a list of people who make up the Advisory Council for CERA, which their website says *"is to act in an advisory and consultative capacity for CERA's Director and staff."* One of the members of this advisory council is Dr. Jerry Hjelle, Ph.D. Take a guess as to whom he works for. Can you guess? C'mon. Take a guess. Yep. **Monsanto!** Dr. Hjelle is Monsanto's VP for Science Policy. So, let me get this straight. One of the advisors for the organization that "researches" the safety of GMO also works for one of the largest companies that manufacture GMO. Are you kidding me? This takes *"the fox is guarding the henhouse"* to another level!

Of course, this is pretty typical with Monsanto. As a matter of fact, because of Monsanto, the only "testing" for safety that is required is for the GMO producer to submit a self-authored report on the safety of the new GMO. This scam was devised by Michael Taylor, a former FDA lawyer who established the "no testing" policy by reasoning that GMO are "substantially equivalent" to food, and food has already been determined to be safe. Taylor (second cousin to Tipper Gore) is notorious for his "revolving door" employment within the US government and Monsanto and was chosen by Obama as the FDA Deputy Commissioner for foods (aka the "food safety czar") in July 2009. While at Monsanto, Taylor's main responsibility was gaining regulatory approval of the GMO cancer-causing bovine growth hormone (rBGH).

And then we have Margaret Miller, a former Monsanto researcher who wrote a report on whether rBGH was safe. Soon after the report was completed, the FDA came knocking on her door. *"Maggie, how would you like a job?"* they asked. Miller was hired by the FDA as the Deputy Director of the Office of New Animal Drugs. Can you take a guess at what her first "job" at the FDA was? Yes indeed, her first job was to "approve" the very report that she authored while at Monsanto. Effectively, in the area of American food safety, we now have the "fox" guarding the "henhouse."

I'm shocked! (Not really.) Especially in light of the fact that Monsanto is the same company that manufactured DDT, Agent Orange, PCB, and dioxin. Cancer is being linked to PCB exposure. Thousands of US soldiers as well as Vietnamese civilians have cancer because of being exposed to Agent Orange during Vietnam. These people are suffering the horrible consequences of this chemical being sprayed in the jungles, leaching toxic and deadly chemicals into the water, soil and the air.

Children are being born with birth defects, and thousands are dying of cancer caused by the exposure. The controlled mainstream media and Medical Mafia have both participated in many cover-ups and lies about the toxic effects of these chemicals. But hey, what do you expect? Many of them are criminals! And the mainstream media has long since been "bought and paid for" by the banksters that own the Fed.

Even though 93% of Americans believe that GMO should be labeled, proponents of GMO labeling are facing a bruising "food fight," given that the Big Agra and the biotech industry have spent massive amounts of money to combat prior GMO-labeling proposals. For example, California's "Proposition 37" was narrowly defeated in 2012 after companies such as Monsanto, Pepsico, and Kraft poured $46 million into lobbying against it. Then, in 2013, the same companies spent over $27 million into lobbying against Washington's "Initiative 522," which was also defeated. So this begs the question: If GMO are so "good for you," then why is Big Agra spending tens of millions of dollars to keep us in the dark about whether or not GMO are on our dinner plate or in our kids' lunchboxes?

GMO "TESTING"

As I previously mentioned, they have not been adequately tested. One of the most glaring faults in the current regulatory GMO "testing" regime is the short duration of animals feeding studies. The industry limits trials to 90 days at most, with some less than a month. Short studies could easily miss many serious effects of GMO. It is well established that some pesticides and drugs, for example, can create effects that are passed on through generations, only showing up decades later. Nearly all GMO crops are described as "pesticide plants" because they either tolerate doses of weed killer (such as Roundup®), or produce an insecticide like Bt toxin. When regulators evaluate the toxic effects of pesticides, they typically require studies using three types of animals, with at least one feeding trial lasting 2 years or more. Typically, at least 1/3 (or more) of the side effects produced by these toxins will show up *only* in the longer study and *not* the shorter ones.

Case in point: Scientists in France, led by Séralini (mentioned earlier) of the University of Caen, recently conducted feeding tests in rats over a period of two years. They fed the animals GMO corn sprayed with Roundup®. In the late summer of 2012, I remember when the results of the study (along with the photos of the rats with grotesque tumors) were published in the journal *Food and Chemical Toxicology*. Some of the tumors were so large the rats even had difficulty breathing. The authors stated: "*Scientists found that rats exposed to even the smallest amounts, developed mammary tumors and severe liver and kidney* *damage as early as four months in males, and seven months for females ... the animals on the GM diet suffered mammary tumors, as well as severe liver and kidney damage."* According to Dr. Michael Antoniou (molecular biologist), *"This research shows an extraordinary number of tumors developing earlier and more aggressively - particularly in female animals. I am shocked by the extreme negative health impacts."*

No, the Séralini study has not been debunked. Remember, any time you challenge mainstream dogma, you will be attacked. And so was Séralini. So let's debunk the debunkers, shall we? According to my friend Mike Adams ("the Health Ranger"), *"Not long after being published, Séralini's study was maliciously ripped apart by 'skeptics,' the media and many industry-backed institutions that claimed it was a badly-designed cancer study. But the truth is that Séralini's study was actually a chronic toxicity study, and one that met or exceeded all accepted scientific standards. ... The chorus of whining that ensued about how Séralini's study allegedly contradicted all other similar studies is also invalid, as no other similar studies have ever been conducted – Séralini's study is the only long-term study involving Monsanto's NK603 GM corn that has ever been conducted. Another popular criticism involves the Sprague-Dawley (SD) variety of rat used by Séralini in his study. This same variety has been used by Monsanto on many occasions in its 90-day 'safety' studies on GMO."*

Simply put, Séralini used the **same** type of rats and the **same** type of GMO corn that had been used in the previous Monsanto tests. The only difference was that, rather than pulling the plug at 90 days like Monsanto had done, Séralini continued the study for one year. And guess what. At between 120 and 150 days, the rats started developing tumors. Hmmm ... do you think Monsanto knew this might happen? Do you think this is why they always pulled the plug at 90 days?

Unbelievably, many people still don't want to know the truth about GMO. I suppose they'd rather live in their dreamland in the sand than believe the studies. So, if you're one of those folks who still want your GMO, please ... don't listen to me. Don't listen to Séralini. Don't listen to Mike Adams or Liam Scheff or Robert Scott Bell or Dr. Joseph Mercola or Jeffrey Smith. The solution is to educate your family, educate friends, and especially educating farmers is crucial. The easiest way to avoid ending up with GMO foods in your shopping cart is to do some pre-planning using the free non-GMO shopping guide, available at the following website: www.NonGMOshoppingGuide.com.

Thanks to Jeffrey Smith, the world's most staunch fighter and exposer of GMO, who developed this free guide. You can find boat loads of information about GMO at www.ResponsibleTechnology.org.

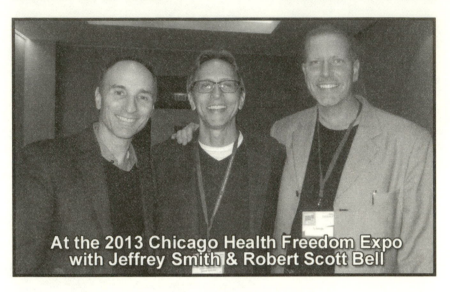

At the 2013 Chicago Health Freedom Expo with Jeffrey Smith & Robert Scott Bell

As a general rule, you should avoid products made with any of the crops that are GMO, such as:

> CORN – corn flour, meal, oil, starch, gluten, and syrup
> SOY – soy flour, lecithin, protein isolate, and isoflavones
> CANOLA – canola oil (aka rapeseed oil)
> COTTON – cottonseed oil
> SUGAR – avoid anything not listed as 100% cane sugar, evaporated cane juice, or organic sugar
> PAPAYA – over 80% of papaya is GMO

Certified organic products are not allowed to contain any GMO. Therefore, when you purchase products labeled *"100% organic,"* *"organic,"* or *"made with organic ingredients,"* these products are completely non-GMO.

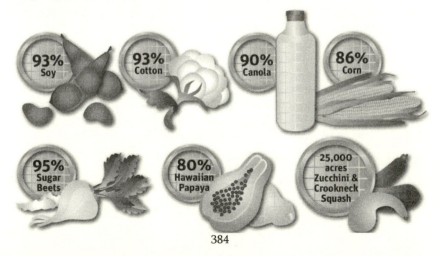

PART 4

FACTS

FICTIONS

&

FRAUDS

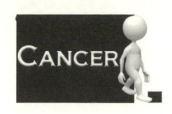
CHAPTER 15
ASPARTAME

FRAUD:
ASPARTAME HELPS YOU LOSE WEIGHT & HAS NO
NEGATIVE SIDE EFFECTS.

FACT:
ASPARTAME IS A NEUROTOXIN, HAS BEEN LINKED TO
BRAIN CANCER, GRAND MAL SEIZURES, AND SEVERAL
OTHER CENTRAL NERVOUS SYSTEM DISORDERS.

How about a diet soda? Diet sodas are harmless, right? Diet sodas will help you lose weight, right? **Wrong.** A worldwide epidemic is raging. The cause is a poisonous chemical sweetener called aspartame (marketed as NutraSweet®, Equal®, and AminoSweet®), which is the most controversial food additive ever approved. This additive, which we have been led to believe is completely safe, is in reality a drug which interacts with other drugs and changes brain chemistry and causes multiple types of chronic illness, including cancer.

I briefly mentioned aspartame a couple of times earlier in the book, but due to the fact that it is extremely toxic, the fact that it is an ingredient in so many foods and drinks, and the sordid history of how it obtained FDA approval, I have devoted an entire chapter of the book. As I mentioned, aspartame is an excitotoxin, which simply means that it excites your brain cells to death. Dr. Russell Blaylock states that *"the ingredients (in aspartame) stimulate the neurons of the brain to death causing brain damage of varying degrees."* (<u>Excitotoxins: The Taste that Kills</u>, 1994)

So what's in aspartame? Aspartame is made of three components, 50% phenylalanine, 40% aspartic acid, and 10% methanol (*wood alcohol*). The methanol is widely distributed throughout the body including brain, muscle, fat and nervous tissue. This is important: when the temperature of aspartame exceeds 86° Fahrenheit, the methanol coverts to formaldehyde (embalming fluid) and formic acid. What is the normal body temperature again? If I remember correctly, it's 98.6°, isn't it? So, when you ingest aspartame, it heats up above 86° and the methanol turns to formaldehyde, which enters the cells and binds to the proteins and DNA.

Phenylalanine is an amino acid typically found in the brain. Persons with the hereditary disorder phenylketonuria (PKU) are unable to metabolize phenylalanine. This results in dangerously high levels of phenylalanine in the brain, which is sometimes fatal. It has been shown that ingesting aspartame (especially along with carbohydrates) can lead to excess levels of phenylalanine in the brain even in persons who do not have PKU. In his testimony before the US Congress, Dr. Louis J. Elsas showed that high blood phenylalanine can be concentrated in parts of the brain and is especially dangerous for infants and fetuses. He also indicated that since it is metabolized much more efficiently by rodents than humans, testing and research on rats alone is not sufficient enough to denounce the dangers of aspartame for human consumption. Phenylalanine also depletes serotonin; thus, it triggers all kinds of psychiatric and behavioral problems, including depression. I have heard it said that many mental institutions are full of patients who are nothing but aspartame victims. Remember the character Marty McFly in "Back to the Future"? Were it not for the phenylalanine in aspartame, which interferes with the brain's uptake of L-Dopa, Michael J. Fox, a former Diet Pepsi spokesman, would likely never have been diagnosed with Parkinson's disease at age 30. It's very possible that he would be healthy today and still making movies ("*Back to the Future Part 27*") were it not for his consumption of Diet Pepsi.

Aspartic acid is also a component of aspartame. My friend, Dr. Russell L. Blaylock, MD, a professor of neurosurgery at the Medical University of Mississippi, recently published a book thoroughly detailing the damage that is caused by the ingestion of excessive aspartic acid from aspartame. Dr. Blaylock makes use of almost 500 scientific references to show how excess free excitatory amino acids such as aspartic acid and glutamic acid (about 99% of MSG is glutamic acid) in our food supply are causing serious chronic neurological disorders and a myriad of other acute symptoms. Much like nitrates and MSG, aspartic acid can cause amino acid imbalances in the body and result in the interruption of normal neurotransmitter metabolism of the brain.

Methanol (wood alcohol) is a toxic poison. Some people may remember methanol as the poison that has caused some "skid row" alcoholics to end up blind or dead. Methanol is gradually released in the small intestine when the methyl group of aspartame encounters the enzyme chymotrypsin. Methanol breaks down into formic acid and formaldehyde ("embalming fluid") in the body. According to the EPA, methanol *"is considered a cumulative poison due to the low rate of excretion once it is absorbed. In the body, methanol is oxidized to formaldehyde and formic acid; both of these metabolites are toxic."*

The EPA's recommended limit of consumption of methanol is 7.8 milligrams per day, but a one liter bottle of a beverage containing aspartame contains over 50 mg of methanol. How many folks do you know that drink a liter of soda pop each day? Heck, I know folks who drink 2 or 3 liters per day! According to a 1990 report by Kathleen Nauss and Robert Kavet entitled, *"The Toxicity of Inhaled Methanol Vapors"* (published in *Critical Reviews in Toxicology*), chronic, low-level exposure to methanol has been seen to cause headaches, dizziness, nausea, memory lapses, blurred vision, ear buzzing, gastrointestinal issues, weakness, vertigo, chills, numbness, behavioral disturbances, insomnia, neuritis, tunnel vision, depression, heart problems, and pancreatic inflammation.

But don't many fruits and vegetables contain some methanol? Yes, they do, but they also contain a large amount of ethanol, which acts as a buffer and neutralizes methanol, thus preventing the conversion of methanol to formaldehyde. In aspartame, there is no such buffer.

Diketopiperazine (DKP) is a byproduct of aspartame metabolism and has been implicated in the occurrence of brain tumors. G.D. Searle conducted animal experiments on the safety of DKP. The FDA found numerous experimental errors occurred, including *"clerical errors, mixed-up animals, animals not getting drugs they were supposed to get, pathological specimens lost because of improper handling,"* and many other errors. These sloppy laboratory procedures may explain why both the test and control animals had 16 times more brain tumors than would be expected in experiments of this length.

Aspartame was accidentally discovered in 1965 by James Schlatter, a chemist at G.D. Searle Company (Searle), who licked some of a new ulcer drug from his fingers and discovered the sweet taste of aspartame. **Eureka!** Selling this chemical as a food additive to hundreds of millions of healthy people every day would mean many more dollars than limited sales to the much smaller group of ulcer sufferers. So, in 1967, Searle began the safety tests on aspartame which were necessary for applying for FDA approval of food additives. Early tests of the substance showed it produced microscopic holes and tumors in the brains of experimental mice, epileptic seizures in monkeys, and was converted by animals into hazardous substances, including formaldehyde.

In 1969, Searle hired Dr. Harold Waisman, a biochemist at the University of Wisconsin, to conduct aspartame safety tests on seven infant monkeys, who were fed aspartame mixed with milk. After 300 days, five of the monkeys had grand mal seizures and one died. (Remember the sprinter, Flo Jo, who drank Diet Coke and died of a grand mal seizure?) Dr. Waisman died before all of his studies were completed. In the spring of 1971, Dr. John Olney (a neuroscientist) informed Searle that his studies showed that aspartame caused holes in the brains of infant mice. Later that year, one of Searle's own researchers confirmed Dr. Olney's findings in a similar study. But Searle didn't care...they were after their cash cow!

In 1973, Searle applied for FDA approval and submitted over 100 studies they **claimed** supported the safety of aspartame. One of the first FDA scientists to review the aspartame safety data stated that *"the information provided (by Searle) is inadequate to permit an evaluation of the potential toxicity of aspartame."* According to the late Dr. Andrian Gross, Searle *"...took great pains to camouflage these shortcomings of the study. As I say filter and just present to the FDA what they wished the FDA to know, and they did other terrible things. For instance, animals would develop tumors while they were under study. Well, they would remove these tumors from the animals."* Nevertheless, on July 26, 1974, the FDA approved aspartame for limited use in dry foods, making available to the public for the first time the data supporting their decision. This data was subsequently reviewed by renowned brain researcher John Olney from Washington University in St. Louis, who filed the first objection against aspartame's approval.

Two years later in 1976, triggered by Olney's objection, the FDA began an investigation of Searle's laboratory practices. The investigation found their testing procedures shoddy, full of inaccuracies and *"manipulated"* test data. The investigators reported that they *"had never seen anything as bad as Searle's testing."* Then in 1977, a governmental task force uncovered that Searle had falsified data by submitting inaccurate blood tests. In another study, a closer look revealed that uterine tumors had developed in many of the test animals, and Searle admitted that these tumors were related to the ingestion of aspartame. The FDA formally requested that the U.S. Attorney's office begin grand jury proceedings to investigate whether indictments should be filed against Searle for knowingly misrepresenting findings and *"concealing material facts and making false statements"* in aspartame safety tests.

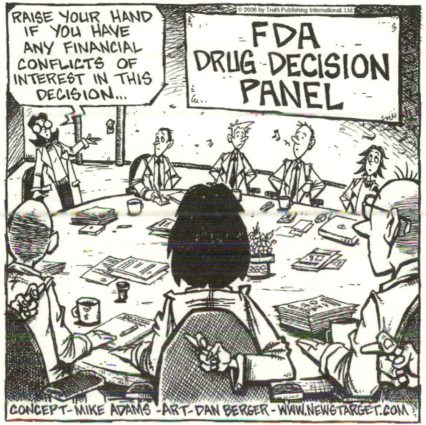

Thanks to Mike Adams and *www.NaturalNews.com* for the cartoon above.

While the grand jury probe was underway, Sidley & Austin, the law firm representing Searle, began job negotiations with the U.S. Attorney in charge of the investigation, Samuel Skinner. In July 1977, Skinner resigned and took a job with Searle's law firm. The resignation of Skinner stalled the grand jury investigation for so long that the statute of limitations lapsed. Eventually, the grand jury investigation was dropped.

In 1979, the FDA established a Public Board of Inquiry (PBOI) to rule on safety issues surrounding aspartame. A year later, the PBOI concluded that aspartame should not be approved pending further investigations of brain tumors in animals, and based on its limited review, the PBOI blocked aspartame marketing until the tumor studies could be explained. Unless the FDA commissioner overruled the board, the matter was closed. But in 1980, Ronald Reagan was elected President of the United States, and his transition team included Donald Rumsfeld, CEO of G. D. Searle. According to a former G.D. Searle salesperson, Patty Wood-Allott, Rumsfeld told his sales force that, if necessary, "*he would call in all his markers and that no matter what, he would see to it that aspartame would be approved that year.*" (Gordon 1987, page 499 of U.S. Senate, 1987) Not surprisingly, the transition team picked Dr. Arthur Hull Hayes Jr. to be the new FDA Commissioner. Hayes was widely profiled as a man who believed that approval for new drugs and additives was too slow because "*the FDA demanded too much information.*"

In May of 1981, three of six in-house FDA scientists who were responsible for reviewing the brain tumor issues advised against approval of aspartame, stating on the record that the Searle tests were unreliable and not adequate to determine the safety of aspartame. However, in July of that same year, in one of his first official acts, Dr. Hayes, the new FDA commissioner, overruled the PBOI and officially approved aspartame for all dry products. In 1982, Searle filed a petition that aspartame be approved as a sweetener in carbonated beverages and other liquids.

Almost immediately, the National Soft Drink Association *(NSDA)* urged the FDA to delay approval of aspartame for carbonated beverages pending further testing because aspartame is very unstable in liquid form. As I have already mentioned, when liquid aspartame is stored in temperatures above 86° Fahrenheit, it breaks down into formic acid and formaldehyde, both of which are known toxins. Despite the public outcry, in 1983, the FDA approved aspartame for soft drinks and the first carbonated beverages containing aspartame were sold for public consumption.

Shortly after aspartame was approved for beverages, complaints began to arrive at the FDA. Reactions such as dizziness, blurred vision, memory loss, slurred speech, headaches, and seizures were common with consumption of drinks containing aspartame. The complaints were more serious than the agency had ever received on any food additive. In just the first several years after aspartame was approved for beverages, the FDA received over 10,000 complaints about aspartame. In February of 1994, the U.S. Department of Health and Human Services released the listing of adverse reactions reported to the FDA. Amazingly, aspartame accounted for more than 75% of all adverse reactions reported to the FDA's Adverse Reaction Monitoring System. By the FDA's own admission, fewer than 1% of consumers who have adverse reactions to products ever report it to the FDA. This balloons the 10,000 complaints to around a million!

In 1985, Dr. Adrian Gross told Congress that because aspartame was capable of producing brain tumors and brain cancer, the FDA should not have been able to set an "allowable" daily intake of the substance at any level. His last words to Congress were, *"And if the FDA violates its own law, who is left to protect the public?"* (August 1, 1985, *Congressional Record*, SID835:131)

From 1985 to 1995, researchers did about 400 aspartame studies. Dr. Ralph G. Walton reviewed all the studies on aspartame and found 166 with relevance for human safety. Of those 166 studies, 74 were funded by Searle, 85 were independent, and 7 were funded by the FDA. The results will amaze you, but probably won't surprise you. Of the 74 studies funded by Searle, all of them gave aspartame a clean bill of health. However, of the 85 studies that were **not** funded by Big Pharma or the FDA, 84 of them found aspartame to be dangerous to one's health. These studies reported a range of side effects including fibromyalgia, brain tumors, memory loss, lymphoma, leukemia, and peripheral nerve cancer.

In the most comprehensive, longest-ever running study on aspartame as a human carcinogen (over two million person-years), researchers analyzed data from the Nurses' Health Study and the Health Professionals Follow-Up Study for a 22-year period. This landmark study was published in late 2012. Over 77,000 women and over 47,000 men were included in the analysis, for a total of almost 2.3 million person-years of data. Apart from sheer size, what makes this study superior to other past studies is the thoroughness with which aspartame intake was assessed. Every two years, participants were given a detailed dietary questionnaire, and their diets were reassessed every four years. Previous studies which found no link to cancer only assessed participants' aspartame intake at one point in time, as opposed to every two years (for two decades) in this study.

The findings were alarming, so say the least. **One diet soda** a day increases leukemia risk by 42% (in men and women), multiple myeloma risk by 102% (men only), and non-Hodgkin lymphoma risk by 31% (men only).

A 2012 University of Miami study, which was published in the *Journal of General Internal Medicine*, admitted that drinking **one diet soda** a day increases the risk of heart attack and strokes by a whopping 44%. This was no small study. The research involved over 2,500 participants over a period of ten years. Of course, this has been known for decades and is discussed in Dr. H. J. Roberts, M.D.'s medical textbook, <u>Aspartame Disease: An Ignored Epidemic</u>. Are you still craving that diet soda now? How about a stick in the eye? Or better yet, how about eating a bag of feces? Why do I mention poop? Because the patent for aspartame is available online and it confirms that the sweetener is made from the waste (i.e. "poop") produced by genetically modified E. coli bacteria! Yuck!

As if being "fecal matter" weren't enough to turn your stomach, aspartame is also considered to be an "excitotoxin." Since humans lack a blood-brain barrier in the hypothalamus, excitotoxins are able to enter the brain and cause damage by reacting with specialized receptors (neurons) in such a way as to lead to the destruction of certain types of brain cells. In other words, they excite your brain cells to death! Aspartame accounts for over 75% of the adverse reactions to food additives reported to the FDA. Many of these reactions are very serious, including seizures and death.

The truth of the matter is that the FDA has always known aspartame is a carcinogen. The late Dr. Adrian Gross (FDA toxicologist) told Congress that without a shadow of a doubt aspartame triggers brain tumors and brain cancers and violates the Delaney Amendment which forbids putting anything in food you know will cause cancer. As Dr. James Bowen told the FDA, the manufacturers of aspartame have damaged a generation of children and should be criminally prosecuted for genocide for the mass poisoning of the USA and hundreds of other countries of the world.

In early 2010, aspartame producer Ajinomoto launched a new initiative to rebrand this toxic sweetener as "AminoSweet®," to remind us that it is made from amino acids, the building blocks of proteins. Oh, isn't that special? People will feel all warm and fuzzy and believe that it must be healthy. After all, amino acids are good, aren't they?

Don't fall for the slick marketing ploy. This is deception at its finest: Begin with a shred of truth, and then "spin it" to fit your own agenda, which in this case appears to be to convince us that this is just a "healthy sweetener" made from amino acids which are already present in our bodies. But whether you call it NutraSweet® or Equal® or AminoSweet®, the aspartic acid in aspartame is a well-documented "excitotoxin." And as I mentioned previously, aspartame was once on a Pentagon list of biowarfare chemicals submitted to Congress!

Truth be told, aspartame triggers every kind of birth defect from autism to cleft palate, and it is also an "abortifacient," which is defined as a drug that induces abortion. It's normal for young girls to look forward to marriage and children. However, many young girls sip on diet soda not realizing that aspartame is an endocrine disrupting agent which changes the menstrual flow and causes infertility. Sadly, many ladies who grew up drinking diet soda never know why they were unable to have children. And if that's not enough reasons to avoid aspartame, studies have shown that aspartame is toxic to the liver, makes you crave carbohydrates, precipitates diabetes, and actually makes you gain weight! www.mpwhi.com

So, when the FDA tells us that aspartame has been proven to be safe, rest assured that it is basing its findings on the fraudulent Searle studies (*i.e.,* they are "lying through their teeth"). Then, when the *JAMA*, examining the FDA findings (which are based on the fraudulent Searle studies), announces that "*the consumption of aspartame poses no health risk for most people,*" don't believe it!

Aspartame kills.

I highly recommend that you watch "Sweet Misery" (a documentary on aspartame). You can see the trailer and the first five minutes here: http://aspartamekills.com. Despite the fact that the FDA claims that aspartame is safe, the toxic effects of aspartame are documented by the FDA's own data. In 1995, the FDA was forced, under the Freedom of Information Act, to release a list of 92 aspartame symptoms reported by thousands of victims. It appears this is only the tip of the iceberg. Dr. H. J. Roberts published the medical text "*Aspartame Disease: An Ignored Epidemic*" which contains over 1,000 pages of symptoms and diseases triggered by this excitotoxin, including the sordid history of its approval.

Oh yes, I almost forgot the "icing on the corruption cake." In 1985, G.D. Searle was absorbed by Monsanto. Donald Rumsfeld reportedly received a $12 million bonus. Who said that the wicked never prosper?

Got a sweet tooth? I recommend stevia, an herbal sweetener, as a healthy alternative.

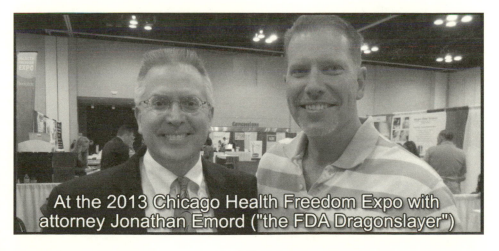
At the 2013 Chicago Health Freedom Expo with attorney Jonathan Emord ("the FDA Dragonslayer")

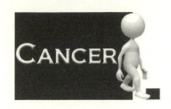

CHAPTER 16

FLUORIDE

> ## FRAUD:
> FLUORIDE IS A HARMLESS ADDITIVE FOUND IN
> TOOTHPASTE AND OUR WATER SUPPLY. IT PREVENTS
> CAVITIES, HELPS MAINTAIN HEALTHY TEETH, AND IS AN
> ESSENTIAL MINERAL.
>
> ## FACT:
> FLUORIDE IS A CUMULATIVE TOXIC WASTE, BANNED IN
> AT LEAST 13 COUNTRIES. FLUORIDE CAN CAUSE BIRTH
> DEFECTS, CANCER, OSTEOPOROSIS, AND MULTIPLE
> OTHER HEALTH PROBLEMS.

There's nothing like a glass of cool, clear water to quench your thirst. But the next time you turn on the tap, you might want to question whether that water is in fact, too toxic to drink. If your water is fluoridated, the answer is likely "**yes**." For decades, we have been told a lie, a lie that has led to the deaths of hundreds of thousands of Americans and the weakening of the immune systems of tens of millions more. **This lie is called fluoridation**. A process we were led to believe was a safe and effective method of protecting teeth from decay is in fact a fraud. In the words of Dr. Robert Carton, former scientist for the EPA, "*Fluoridation is the greatest case of scientific fraud of this century, if not of all time.*"

WHAT IS FLUORIDE?

Fluoride is any combination of elements containing the fluoride ion. In its elemental form, fluorine is a pale yellow, highly toxic and corrosive gas. In nature, fluorine is found combined with minerals as "fluorides."

Fluorine compounds ("fluorides") are listed by the US Agency for Toxic Substances and Disease Registry as among the top 20 of 275 substances that pose the most significant threat to human health. They are cumulative toxins.

The fact that fluorides accumulate in the body is the reason that US law requires the Surgeon General to set a "maximum contaminant level" (MCL) for fluoride content in public water supplies as determined by the EPA. It boggles my mind that thousands of brainwashed dentists proudly proclaim fluoride to be the "wonder nutrient" that prevents cavities and promotes healthy teeth and gums. Let me ask you a question. How can a toxic waste product and a cumulative toxin be described as a "nutrient?"

It is well-known that fluoride prevents iodine absorption and causes thyroid disorders. Did you know that endemic "dental fluorosis" areas have been shown to be the same as those affected with iodine deficiency? Iodine deficiency causes brain disorders, miscarriages and goiter, among many other diseases.

FLUORIDE'S SORDID HISTORY

What if you found out that fluoride is a neurotoxic industrial waste? What if you found out that it damages the immune, digestive, and respiratory systems as well as the kidneys, liver, brain, and thyroid? What if you discovered that there is no scientific evidence that fluoride is a beneficial additive to water, and in fact that there is overwhelming scientific evidence that proves, without a doubt, that fluoride is harmful? What if you found out that all federal health agencies have known these facts for years, but have been controlled by the political interests of the nuclear arms, aluminum, and phosphate manufacturers to keep it a secret?

The fluoridation of our public water is something that has been highly debated for decades, yet the practice continues today, despite strong evidence which indicates that fluoridation causes human suffering and disease. The history of water fluoridation goes back almost 90 years. In the 1920s, aluminum manufacturing, due largely to the thriving canning industry, was booming. But it was also a big producer of toxic fluoride waste. The biggest dilemma was the cost to safely dispose of this hazardous waste, since it was extremely expensive. A company in Pittsburgh, ALCOA, had some revolutionary ideas on how to cut the costs of disposal. At that time, the U.S. Public Health Service (PHS) was under the jurisdiction of Treasury Secretary Andrew W. Mellon, who just happened to be the founder and major stockholder of ALCOA.

In 1931, a PHS dentist named H. Trendley Dean (aka the "father of fluoridation") was dispatched to over 300 small towns in Texas where water wells contained high concentrations of fluoride, which was most likely calcium fluoride (CaF_2). His mission was to determine how much fluoride people could tolerate without sustaining obvious damage to their teeth. What he found was startling: teeth in these high-fluoride towns were often discolored and mottled. However, he also theorized that there *"appeared to be"* a lower incidence of cavities in communities having about one part per million (1 PPM) fluoride in the water.

Dean used a strategy called "selective use of data" to try to prove his theory. He chose to use the data from only 21 communities to "*back into his number.*" That's what we call it in the accounting world when you know the desired answer and use only numbers which will support your desired answer, and then you reach your predetermined conclusion. Dean totally disregarded the other 270+ localities that showed no correlation between fluoride and cavities. Later, in 1955, Dean admitted (under oath) that fluoride does **not** work as a remedy for tooth decay (*Fluoride*, Vol. 14, No. 3, July 1981). Then in 1957, he had to admit at AMA hearings that even water which contained a mere .1 (1/10th) PPM could **cause** dental fluorosis. Moreover, there has never been a single double-blind study to indicate that fluoridation is effective in reducing cavities. Not one!

But ALCOA didn't let the facts get in their way! ALCOA-funded scientist Gerald J. Cox learned of Dean's findings, and devised a way for ALCOA to actually profit from fluoride. He proposed that this "*apparently worthless by-product*" **might** reduce cavities in children (despite no evidence). He haughtily declared that fluoride was good for your teeth, and in 1939, he proposed that the USA should fluoridate its water supplies. That's right, not by a doctor, not by a dentist, but by a scientist who was working for the largest producer of fluoride in the entire USA.

The aluminum industry had already been marketing their toxic fluoride waste as an **insecticide** and **rat poison**, but they wanted a much larger market. But they had a minor roadblock. In the 1944 *Journal of the American Dental Association*, the ADA warned that "*the potentialities for harm (from fluoridation) far outweigh those for the good.*" In 1945, two Michigan cities were selected for an official "fifteen-year" comparison study to determine if fluoride could safely reduce cavities in children, and fluoride was pumped into the drinking water of Grand Rapids. In 1946, despite the fact that the official fifteen-year experiment in Michigan had barely begun, six more American cities were allowed to fluoridate their water. The two-city Michigan experiment was abandoned before it was half over, with the results "inconclusive." This is the only scientifically objective test of fluoridation's safety and benefits that was ever performed.

In 1947, Oscar R. Ewing, a long-time ALCOA lawyer, was appointed head of the Federal Security Agency, a position that placed him in charge of the PHS. Under Ewing, a national water fluoridation campaign began. The public relations strategist for the water fluoridation campaign was none other than Sigmund Freud's nephew Edwin L. Bernays, known as the "Father of Spin." Bernays pioneered the application of Freud's theories to advertising and government "half truths." In his book Propaganda, Bernays argued that scientific manipulation of public opinion is the key. He stated, *"A relatively small number of persons pull the wires which control the public mind."* The government's fluoridation campaign was one of his most enduring successes.

Bernays' techniques were simple. Pretend there is some favorable research by using phrases like *"Numerous studies have shown..."* or *"Research has proven..."* or *"Scientific investigators have found..."* but then never really cite anything (since they had zero scientific studies to cite). Say it long enough and loud enough, and eventually people will believe it. If anyone doubts or questions the lies, attack their character and/or their intellect. On a side note, a few years later, Bernays helped popularize the notion of women smoking cigarettes. Not being one to turn down a challenge, Bernays set up the advertising format which lasted for almost 50 years "proving" that cigarettes are "beneficial" to health.

Bernays never strayed from his fundamental axiom to *"control the masses without their knowing it."* He believed that the best brainwashing takes place when the people are unaware that they are being manipulated. So, under Bernays' spell, the popular image of this insecticide and rat poison was transformed into a beneficial provider of gleaming smiles, absolutely safe, and good for children. This was a brilliant marketing move by ALCOA! Rather than having to pay extremely high costs to safely dispose of this toxic waste, ALCOA (and other aluminum manufacturers) could now **sell it** to municipalities for a **huge profit!** Any opponents were quickly and permanently engraved on the public mind as crackpots, quacks, and lunatics.

"BAIT & SWITCH"

Calcium **fluor**ide (CaF_2), also known as fluorite, is found naturally in plants and water. However, the fluoride which is added to the water supply (and toothpaste) is not calcium fluoride. No, the water and toothpaste additive is either sodium **fluor**ide (NaF), hydro**fluor**osilicic acid (H_2SiF_6), or sodium silico**fluor**ide (Na_2SiF_6), all three of which are **toxic wastes.** Just because the substance contains the letters "*fluor*" doesn't mean that it's the same as naturally occurring calcium fluoride. But the Medical Mafia tells us that the fluoride in our water and toothpaste is good for us. You see, they pulled the classic "bait and switch" on us, relying on the American "sheeple" to believe anything they are told. Have you ever read the labels on your toothpaste? I suggest that you do so. The

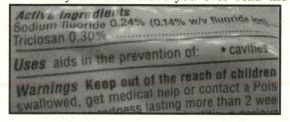

warning says to keep away from children. I wonder why. Perhaps it is because if an entire tube of toothpaste were ingested by a small child, the dosage would likely be **fatal**!

According to the CDC, the most common "fluoride" used in the US water supply is hydrofluorosilicic acid (63%), followed by sodium silicofluoride (28%) and sodium fluoride (9%). Hydrofluorosilicic acid is an EPA regulated toxic waste produced in the smoke-stacks of various industrial chemical producers. This form of "fluoride" represents such a health hazard that it is regulated by the EPA, and must be disposed of as a toxic waste. In other words, it is illegal to take this hydrofluorosilicic acid and bury it in the ground or dump it in rivers or streams in this country, but it is perfectly legal (even mandated) to sell it to municipalities that drip it into the water supply so that people will drink it. According to Dr. William Hirzy from the EPA, "*if it goes into the air, it's a pollutant. If it goes into the local water, it's pollution. But if the public water utilities buy it and pour it in our drinking water, it's no longer a pollutant. All of a sudden like magic it's a beneficial public health measure.*"

Of course, what goes in must come out, so we eventually pass the fluoride (at least some of it) through our bodies and directly into the rivers and streams. Thus, it brings us to this bizarre reality of fluoridation: this environmentally hazardous, toxic substance is illegal to dump into rivers and streams, unless it passes through the bodies of human beings first, in which case it's not only perfectly legal, but it's actually mandated by dentists. Pretty weird, huh? Of course, these are the same people who are still putting mercury in our mouths, so what do you expect?

Fluoride is more toxic than lead, and there are more than 500 peer-reviewed studies documenting adverse effects of fluoride ranging from cancer to brain damage. Yet municipalities throughout the USA actually purchase this product and then drip it into the public water supply. Not only does fluoride **not** protect our teeth, but it has also been shown to cause dental fluorosis and lowered IQ. Numerous studies have shown that fluoride causes genetic damage at concentrations as low as one part per million. Can you guess what the average level of fluoridation is in our water supply? That's right...one part per million.

The first occurrence of fluoridated drinking water was found in Germany's concentration camps. The Gestapo had little concern about fluoride's supposed effect on children's teeth. Their alleged reason for mass-medicating water with sodium fluoride was to **sterilize** humans and **force** the people in their concentration camps into calm submission. (Joseph Borkin, <u>The Crime and Punishment of I.G. Farben</u>) Interesting to note, sodium fluoride is also one of the basic ingredients in both Prozac® (FLUoxetene Hydrochloride) and Sarin Nerve Gas (Isopropyl-Methyl-Phosphoryl FLUORIDE).

THE NAZI-CANCER-ALZHEIMER'S CONNECTION

Charles Elliot Perkins, research scientist sent by the U.S. government to take charge of the I.G. Farben drug/chemical plants in Germany, confirmed this fact when he discovered that *"the real purpose behind water fluoridation is to reduce the resistance of the masses to domination, control and loss of liberty."* In his report to the Lee Foundation for Nutritional Research in October of 1954, he said, *"Repeated doses of infinitesimal amounts of fluoride will in time reduce an individual's power to resist domination, by slowly poisoning and narcotizing a certain area of the brain, thus making him submissive to the will of those who wish to govern him."*

Some of the most harmful attributes of fluoride are that it inhibits enzyme activity, paralyzes white blood cells, and causes collagen to break down. Enzymes, the immune system's leukocytes, and collagen are all fundamental in fighting cancer. And all three are adversely affected by fluoride. Dr. John Yiamouyiannis, a biochemist and president of the Safe Water Foundation, was one of two researchers who first determined the fluoride-cancer link. Yiamouyiannis warns: *"Fluoride is a poison! . . . It has been used as a pesticide for mice, rats and other small pests. A 10-pound infant could be killed by 1/100 of an ounce, and a 100-pound adult could be killed by 1/10 of an ounce of fluoride. The Akron Regional Poison Center indicates that a 7-ounce tube of toothpaste contains 199 mg. of fluoride, more than enough to kill a 25-pound child."*

In 1977, epidemiological studies by Dr. Dean Burk, former head of the National Cancer Institute's cell chemistry section, and Dr. Yiamouyiannis showed that fluoridation is linked to about 10,000 cancer deaths yearly. According to Dr. Burk, *"Fluoride causes more human cancer, and causes it faster, than any other chemical."* (<u>Fluoride, The Aging Factor</u>, 1986)

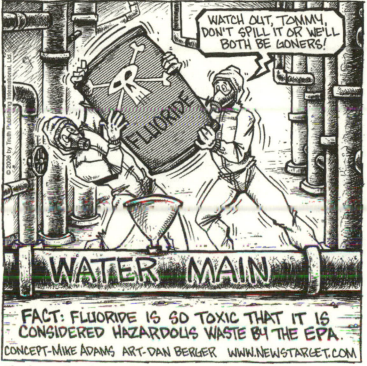

Thanks to Mike Adams and *www.NaturalNews.com* for the cartoon above.

Fluoride has also been linked to Alzheimer's disease, since the aluminum binds with fluoride to form aluminum fluoride, which is able to pass the blood-brain barrier. In January 1987, experiments performed at the Medical Research Endocrinology Department (Newcastle upon Tyne, England) and the Physics Dept of the University of Ruhana, Sri Lanka, showed that fluoridated water at one part per million (when used in cooking in aluminum cookware) concentrated the aluminum up to 600 times, whereas water without fluoride did not. (*Science News*, 131:73)

FLOURIDE "EXPERTS"

One of the things I find so interesting about this debate on fluoride is that dentists and doctors will leap to defend this practice at every opportunity. Why? Is it because there's good scientific evidence that fluoridation is somehow beneficial to the public? **NO**. It's because they've been told to support it by the Medical Mafia (specifically the AMA and ADA). All of this is so bizarre that a reasonable person can only conclude these doctors and dentists are operating on auto-pilot. They are parroting whatever "talking points" that they are given.

And to top it off, they are typically extremely arrogant about the whole thing. They act as if they are qualified to talk about this one single nutritional deficiency and its effects on the entire human body because they are dentists. In fact, dentists have no qualifications to talk about the effects of fluoride on the human nervous system, the blood supply, chronic disease, behavioral disorders, or other physiological effects. Dentists are really only qualified to talk about what's happening with your teeth – not drugs or chemicals that you ingest and that have a systemic effect. Neither are medical doctors qualified to talk about nutrition. As I've already mentioned, at best they have a few hours of education on nutrition and are largely illiterate about the relationship between nutritional deficiencies and chronic disease. The bottom line is that you have a whole group of so-called *"experts"* that know **nothing** about the subject, yet grandstand and claim to be the authorities on it.

FLOURIDE STUDIES

In the mid 1980s, the largest study ever conducted on fluoridation and tooth decay was performed, using data from 39,000 school children in 84 areas around the country. The results showed no statistically significant difference in rates of tooth decay between fluoridated and non-fluoridated cities. Surprised? I'm not. But that's not all. A 1989 study by the National Institute for Dental Research concluded that 12% of children living in areas artificially fluoridated (between one and four parts per million) developed dental fluorosis, which is a permanent discoloration and brittling of the teeth.

A 2005 Harvard School of Dental Health study found that fluoride in tap water directly contributes to osteosarcoma (bone cancer) in young boys; *"boys exposed to fluoride between the ages of five and 10 will suffer an increased rate of osteosarcoma – bone cancer – between the ages of 10 and 19,"* according to a *London Observer* article about the study. Interestingly, Harvard Professor Chester Douglass initially downplayed the connection, stating that there was *"no relationship."*

However, Douglass was investigated for scientific misconduct when it was discovered that he was, in fact, the editor-in-chief of *The Colgate Oral Health Report*, a quarterly newsletter funded by Colgate-Palmolive Company, which, by the way, just happens to make fluoridated toothpaste. Purely coincidence, I'm sure. No conflict of interest, there, right? Eventually, Douglass published a letter stating, *"We are also finding some positive associations between fluoride and osteosarcoma."* Wow, that's diametrically opposed from *"no relationship,"* isn't it? I guess he was forced to tell the truth once the bloodhounds were on his scent.

In early 2010, two separate stories out of India reveal that children are being blinded and crippled partly as a result of fluoride being artificially added to their drinking water. In the Indian village of Gaudiyan, well over half of the population has bone deformities, making them physically handicapped. Children are born normally, but after they start drinking the fluoridated water, they begin to develop crippling defects in their hands and feet.

"Due to the excess fluoride content in drinking water, the calcium intake is not absorbed in the body, causing disabilities and deformities," said Dr. Amit Shukla, a neurophysician. However, in a supercilious manner that would make the Medical Mafia proud, Indian government doctors have denied that fluoridation of drinking water has any connection to the disabilities and have refused to test the water, insisting such tests are *"not necessary."* Meanwhile, in the village of Pavagada, children are going blind after being diagnosed with Lamellar Congenital cataract (a condition wherein the eye lenses are damaged). The local doctors attribute the child blindness to two factors – consanguineous marriages and the "fluoride content" of the water. www.infowars.com/indian-children-blinded-crippled-by-fluoride-in-water

Quoting Albert Einstein's nephew, Dr. E.H. Bronner (a chemist who had also been a prisoner of war during World War II) in a letter printed in *The Catholic Mirror*, Springfield, MA, January 1952, excerpts follow, separated by ellipses: *"There is a sinister network of subversive agents, Godless 'intellectual' parasites, working in our country today whose ramifications grow more extensive, more successful and more alarming each new year and whose true objective is to demoralize, paralyze and destroy our great Republic – from within if they can, according to their plan – for their own possession. ...Fluoridation of our community water systems can well become their most subtle weapon for our sure physical and mental deterioration. ... As a research chemist of established standing, I built within the past 22 years, 3 American chemical plants and licensed 6 of my 53 patents. Based on my years of practical experience in the health-food and chemical field, let me warn: fluoridation of drinking water is criminal insanity, sure national suicide. Don't do it ... Even in small quantities, sodium fluoride is a deadly poison to which no effective antidote has been found. Every exterminator knows that it is the most efficient rat-killer ... Sodium fluoride is entirely different from organic calcium-fluoro-phosphate needed by our bodies and provided by nature, in*

God's great providence and love, to build and strengthen our bones and our teeth. This organic calcium-fluoro-phosphate, derived from proper foods, is an edible organic salt, insoluble in water and assimilable by the human body, whereas the non-organic sodium fluoride used in fluoridating water is instant poison to the body and fully water soluble. The body refuses to assimilate it."

Dr. Bronner continues, *"Careful, bonafide laboratory experimentation by conscientious, patriotic research chemists, and actual medical experience, have both revealed that instead of preserving or promoting 'dental health,' fluoridated drinking water destroys teeth, before adulthood and after, by the destructive mottling and other pathological conditions it actually causes in them, and also creates many other very grave pathological conditions in the internal organisms of bodies consuming it ... That any so-called 'doctors' would persuade a civilized nation to add voluntarily a **deadly poison** to its drinking water systems is unbelievable. It is the height of criminal insanity. ... Are our Civil Defense organizations and agencies awake to the perils of water poisoning by fluoridation? Its use has been recorded in other countries. Sodium fluoride water solutions are the cheapest and most effective rat killers known to chemists: colorless, odorless, tasteless; no antidote, no remedy, no hope: Instant and complete extermination of rats ... fluoridation of water systems can be slow national suicide, or quick national liquidation. It is criminal insanity – treason!"* www.rense.com/general79/hd3.htm

In 1950, despite no scientific evidence to support the use of fluoride in our public water supply, the US government officially endorsed fluoridation. Since then, over 75% of the nation's reservoirs have been fluoridated and 150,000 tons of toxic fluoride is pumped annually to keep them that way. On the flip side of the coin, despite pressure from brainwashed dentists, over 90% of Europe has rejected, banned, or stopped fluoridation due to environmental, health, legal, or ethical concerns.

On April 12, 2010, *Time* Magazine listed fluoride as one of the "Top Ten Common Household Toxins" and described fluoride as both *"neurotoxic and potentially tumorigenic if swallowed."* Truth be told, in almost every country in the world (including the USA), it's against the law to "mass medicate" an entire population with a substance that everyone admits is toxic. However, in the USA, we do it anyway...

In an illuminating article published on NaturalNews.com in September of 2013, Mike Adams revealed some shocking information about fluoride. There was a story published in UK's *The Independent* which was entitled, *"Revealed: Government let British company export nerve gas chemicals to Syria."* In the article, it was reported that *"The*

Government was accused of 'breathtaking laxity' in its arms controls last night after it emerged that officials authorised the export to Syria of two chemicals capable of being used to make a nerve agent such as sarin a year ago." What, exactly, are those two dangerous chemicals that need to be controlled via "arms control" regulations to prevent the manufacture of sarin gas? Well ... ummm ... they would be ... drum roll please ... **sodium fluoride** and potassium fluoride!

So, yes, it appears that we do indeed live in the "medical matrix, because the same toxic chemical (sodium fluoride) that is force fed to the US population in what the CDC and FDA refer to as a "public health victory" is openly and frequently referred to as a "chemical weapon" when sold to Syria. Mike Adams states: *"According to US Secretary of State John Kerry, any government "regime" that uses chemical weapons against its own people should be bombed / invaded / overthrown by a coalition of other United Nations members. By his own definition, then, the United States of America should now be invaded by the UN because the government uses a deadly chemical weapon – sodium fluoride – on its own people. By implication, then, John Kerry is now calling for the UN to bomb the USA. As the international media now confirms, **sodium fluoride is a chemical weapon**, and this chemical weapon is used against the American people every single day in the water supply, a favorite attack vector for terrorists."* Well said, Health Ranger!

What should you do to protect yourself from fluoride? First off, you should never use products that contain fluoride, such as fluoridated toothpaste or mouthwash. Also, don't purchase bottled water that has added fluoride in it. I think that's a ludicrous product to have on the shelves. And don't drink from the public water supply unless you have a good fluoride filter. Visit http://apps.nccd.cdc.gov/MWF/Index.asp to see if your water supply is being poisoned with deadly fluoride.

I highly recommend Christopher Bryson's book entitled <u>The Fluoride Deception</u>. In this book, Bryson (award winning journalist and former BBC producer) describes the entangled interests that existed in the 1940s and 1950s between the aluminum industry, the US nuclear weapons program, and the dental industry, which resulted in fluoride being declared not only safe, but *"beneficial to human health."* I also recommend the article "50 Reasons to Oppose Fluoridation" at www.fluoridealert.org/50reasons.htm.

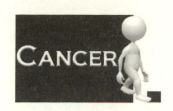
CHAPTER 17
VACCINATIONS

FRAUD:
VACCINATIONS ARE SAFE, EFFECTIVE, AND BASED ON SOUND SCIENTIFIC STUDIES & EVIDENCE, AND ARE RESPONSIBLE FOR THE DECREASE IN MANY INFECTIOUS DISEASES.

FACT:
VACCINATIONS ARE BASED ON FLAWED SCIENCE & FRAUDULENT DATA. THEY CAUSE DISEASE, DISABILITY, & EVEN DEATH. HYGIENE & SANITATION, NOT VACCINATIONS, HAVE RESULTED IN THE DECREASE OF NEARLY EVERY INFECTIOUS DISEASE OVER THE PAST CENTURY.

Don't vaccinations **prevent** disease? Aren't they safe and effective? Health authorities credit vaccines for disease declines and assure us of their safety and effectiveness. Yet these assumptions are directly contradicted by government statistics, published medical studies, FDA and CDC reports, and the opinions of credible research scientists from around the world.

Vaccines are the sacred cow of modern medicine, or as my friend, Robert Scott Bell, often declares, "*The Church of Biological Mysticism.*" The first vaccines (smallpox) were derived from pus and blood scraped from sores on cows and horses, then put on a lancet, scalpel, or needle, then jabbed into someone's arm. "*Blood and pus, anyone? How about some feces?*"

Do you think that it's a good idea to inject our bodies with blood and pus from infected animals? That's not only disgusting, it borders on insane. But that's where the modern practice of vaccination came from. And it's only gotten more repulsive and more insane since the smallpox vaccine.

The fact is that vaccines have emerged as one of the most sinister monumental myths ever fabricated by the modern Medical Mafia. The absurd ideas that vaccines protect you from infectious diseases and increase immunity are blatantly false. Health "authorities" credit vaccines for disease declines and assure us of their safety and effectiveness, yet these assurances are directly contradicted by government statistics, published medical studies, FDA and CDC reports, and the opinions of credible research scientists from around the world.

Now, for the nasty stuff. Vaccines must be "grown" in a "substrate," which simply means that it takes living tissue to grow the microscopic vaccine ingredients. So where do they get the living tissue? Lots of places. Animal brains, kidneys, blood, pus, testicles, and the likes. Yummy. Oh yes, and here's a real favorite with my Christian brothers and sisters – tissue from aborted babies. That's right! The government is allowing Big Pharma companies to sell vaccines which contain aborted fetal tissue. Have you ever wondered why abortion is so widely accepted and often encouraged? The abortion industry gets paid by Big Pharma and the government in exchange for deceased human beings in a syringe! **Question:** in light of this fact, how can you be a Christian who is both "pro-life" and "pro-vaccine"?

VACCINES & INFANT DEATH

An alarming medical study (recently published in a medical journal) has found a direct statistical link between higher vaccine doses and infant mortality rates. **Translation:** Vaccines Kill Infants! The study was conducted by Neil Z. Miller and Gary S. Goldman and was published in the reputable *Journal of Human and Experimental Toxicology*, which is indexed by the National Library of Medicine.

Who are the authors? According to his biography, *"Goldman has served as a reviewer for the Journal of the American Medical Association (JAMA), Vaccine, AJMC, ERV, ERD, JEADV,and British Medical Journal (BMJ). He is included on the Editorial Board of Research and Reviews in BioSciences."* Miller, a medical research journalist and the Director of the Thinktwice Global Vaccine Institute, has been studying the dangers of vaccines for 25 years.

The table on the top of the next page shows the countries with the lowest infant deaths at the top of the left side, while the countries with the lowest number of vaccines administered are at the top of the right side.

Table 1. 2009 Infant mortality rates, top 34 nations[8]

Rank	Country	IMR
1	Singapore	2.31
2	Sweden	2.75
3	Japan	2.79
4	Iceland	3.23
5	France	3.33
6	Finland	3.47
7	Norway	3.58
8	Malta	3.75
9	Andorra	3.76
10	Czech Republic	3.79
11	Germany	3.99
12	Switzerland	4.18
13	Spain	4.21
14	Israel	4.22
15	Liechtenstein	4.25
16	Slovenia	4.25
17	South Korea	4.26
18	Denmark	4.34
19	Austria	4.42
20	Belgium	4.44
21	Luxembourg	4.56
22	Netherlands	4.73
23	Australia	4.75
24	Portugal	4.78
25	United Kingdom	4.85
26	New Zealand	4.92
27	Monaco	5.00
28	Canada	5.04
29	Ireland	5.05
30	Greece	5.16
31	Italy	5.51
32	San Marino	5.53
33	Cuba	5.82
34	United States	6.22

Table 2. Summary of International Immunization Schedules: vaccines recommended/required prior 34 nations

Nation	Vaccines prior to one year of age	Total[b] doses
Sweden	DTaP (2), Polio (2), Hib (2), Pneumo (2)	12
Japan	DTaP (3), Polio (2), BCG	
Iceland	DTaP (2), Polio (2), Hib (2), MenC (2)	12
Norway	DTaP (2), Polio (2), Hib (2), Pneumo (2)	12
Denmark	DTaP (2), Polio (2), Hib (2), Pneumo (2)	12
Finland	DTaP (2), Polio (2), Hib (2), Rota (3)	13
Malta	DTaP (3), Polio (3), Hib (3)	15
Slovenia	DTaP (3), Polio (3), Hib (3)	15
South Korea	DTaP (3), Polio (3), HepB (3)	15
Singapore	DTaP (3), Polio (3), HepB (3), BCG, Flu	17
New Zealand	DTaP (3), Polio (3), Hib (2), HepB (3)	17
Germany	DTaP (3), Polio (3), Hib (3), Pneumo (3)	18
Switzerland	DTaP (3), Polio (3), Hib (3), Pneumo (3)	18
Israel	DTaP (3), Polio (3), Hib (3), HepB (3)	18
Liechtenstein[a]	DTaP (3), Polio (3), Hib (3), Pneumo (3)	18
Italy	DTaP (3), Polio (3), Hib (3), HepB (3)	18
San Marino[a]	DTaP (3), Polio (3), Hib (3), HepB (3)	18
France	DTaP (3), Polio (3), Hib (3), Pneumo (2), HepB (2)	19
Czech Republic	DTaP (3), Polio (3), Hib (3), HepB (3), BCG	19
Belgium	DTaP (3), Polio (3), Hib (3), HepB (3), Pneumo (2)	19
United Kingdom	DTaP (3), Polio (3), Hib (3), Pneumo (2), MenC (2)	19
Spain	DTaP (3), Polio (3), Hib (3), HepB (3), MenC (2)	20
Portugal	DTaP (3), Polio (3), Hib (3), HepB (3), MenC (2), BCG	21
Luxembourg	DTaP (3, Polio (3), Hib (3), HepB (2), Pneumo (3), Rota (3)	22
Cuba	DTaP (3), Polio (3), Hib (3), HepB (4), MenBC (2), BCG	22
Andorra[a]	DTaP (3), Polio (3), Hib (3), HepB (3), Pneumo (3), MenC (2)	23
Austria	DTaP (3), Polio (3), Hib (3), HepB (3), Pneumo (3), Rota (2)	23
Ireland	DTaP (3), Polio (3), Hib (3), HepB (3), Pneumo (2), MenC (2), BCG	23
Greece	DTaP (3), Polio (3), Hib (3), HepB (3), Pneumo (3), MenC (2)	23
Monaco[a]	DTaP (3), Polio (3), Hib (3), HepB (3), Pneumo (3), HepA, BCG	23
Netherlands	DTaP (4), Polio (4), Hib (4), Pneumo (4)	24
Canada	DTaP (3), Polio (3), Hib (3), HepB (3), Pneumo (3), MenC (2), Flu	24
Australia	DTaP (3), Polio (3), Hib (3), HepB (4), Pneumo (3), Rota (2)	24
United States	DTaP (3), Polio (3), Hib (3), HepB (3), Pneumo (3), Rota (3), Flu (2)	26

Notice a pattern? The study showed that the USA, which administers **more** childhood vaccines than any other country in the developed world (26), also has the **highest** number of infant deaths per 1000 births in the developed world (6.22). It also showed that Japan and Sweden, which require the **fewest** vaccinations, have the **lowest** mortality rates. I have been preaching this message for years. In light of the voluminous amount of research which proves that vaccines are deadly, those who advocate vaccines are either ignorant or evil. There is no other choice.

CHECK OUT THE GRAPHS!

If you look at the graph on the next page, it will be crystal clear that the decline in deaths from pertussis ("whooping cough") occurred **before** the introduction of the related vaccine. The same goes for diphtheria, and measles. According to the *British Association for the Advancement of Science*, childhood diseases decreased 90% between 1850 and 1940, paralleling improved sanitation and hygienic practices, well before mandatory vaccination programs. Deaths from infectious disease in the USA and England declined steadily by an average of about 80% during the same period.

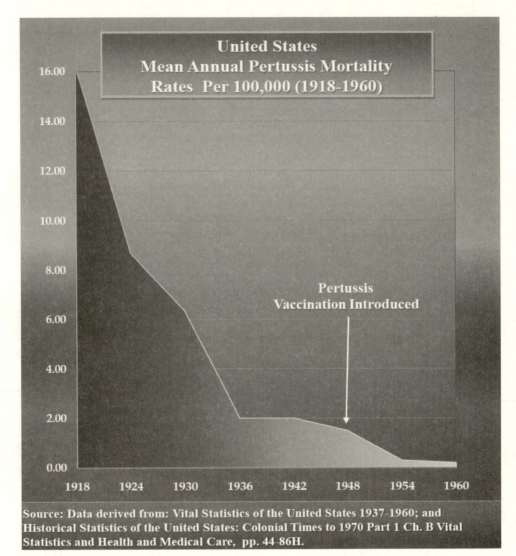

The pertussis vaccine has also been implicated in sudden infant death syndrome ("SIDS"). So, I took a close look at the Sanofi Pasteur DTaP vaccine (Diphtheria, Tetanus, Pertussis).

See the image on the next page.

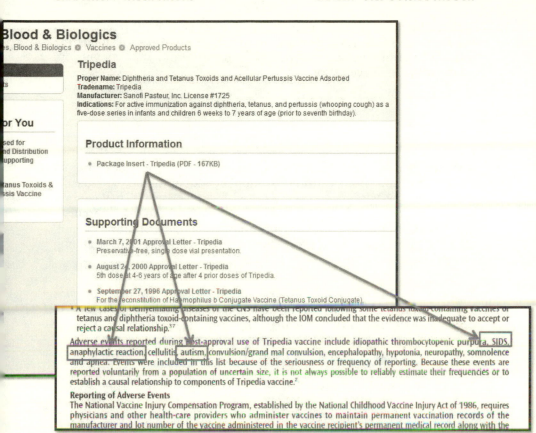

I was astonished to discover that **anaphylactic reaction, autism,** and **SIDS** are listed as "*adverse events reported during post-approval use ... Events were included in this list because of the seriousness or frequency of reporting.*" Wow!

The CDC, the FDA, Paul Offit, and every Medical Mafia "flunky" swear up and down the aisle that vaccines are perfectly safe and don't cause autism or SIDS. Yet those conditions are **actually** listed on the DTaP package insert with the statement that they are included because such vaccine adverse reactions are serious and frequent. Despite these facts, the mainstream media bobble-heads are making a full court press with news stories everywhere to convince the public that vaccines are totally safe and it is our moral obligation to accept them.

They are so far down the road of denial and dishonesty that they are incapable or unwilling to acknowledge the fact prominently displayed on the DTaP package insert: **Autism** and **SIDS** are associated with this vaccine. This is a powerful indictment of the CDC, Big Pharma, vaccine manufacturers, and Medical Mafia "talking heads" like Offit. As you can see from the DTaP package warning insert above, it also includes the following serious adverse events: convulsion/grand mal convulsion, neuropathy, and encephalopathy.

"TOXIC COCKTAILS"

I have heard vaccinations described as *"toxic cocktails"* of the most toxic substances on earth. They are combined with live and dead animal viruses that have been cultured in monkey kidney tissue, cow tissue, goat tissue, pig tissue, and even aborted human fetuses. They contain any combination of the following: thimerosal (ethyl mercury), aluminum, formaldehyde (carcinogenic embalming fluid), phenol, ethylene glycol (antifreeze), live viruses, bacteria, and acetone, among other things.

In his book, Official Stories, my friend, Liam Scheff, states: *"Vaccines are not conjured at Hogwarts by honest wizards. Willy Wonka doesn't brew them in his chocolate factory. They are not magical and there is a reason, or many, why some people oppose them too strongly. Vaccines are toxic, by their very nature."*

University of Kentucky professor Dr. Boyd Haley asserts: *"You couldn't even construct a study that shows thimerosal is safe. It's just too darn toxic. If you inject thimerosal into an animal, its brain will sicken. If you apply it to living tissue, the cells die. If you put it in a petri dish, the culture dies. Knowing these things, it would be shocking if one could inject it into an infant without causing damage."*
www.rollingstone.com/politics/story/7395411/deadly_immunity

What if I were to take some mercury, formaldehyde, aluminum, antifreeze, and live viruses cultured in dead animal tissue, then mix them together with some peanut butter and spread it on a piece of bread for my children to eat for a snack? Would you think I was a good parent? What if I said, *"This will keep them from getting sick"*? Would you question my sanity? The odds are that I would likely be arrested for child abuse. However, when doctors inject our children with the same ingredients (less the peanut butter) and tell us *"this will keep them from getting sick,"* most of us don't even give it a second thought. What if you call your physician and tell him that you are going to inject your baby with mercury, aluminum, and formaldehyde, and that you are wondering what the "safe dosage" was for these ingredients? Well, right after he calls Child Protective Services, he will probably call the police! You see, there is **no safe dosage** because these are all toxic.

Mercury derivatives, aluminum, and formaldehyde are ingredients in most vaccinations. How is it possible that they are safe? The answer depends upon who is injecting them. If you or I inject our child with mercury or formaldehyde, we are going to jail. But if a drug company and a doctor inject the same toxic poisons, then they are perfectly safe. What's wrong with this picture? Unfortunately, most Americans follow the masses, believe what we're told, don't ask questions, and place blind faith in our doctors. But where do doctors get their medical training? That's right...in medical school.

Medical schools, which are largely subsidized by Big Pharma, brainwash students into believing that vaccinations are safe and prevent the spread of infectious diseases. Not surprisingly, there is a huge financial incentive for Big Pharma to *"peddle"* vaccinations, as they make a fortune on the sale of these toxic cocktails. Once these medical students graduate and become physicians, they are offered large commissions to sell more vaccinations to patients and continue their blind faith in the necessity of these poisons.

Then, most people acquiesce to the poisoning of their children because they simply cannot believe (or **refuse** to believe) that their "omniscient" physician could possibly be wrong. What we have is blind faith in doctors, who have blind faith in what they learned in medical school, which are governed by the AMA, which is "in bed" with Big Pharma, which is interested in shareholder profits, **not** in the safety of our children.

JENNER & SMALLPOX

England's Edward Jenner, born in 1749, is credited with being the "Father of Vaccines." He believed the superstition among the dairymaids that a person who had suffered cowpox could not contract smallpox. In 1786, for his initial "human guinea pig" test, Jenner scraped pus from the lesions from a dairymaid and injected this pus into James Phipps, an eight year old boy. A short time afterwards, he inoculated the boy with small-pox, and the small-pox did not take. Jenner believed that he had found the cure to smallpox. Over the next twelve years, Phipps was inoculated over a dozen times and eventually died of tuberculosis at the age of twenty. Jenner's own son also served as one of his guinea pigs and also died of tuberculosis at the age of twenty-one. Since that time, researchers have linked tuberculosis to the smallpox vaccine. (Eleanor McBean, The Poisoned Needle)

Over the next few years, Jenner gathered the "proof" that his smallpox vaccine worked, and then he presented it to Parliament. He was sure to report only the data which supported his theory, and to never mention the multitudes of people who would disprove his theory (*i.e.*, those people who contracted cowpox and then contracted smallpox afterwards). He was careful to mention only the cases of a dozen old men who had cowpox and did not contract smallpox afterwards, while conveniently omitting the hundreds of cases who had had both. Eventually, after years of manipulating data and "tweaking" his smallpox vaccination formula, he "sold" his theory of vaccinations to the intellectual elite and governmental officials alike.

Despite Jenner's efforts, widespread vaccination did not really catch on. As of 1807, only 1.5% of the Brits had been vaccinated. Up until 1823, the year that Jenner died, there were only regional outbreaks of smallpox in England, nothing that would be considered an epidemic. For the next thirty years, smallpox was under control. However, vaccinations became mandatory in England in 1853, and by 1857, fines and imprisonment awaited people who refused to be vaccinated against smallpox.

Once smallpox vaccination became mandatory in England, massive epidemics began to occur. Between 1857 and 1859, there were over 14,000 deaths from smallpox. Then, between 1863 and 1865, there were over 20,000 smallpox deaths. A few years later, there were almost 45,000 smallpox deaths between 1870 and 1872. According to official estimates, 97% of the population had been vaccinated. (Anne Riley Hale, The Medical VooDoo) Japan introduced compulsory vaccinations in 1872. In 1892 there were 165,774 cases of smallpox with 29,979 deaths despite the vaccination program. **Bottom line**: the smallpox vaccine does **not** work.

"OUTBREAKS ALWAYS OCCUR IN NON-VACCINATED PEOPLE, RIGHT?"

You see, we're constantly inundated with false information (lies) about vaccines. One tidbit of information that is conveniently swept under the rug is how often (and badly) vaccines fail. Ask yourself, "*Why don't these vaccine failures regularly make the news?*" If you can imagine in your mind's eye, for a moment, the cash register "ka-chinging" while Big Pharma is pulling out a wad of cash, I think you may be getting close to the real answer. There's big money in making sure the vaccine program is perceived as a success by you.

The fact is that most outbreaks of disease occur in vaccinated populations. Here are just a few examples. There are literally dozens more. In early 2010, there was an outbreak of mumps among more than 1,000 people in New York and New Jersey. What's interesting is that in Ocean County, New Jersey, county spokeswoman Leslie

Terjesen told *CNN* that 77% of those who caught mumps had already been vaccinated against mumps. If mumps vaccines actually worked, then what you should see instead is mumps spreading among those who refused the vaccines, right? That is logical, isn't it? But, in this case, reality tells a different story.

An objective analysis must conclude that it is the vaccinated people who caused this outbreak of mumps. In 1967, the WHO declared Ghana to be "measles free" after 96% of its population was vaccinated. However, in 1972, Ghana experienced one of its worst measles outbreaks with its highest ever mortality rate. The November 21, 1990, issue of the *Journal of the American Medical Association* stated, *"Although more than 95% of school-aged children in the US are vaccinated against measles, large measles outbreaks continue to occur in schools, and most cases in this setting occur among previously vaccinated children."*

An article published in the March 1987 issue of the *New England Journal of Medicine (NEJM)* indicated that an outbreak of measles occurred in a 99% vaccinated school population in Corpus Christi, Texas.

Check out the graph below.

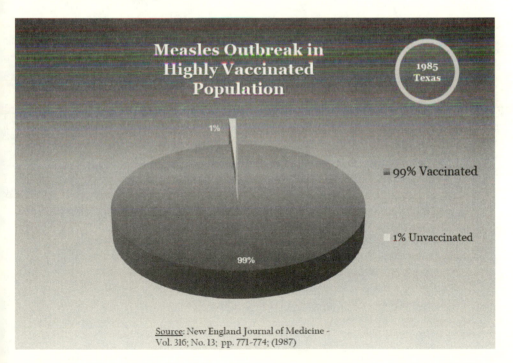

Measles Outbreak in Highly Vaccinated Population

1985 Texas

1%

■ 99% Vaccinated

■ 1% Unvaccinated

99%

Source: New England Journal of Medicine –
Vol. 316; No. 13; pp. 771-774; (1987)

Here are a few more examples represented by the following graphs.

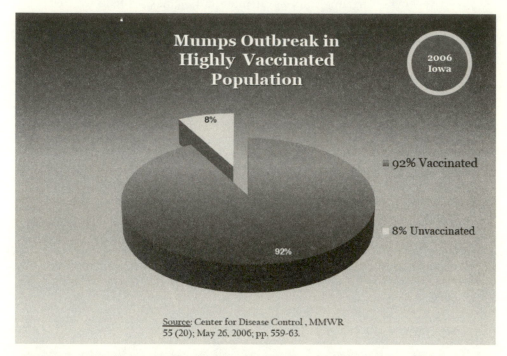

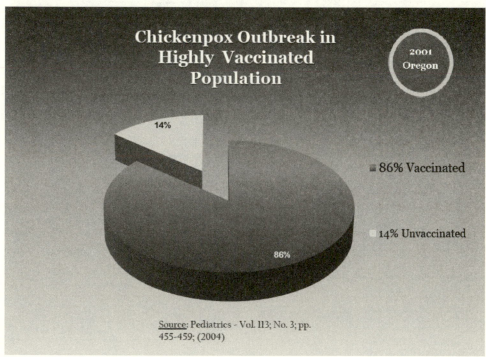

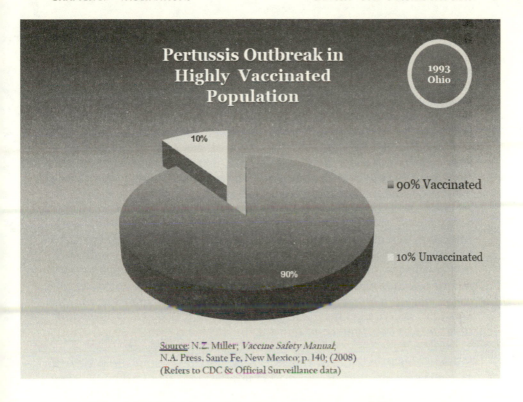

Pertussis Outbreak in Highly Vaccinated Population

1993 Ohio

10%

■ 90% Vaccinated

■ 10% Unvaccinated

90%

Source: N.Z. Miller; *Vaccine Safety Manual*, N.A. Press, Sante Fe, New Mexico; p. 140; (2008) (Refers to CDC & Official Surveillance data)

"AT LEAST WE KNOW THAT THE FLU SHOT IS SAFE AND EFFECTIVE!"

Well, not exactly. But before we debunk the myths surrounding the flu shot, first let's learn how they make the flu shot. In January or February of each year, health "authorities" travel to Asia to determine which strains of the flu are currently active. Based on their findings in Asia, they assume that the same strains of viruses will spread to the USA by fall. In other words, they guess at the strain of flu that will hit the USA. If the viral strains circulating in the USA are not identical to those in Asia (which they never are since the flu virus mutates), then the vaccine you receive will be a complete dud (at best).

According to the CDC, the majority of flu vaccines contain thimerosal. Some contain as much as 25 micrograms of mercury per dose. This means that it may contain more than **250 times** the Environmental Protection Agency's safety limit for mercury. That's one good reason to avoid the flu shot, isn't it?

For those of you, who are still unconvinced, know that there's plenty of scientific evidence available to back up the recommendation to avoid flu vaccines. A study published in the October 2008 issue of the *Archives of Pediatric & Adolescent Medicine* found that vaccinating young children against the flu had **no impact** on flu-related hospitalizations or doctor visits during two recent flu seasons. The researchers concluded that "*significant influenza vaccine effectiveness could not be demonstrated for any season, age, or setting.*" Research published in the September 2008 issue of the *American Journal of Respiratory and Critical Care Medicine* also confirms that there has been **no decrease** in deaths from influenza and pneumonia in the elderly, despite the fact that vaccination coverage among the elderly has increased from 15% in 1980 to 65% now.

In 2007, researchers with the National Institute of Allergy and Infectious Diseases, and the National Institutes of Health published this conclusion in the *Lancet Infectious Diseases*: "*We conclude that frailty selection bias and use of non-specific endpoints such as all-cause mortality, have led cohort studies to greatly exaggerate vaccine benefits.*" Did you get that? Please allow me to translate. "*We conclude that the tests are rigged and that the flu vaccine is worthless.*"

Still not convinced? Check this out. A large-scale, systematic review of 51 studies involving over 260,000 children, published in the Cochrane Database of Systematic Reviews in 2006, found **no evidence** that the flu vaccine is any more effective than a placebo in children between the ages of 6 months and two years. **Zero percent effective!** In a review of 64 studies covering over 40 years, the Cochrane Database also reported that, for elderly living in nursing homes, flu shots provided "**little or no effectiveness**" at preventing the flu.

But it's good for pregnant women, right? The CDC even states on their own website (www.cdc.gov): "*If you're pregnant, a flu shot is your best protection against serious illnesses caused by the flu … A flu shot can protect pregnant women, their unborn babies, and even the baby after birth.*" Au contraire! Documentation from the National Coalition of Organized Women (NCOW) demonstrated that between 2009 and 2010 the mercury-laden flu vaccines increased Vaccine Adverse Events Reporting Systems (VAERS) fetal death reports by **4,250%** in pregnant women. The director of NCOW, Eileen Dannemann, indicated that despite these figures being known to the CDC, they still recommend the flu vaccine containing mercury (Thimerosal) to pregnant women as a "safe" vaccine.

Want more? OK. There was the 2012 study published in *The Lancet*, which (according to the vaccine-pushing CDC bureaucrats) established that the flu vaccine is 60% effective. But, is it really? My friend, Mike

Adams (aka the "Health Ranger") had the audacity to actually read the *Lancet* study and crunch the actual numbers. How dare he! What did he determine about the study? The "60% effectiveness" claim is a total lie.

In his own words, *"What we found is that the '60% effectiveness' claim is utterly absurd and highly misleading. For starters, most people think that '60% effectiveness' means that for every 100 people injected with the flu shot, 60 of them won't get the flu! Thus, the '60% effectiveness' claim implies that getting a flu shot has about a 6 in 10 chance of preventing you from getting the flu. This is utterly false. In reality ... only about 2.7 in 100 adults get the flu in the first place! ... The 'control group' of adults consisted of 13,095 non-vaccinated adults who were monitored to see if they caught influenza. Over 97% of them did not. Only 357 of them caught influenza, which means only 2.7% of these adults caught the flu in the first place."*

Mike continues, *"The 'treatment group' consisted of adults who were vaccinated with a trivalent inactivated Influenza vaccine. Out of this group, according to the study, only 1.2% did not catch the flu. The difference between these two groups is 1.5 people out of 100. So even if you believe this study, and even if you believe all the pro-vaccine hype behind it, the truly 'scientific' conclusion from this is rather astonishing: Flu vaccines only prevent the flu in 1.5 out of every 100 adults injected with the vaccine!"* www.NaturalNews.com

Honestly folks, this is **truly** amazing. Flu shots are **1.5%** effective? Are you kidding me? That means that they have approximately the same efficacy as waving a magic wand, wearing a lucky hat, wishing on a four-leaf clover, or rubbing a rabbit's foot. Hey, let's not forget to pick up that lucky penny ... and maybe toss some salt over our shoulder.

What many people do not know is that death caused directly by the flu virus is very rare, despite the fact that the CDC has been telling the public for a decade that there are more than 200,000 estimated hospitalizations and 36,000 estimated deaths from influenza in the USA each and every year.

Here's how it happened. In 2003, CDC employees used a convoluted statistical modeling scheme to "guesstimate" that 36,000 people die from influenza in the USA every year. The problem was that they counted not just deaths from influenza, but also threw in other respiratory, circulatory, cardiac, and pulmonary deaths they thought **might** have been associated with influenza.

Barbara Fisher, Co-Founder and President of the National Vaccine Information Center (NVIC), analyzed the vital statistics data and concluded flu deaths peaked in 1941 at 21,047 and have been dropping ever since. Over the past decade, deaths from influenza ranged from a low of 494 (in 2010) to a high of 1,722 (in 2008).

Meanwhile, on their own website, doctors at the CDC now sheepishly admit that the *"CDC does not know exactly how many people die from seasonal flu each year."* Having gotten that cradle to the grave flu shot recommendation firmly in place, they are backing away from the 36,000 influenza annual death figure. CDC now says that *"only 8.5% of all pneumonia and influenza deaths and only 2.1% of all respiratory and circulatory deaths"* are influenza related.

Now compare those statistics to the following facts. As of the end of 2012, there were more than 84,000 reports of reactions, hospitalizations, injuries and deaths following influenza vaccinations made to the VAERS, including over 1,000 related deaths and over 1,600 cases of GBS. **Wow**! Looks like the vaccine is much more dangerous than the virus, doesn't it?

Case in point: On December 2, 2011, seven year-old Kaylynne Matten was taken by her parents for her annual physical. During the physical Kaylynne was given a flu shot. Four days later she was dead. She wasn't even sick when she went to the doctor!

The state health commissioner, Dr. Harry Chen (no, I'm not kidding...this is his real name), was "not convinced" the girl's death was from the flu vaccine, citing the "very rare" incidence of serious reactions to the flu shot and the huge numbers of people who receive them each year. Apparently Dr. Chen is not familiar with the VAERS statistics cited in the previous paragraphs.

That's the problem! Every time a healthy child dies or is seriously injured by a vaccine, those who are responsible for determining the cause of death immediately rule out vaccines because they are "so safe" and serious reactions are "so rare," being completely ignorant of the thousands of injuries and deaths caused by the vaccine. And can we say "conflict of interest"? Dr. Chen's job is dependent on the sale of vaccines. That's what he does. He ensures that all of the people in his state are fully vaccinated. Without vaccines, Dr. Chen would be unemployed, and so would a whole heap of doctors!

In the 2011 report, Dr. Chen was worried that people would "over-react" to Kaylynne's death, and he cautioned about "alarmist" reactions. Excuse me? We are not supposed to be **alarmed**? Clearly, Dr. Chen has become condescending and self-righteous when it comes to young children dropping dead for "no apparent reason."

Dr. Chen is worried that if people become "alarmed" their concerns may lead them to avoid getting a flu shot. If they start looking into the dangers of flu shots, it's a very slippery slope. You know how it goes. Flu shot research is like "the gateway drug" that causes "investigative" parents to become "fanatics." We research the flu vaccine and the true dangers of the flu, and before you know it we start to realize we've been lied to about influenza. From there it's all downhill for Dr. Chen and his cronies. As we become "hooked" on research we learn more and more about vaccines and the more we learn the more we realize that vaccines are dangerous and the risks of infectious diseases are small in comparison.

Heavens! That would be a real tragedy for Dr. Chen, who is another example of the fox guarding the henhouse. How in the world can this vaccine-related death even be questioned? It's like saying *"Jane Doe was crossing the interstate when she was hit by a taxi. Ms. Doe was taken to the hospital where she lapsed into a coma and died 4 days later. Her husband, John Doe, believes that it was the impact from the taxi that killed his wife. However, the coroner (who just happens to be married to the taxi driver) is not quite sure about the cause of death. Autopsy results are pending..."*

According to Hugh Fudenberg, MD, the world's leading immune-geneticist and 13th most quoted biologist of our time (with nearly 850 papers in peer reviewed journals): If an individual has had 5 consecutive flu shots between 1970 and 1980 (the years studied) his/her chances of getting Alzheimer's Disease is **10 times** higher than if he/she had one, two or no shots. As I mentioned earlier, flu shots contain 25 micrograms of mercury. One microgram is considered toxic.

"WHAT ABOUT THE HPV VACCINE?"

A March 2013 publication in the *Annals of Medicine* exposed the true nature of Human papillomavirus (HPV) vaccines such as Gardasil (from Merck) and Cervarix (from GlaxoSmithKline). The researchers reported that there is a lack of evidence that HPV vaccines prevent cervical cancer and there has been no evaluation of health risks associated with the vaccines. The researchers concluded that due to the presentation of "partial and non-factual information" regarding cervical cancer risks and the usefulness (or lack thereof) of HPV vaccines, the current research on HPV is **neither** scientific **nor** ethical.

But this isn't the first study to indicate that, at best, the HPV vaccine is virtually worthless. Research published in the August 2007 *JAMA* sought to determine the usefulness of the HPV vaccine among women who already carry HPV (which includes virtually all women who are sexually active, regardless of their age). This document revealed startling information about the ineffectiveness of the Gardasil vaccine.

It revealed that the HPV vaccine often caused an increase in the presence of HPV strains while utterly failing to clear the viruses in most women. The fact of the matter is that Merck's Gardasil vaccine was studied for less than 3 years in about 12,000 healthy girls and 14,000 healthy boys under age 16 before it was licensed in 2006. Gardasil was **not** studied in children with health problems or in combination with all other vaccines routinely given to American adolescents. Clinical trials did **not** use a true placebo to study safety but compared Gardasil against the reactive aluminum adjuvant in Gardasil.

One major problem is that there are over 100 strains of HPV, yet only 30 of them are even theoretically linked with cervical cancer. In addition, HPV is present in at least half the normal population, yet it almost never causes any disease or problems whatsoever. Truth be told, HPV has never been proven as a pathogen for any disease. As a matter of fact, studies show that over 90% of women have some form of HPV and in almost all those cases, **it goes away by itself**. Heck, even the CDC's own website states, *"In most cases HPV goes away by itself before it causes any health problems."*

Another major problem is the side effects of the HPV vaccines. According to the National Vaccine Information Center (www.NVIC.org), *"after Gardasil was licensed and three doses recommended for 11-12 year old girls and teenagers, there were thousands of reports of sudden collapse with unconsciousness within 24 hours, seizures, muscle pain and weakness, disabling fatigue, Guillain Barre Syndrome, facial paralysis, brain inflammation, rheumatoid arthritis, lupus, blood clots, optic neuritis, multiple sclerosis, strokes, heart and other serious health problems, including death, following receipt of Gardasil vaccine."*

And they want to inject this unproven, uninsurable brew into our children first to *"wait and see if there aren't too many adverse events"*? I say, *"Over our collective cold, dead bodies!"* Let's put on our "math hats." As of the middle of 2013, there have been almost 30,000 reports made to the federal Vaccine Adverse Events Reporting System (VAERS) associated with Gardasil or Cervarix vaccines, including 118 deaths. It is estimated that 90% of adverse events are not reported, so if we extrapolate the total numbers, it's likely that there have been close to 300,000 adverse reactions and over 1,000 deaths!

It turns out that studies actually show that not only does HPV **not** cause cervical cancer, the HPV vaccine itself **does**. Are you ready for this? Gardasil appears to ***increase*** cancer by 44.6% in folks who were already carriers of the same HPV strains used in the vaccine. The FDA actually had this information on its own website, but they removed it. Surprise surprise. But fortunately, Mike Adams anticipated this and saved a copy here: http://www.naturalnews.com/downloads/FDA-Gardasil.pdf.

In other words, it appears that if the vaccine is given to a young woman who already carries HPV in a "harmless" state, it may "activate" the infection and directly cause precancerous lesions to appear. The vaccine, in other words, may accelerate the development of cancer!

In an ABC News interview in September of 2009, Dr. Diane Harper (the leading international developer of the HPV vaccines) admitted that "*the rate of serious adverse events is greater than the incidence rate of cervical cancer. The incidence of cervical cancer in the US is so low that if we get the vaccine and continue PAP screening, we will not lower the rate of cervical cancer in the US … if you vaccinate a child, she won't keep immunity in puberty and you do nothing to prevent cervical cancer.*" http://abcnews.go.com/m/story?id=8356717

WHAT EXACTLY IS "HERD IMMUNITY"?

The "herd immunity" theory was originally coined in the 1930s by a researcher named A.W. Hedrich. He had been studying measles patterns in the USA since 1900 (before any vaccine was ever invented for measles) and he observed that epidemics of the illness only occurred when less than 68% of children had developed a **natural immunity** to it. Hedrich's "herd immunity" theory was, in fact, about natural disease processes and had nothing to do with vaccinations.

Over the next half century, some of those who worship at the altar of "modern medical mysticism" (vaccinologists) adopted the phrase and magically increased the figure from 68% to 95% (with no scientific justification as to why) and then stated that there had to be 95% **vaccine coverage** to achieve immunity. Essentially, they took Hedrich's study and manipulated it to promote their own vaccination programs.

Now, over 80 years since Hedrich developed his theory, the mainstream media and Medical Mafia are attempting to keep vaccination rates high by **mis**using his concept of "herd immunity" and pitting parent against parent. What better way to keep Mr. and Mrs. Jones vaccinating "Junior" than through good old fashioned peer pressure and the fear that their next door neighbor won't let Johnny come over and play because Junior isn't vaccinated. A very powerful influence of behavior is it not? The "guilt trip" method is a common vaccine marketing technique. If a parent is concerned, say about the ingredients in the shot for their child, they are told that they "have to" vaccinate for the greater good of all other children to prevent the spread of disease in the community. What a bunch of bunk. As I have showed with numerous graphs and charts in this chapter, much to the dismay of vaccination proponents, outbreaks still occur in groups of children who have been fully vaccinated.

My friend, Dr. Russell Blaylock MD, a retired neurosurgeon, says the fact that vaccine-induced herd immunity is mostly myth can be proven quite simply. According to Dr. Blaylock, *"When I was in medical school, we were taught that all of the childhood vaccines lasted a lifetime. This thinking existed for over 70 years. It was not until relatively recently that it was discovered that most of these vaccines lost their effectiveness 2 to 10 years after being given. What this means is that at least half the population, that is the baby boomers, have had no vaccine-induced immunity against any of these diseases for which they had been vaccinated very early in life. In essence, at least 50% or more of the population was unprotected for decades. If we listen to present-day wisdom, we are all at risk of resurgent massive epidemics should the vaccination rate fall below 95%. Yet, we have all lived for at least 30 to 40 years with 50% or less of the population having vaccine protection. That is, herd immunity has not existed in this country for many decades and no resurgent epidemics have occurred. **Vaccine-induced herd immunity is a lie used to frighten** doctors, public-health officials, other medical personnel, and the public into accepting vaccinations."*

We have an ever growing (and desperate) propaganda campaign based upon smearing those who refuse to inject themselves or their precious children with toxic (and potentially deadly) poison and blaming every failure on their unwillingness to submit to the needle. Folks who are critical thinkers and thus opposed to vaccinations are referred to as "denialists," "kooks," "quacks," "uneducated," "confused," and "enemies of public safety." This desperation is based upon their fear that the public might soon catch on to the fact that the entire vaccine program is based upon unscientific drivel, nonsense, fear, and concocted fairytales.

If you are a parent who chooses to vaccinate, note that the concept of herd immunity as it is erroneously applied to vaccines is being used to manipulate you into using scorn and fear to pressure family and friends within your circle of influence into accepting vaccination against their will. Without the mantra of "herd immunity," the Medical Mafia dons wouldn't be able to justify forced mass vaccinations.

Please remember: Scientific fraud isn't the exception in modern medicine; *it is the rule.* Most of the "science" you read in today's medical journals is really just corporate-funded "quackery" dressed up in the language of pseudoscience. The fact of the matter is that, in classic Orwellian maneuvering, the journals of the Medical Mafia are actually rewriting history to remove any studies that document the harm caused by vaccines.

But they won't succeed. The truth is slowly trickling out, and doctors across the globe are admitting that vaccines are responsible for a whole host of ailments, diseases, and even death. In a shocking report, the *Global Times* reported that an expert from the Chinese CDC, Dr. Wang Yu, has openly admitted that vaccines can cause severe adverse reactions, swollen organs, epilepsy, the diseases that they were supposed to prevent, and even death! As they say in New Zealand, "*Good on you*," Dr. Yu. The truth shall set you free!

WHAT ABOUT POLIO?

Didn't the polio vaccine save millions? The population of New York in 1950 was fifteen million, and at that time, there were thirteen polio cases and one polio death per 100,000 population. Hardly an epidemic! But based solely on the scant evidence of a polio "epidemic," Dr. Jonas Salk convinced the federal government to inoculate 97% of the American population with a culture grown in dead green monkeys. As the Salk vaccine program expanded, cases of paralytic polio began to increase. In 1959, more than 5,000 paralytic polio cases occurred–50% more than in 1958, and 100% more than in 1957. This trend developed in spite of 300,000,000 doses of Salk vaccine administered in the USA by the end of 1959.

Six New England states reported increases in polio one year after the Salk vaccine was introduced, ranging from Vermont's 100% increase to Massachusetts' astounding increase of 642%. During the Congressional hearings of 1962, Dr. Bernard Greenberg (head of the Department of Biostatistics for the University of North Carolina School of Public Health) testified that not only did the cases of polio increase substantially after mandatory vaccinations, but that the statistics were manipulated by the Public Health Service and CDC to give the opposite impression. (*Hearings before the Committee on Interstate and Foreign Commerce*, House of Representatives, 87th Congress, Second Session on H.R. 10541, May 1962, p.94)

For example, after the introduction of the live polio vaccine in 1958, the CDC changed the definition of "polio." Cases of inflammation of the membrane that protects the brain and spinal neuron cells, causing muscular weakness and pain (but not paralysis) were no longer classified as "polio." They were to be referred to as aseptic meningitis, even if the polio virus was present. Reported cases of aseptic meningitis went from near zero to thousands, and polio cases dropped the same amount. Then, later in 1958, the CDC changed the definition of "polio" again! All cases with classic polio paralytic symptoms were to be called acute flaccid paralysis. In 1960, the CDC triumphantly declared large parts of the world as "polio free," while the newly created acute flaccid paralysis "mysteriously" became quite common.

Almost 20 years after the first polio inoculations, in 1977, Salk testified before a Senate subcommittee that all polio outbreaks since 1961 were caused by the oral polio vaccine. In 1985, the CDC reported that 87% of the cases of polio in the USA between 1973 and 1983 were caused by the vaccine and most of the reported cases occurred in fully immunized individuals. Alarmingly, the CDC has admitted that the polio vaccine is the only known cause of polio in the USA today.

Remember I mentioned that the polio vaccine was initially cultured from dead green monkeys and was contaminated with SV-40 (from 1959 to 1965)? It turns out that SV-40 can be passed horizontally (*i.e.,* between father and mother) and vertically (*i.e.,* between mother and child). In fact, SV-40 is often associated with medulloblastoma, the most prevalent pediatric brain tumor. When scientists injected young hamsters with SV-40, over 80% developed brain cancers. Traces of this virus are commonly found in brain cancers among the millions of people who received polio vaccines contaminated with SV-40. In 1979, Doctors J. Farwell, G. Dohrmann, L. Marrett, and J. W. Meigs wrote a paper entitled "Effect of SV40 Virus-Contaminated Polio Vaccine on the Incidence and Type of CNS Neoplasms in Children: A Population-Based Study." In this paper, they reported a substantial increase in childhood brain tumors, especially medullo-blastoma, when the mothers had been inoculated with vaccines containing SV-40.

VACCINES & AUTISM

Congressman Dan Burton of Indiana began holding hearings on the relationship between vaccinations and autism in the fall of 2001. His grandson became autistic after receiving 49 times the amount of mercury considered safe by the EPA during a visit to his pediatrician who gave him nine vaccines at once. During these hearings, parent after parent told very similar stories of how their normally developing babies had suddenly reversed their development soon after the **MMR** vaccination or the **DPaT** vaccination. (I previously mentioned that **autism** is actually listed as an "adverse event" resulting from the DPaT shot.)

The children spiraled downward into the "vegetable-like" existence of autistic behavior, in which previously happy, bright children suddenly can no longer learn, or communicate, or recognize their parents.

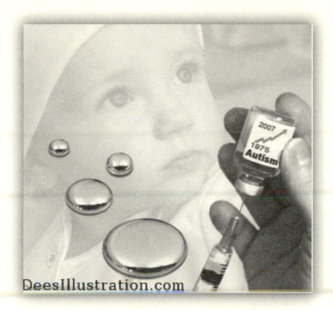

Thanks to David Dees for the picture above.

Astonishing testimony was given by experts in the field of autism. For instance, Dr. Michael Goldberg explained how it was impossible to have an epidemic based solely on genetics. That's the standard excuse the CDC and the NIH have been using to explain how autism has literally exploded in just over 2 decades. Dr. Mary Megson explained how autism has gone from being an unknown in 1978 (with an incidence of one **in 10,000**) to an epidemic in 2000 (with an incidence of **one in 166**). Her research has shown total deficiency of vitamin A in almost all autistic children.

Can you guess what depletes the body of vitamin A? You got it...the MMR vaccination. Amazingly, the Medical Mafia still insists that there is no connection between toxic mercury preservatives in mandated childhood vaccinations and the astounding increase in autism, despite ample scientific evidence to the contrary. Dr. John O'Leary, a world class researcher and molecular biologist from Ireland, using state of the art sequencing technology, showed how he had found measles virus in the gut of **96%** of autistic children, compared to **6.6%** of normal children. Interestingly, this virus did not come from the natural disease; it came from the measles vaccine.

Finally, Dr. V. Singh, an autism specialist from Utah, found that in over 400 cases of autism, the children had experienced an autoimmune episode, in which their own body has been made to attack the lining of the nervous system. He stated that 55% of the families said that autism appeared soon after the MMR vaccination and that 33% of families said it appeared soon after the DPT vaccination. Such neurologic damage is a well-established side effect of the mercury, aluminum, and formaldehyde in these vaccines.

And, yes, mercury is still present as a preservative in most vaccines, including the flu shot. Many people are under the false impression that it was removed from vaccines between 2000 and 2002, but this is not accurate. Thimerosal, or ethyl mercury, is still used in the manufacturing process of almost all vaccines, but it is no longer disclosed on the vaccine labels, since it is no longer an "added" ingredient. As a result of this fact, Congressman Dan Burton, during a congressional hearing held in 2003 regarding this specific issue, asked for criminal sanctions to be brought against the head of the FDA and the FTC. Yet, nothing was done. The media failed to report the story, and mercury continues to be used in the manufacturing process of all vaccines.

On November 26, 2005, President George W. Bush asked a federal claims court to seal documents relating to hundreds of cases of autism allegedly caused by thimerosal, one of the toxic ingredients used in many childhood vaccines. The government's legal action comes on the heels of an insertion into the Homeland Security bill that protects Eli Lilly, the drug company giant that developed thimerosal, from lawsuits involving the additive. The bill removes **all liability** from the pharmaceutical industry and health officials for the injuries and deaths resulting from the preservative.

Interestingly, in March of 2008, the U.S. government conceded that childhood vaccines were responsible for the **autism** in nine-year-old Hannah Poling. More significantly, an explosive investigation by CBS News has found that since 1988, the vaccine court has awarded money judgments, often in the millions of dollars, to over 1,300 families whose children suffered brain damage from vaccines. In many of these cases, the government paid out awards following a judicial finding that vaccine injury lead to the child's autism spectrum disorder.

Yes, our government is corrupt, folks. According to a March 12, 2010, article by F. Wiliam Engdahl, since 2002 the U.S. Center for Disease Control (CDC) has paid Dr. Poul Thorsen, head of a Danish research group, $14.6 million to publish studies that disprove the links between vaccinations and autism, despite the fact that investigations uncovered "research fraud" in previous studies conducted by Thorsen. His partner, Kreesten Madsen, was recently discovered conspiring with CDC officials to fraudulently select only favorable data to "prove" vaccine safety. Danish police are currently investigating Thorsen for criminal fraud charges and claim that he has disappeared along with $2 million in US taxpayer money from the CDC.

CHRISTIAN'S STORY

The following is the story of a dedicated, loving mother who was not willing to accept the fact that her precious two year old son, Christian, was diagnosed with autism. She noticed a change in Christian immediately after he received his six-month and nine-month vaccinations.

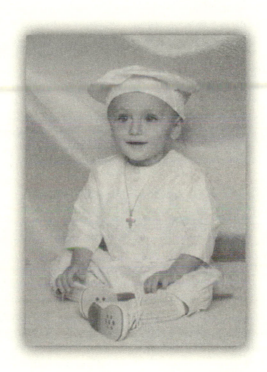

This is Christian's story, as told by his mother:

When my son was six months old, we went in (to the doctor's office) happy and well, and left the office with him screaming so much that after an hour of screaming he fell into a deep sleep for over four hours. I tried to wake him to eat, but all he wanted to do was sleep, and he started to develop a fever that was as high as 104 degrees. That night, we kept calling the doctor/hospital, and they kept telling us this was normal and just to give him some Tylenol. I kept trying to cool down his body with room temperature water; it worked on and off, but it was a very scary night. The next day, I took the baby into the doctor's office, and they said, "We can't do anything about the fever, just give him Tylenol." The next day, the same thing happened, and that day I changed doctors. On the fourth day, I went to a new doctor who told me it was a viral infection and it had nothing to do with his vaccines. He was nice and caring with a good bed side manner, so I believed him and went back for Christian's nine month vaccines. Again, he got sick, but it was not as bad as his six months shots. This time he got a fever up to 102 degrees and was sleepy and out of it for about twenty-four hours but seemed OK soon afterwards.

Children change from day to day when they are so young. Christian started to talk and walk at twelve months old. But by fifteen months, he had lost the ability to speak and could only say "Mama." Before our very eyes, we started to lose him; he would not respond to his name, lost all eye contact, and started crying almost all the time. He would not sleep more than two hours at a time, was always angry and violent, no longer wanted to play with his toys or with others, and just wanted to be alone and watch TV all day. Close to his 2nd birthday, at 20-months old, we took him in to find out what was going on. At first, they told us he had food allergies and we should try a Gluten Free / Casein Free (GF/CF) Diet. Well, we did, but the progress was slow, and by his 2nd birthday, we were told he had PDD/Autism.

That's how it all started. Looking back now, the writing was on the wall, but I just did not know what to look for. To make things worse, the people I trusted and turned to for help lied to my face over and over again. I will never be that foolish again. For a mother that knew nothing about autism, my life became all about autism. I would care for my child during the day and spend nights researching available treatments for my son. For the next two years, we saw five "specialists", over ten therapists, and made a lot of diet changes which included lots of supplements. We were on a GF/CF Diet, then on the SCD Diet, and then on a restrictive-rotating diet. During this time, we saw some improvements, but it was not much. It was expensive, exhausting, overwhelming and difficult all at the same time. For other parents, doing this is enough to see big gains. Even with all this, my son was now four years old, still non-verbal… only speaking thirty words, very little eye contact, would not respond to his name, was in a world of his own, and have at least three major temper tantrums a day. We needed to go in deeper and fine tune what we were doing.

The turning point for me was when I started to take charge and put all the pieces together. I decided to fight back and take control of my son's health. Up until now I was just taking orders and following what the "specialist" would tell me. I decided to start from the basics and work toward healing him completely. I was fortunate enough to find a doctor that was able to run the proper lab test and discovered the core of his health problems not just the symptoms. He found that my son was toxic, under-nourished, and had a weakened immune and metabolic system. We focused on all four issues for the next 12 months and slowly started to see improvements.

With a whole-body approach to healing, his body naturally reactivated the body's magnificent ability to heal itself. I found a diet that his body responded to, which included fresh juices daily. We removed the toxins through chelation. And by restoring his metabolic and immune system, his body was able to heal. Today, my son is fully recovered. At six years old, he is in a mainstream first grade classroom and involved in baseball, swimming, and tennis. Today, he is indistinguishable from his peers. People are often surprised to hear of him ever having an autism spectrum disorder.

This experience has taught me the importance of what you do and in what order you do them. Had I known the order sooner, I would have saved time, money, and frustration, while seeing results sooner.

This is simply an outline that worked for us. Please consult with a doctor before making any changes to your child's care. This protocol is designed to be followed in order at 100% effort with no exceptions. Follow this protocol in this order and you will see improvement within a short period of time... this will help motivate you to stick with it! It took me 2 years to heal my son once I started this protocol, but he was starting at a better place. Meaning he was already making slow progress, and we were already doing parts of it so the transition was easier. Here is the protocol:

10 step Protocol to Healing Autism Naturally

1. **Mentally Preparing...**get organized, make lists of what you need, set a timeline to start and implement changes (If it's too much to do all at once, then do one new change per week)
2. **Clean out...** Kitchen, food, environment, appliances, products, lifestyle-old habits
3. **Clean in...** Water, Kitchen, food, environment, appliances, products, lifestyle, creating new habits
4. **Diet...**no fluoride in drinking water-filter water only, eat 80% alkaline, 20% acidic food, eat superfoods daily, organic food only, nothing in a box, fresh/frozen only, follow the Feingold Program, lots of potassium foods, no salt/sodium, no red meat, avoid fat, eat more RAW fruits and vegetables, avoid allergic

     foods such as wheat, dairy, soy, corn, peanuts, avoid sugar...learn to eat fruits for dessert

5. **The "do's" and "don'ts" about autism...** *find a DAN doctor, run lab tests, and use supplements free of allergies*
6. **Juice and Smoothie**... *(the more the better) Tip: Juice what they won't eat; 1-2 Green juices are nutrient-rich with little time needed for digestion; Carrot-Apple juices are full of vitamins*
7. **Lifestyle changes...** *Green living, organic is best, don't dine out, play & talk to child daily, use sports as therapy (hand-eye coordination, interaction, following directions), kids learn best when having fun and laughing, make a game of everything and let them be silly kids*
8. **Chelation...** *(should be done under the care of a Doctor), lab tests will show the results...if toxic, a chelator is used to move toxins out of body such as DMSA, Sauna, Food and Juices*
9. **Therapies** *...quantity and quality matter, (sit in during therapy and repeat at home), ABA, OT, Speech, Floor time, Sensory*
10. **Living Fearlessly...** *Incorporate these changes into your lives and stick to them. Don't go back to your old habits once your child is healed. He is still rebuilding his body and is not fully healed. Be cautious of toxins and chemicals*

Educated health consumers, including informed parents, are taking matters into their own hands. They are choosing healthy lifestyles and wise health care alternatives that do not rely on constant pharmaceutical product use, including an alternative vaccine schedule. You may feel you are already doing this, but look closely. Are you consistent? Are you making any exceptions? For example, taking your child for speech every week and eating packaged foods or fast food will not produce the same results as a child on an organic, home- made diet free of allergic foods, eating superfoods and drinking healthy fresh juices daily while taking speech. The results are significantly different.

My favorite quote is by Hippocrates, "Let food be thy medicine and medicine be thy food." *As for me, I was desperate and determined to heal my son. Keep working and don't loose your focus on your long term goal which is...*<u>healing your child</u>*. If you need a motivator, start saving for college! It may take you more than 2 years but it will happen if you're completely dedicated and consistent. Remember, every step forward is a step closer to your goal of healing your child.*

"

~ Eleni Prokopeas
<u>www.GreenDivaMom.com</u>

ABIE'S STORY

The following is an inspiring story of a dedicated father who worked diligently to help his son overcome autistic symptoms and live a normal life. This is Abie's story, as told by his father, Dr. Rashid Buttar:

My son Abie lost his ability to speak around the age of 14 months. His limited vocabulary of about 15 or so words rapidly disappeared within a few weeks of his third set of inoculations. His first word, "Abu" (meaning "father" in Arabic) was the first to disappear. His mother and I had decided we would not inoculate our son due to the presence of thimerosal (ethyl mercury) in vaccinations, which as mentioned, is used as a preservative. As I was considered one of the up-and-coming leading authorities in metal toxicology, there was no way my son would be exposed to mercury. Unbeknownst to me, however, my now ex-wife had gotten Abie the regularly scheduled vaccines because she had listened to the fear-evoking propaganda fed to her by the pediatricians and the doctors at the hospital when she delivered. She had gone back and gotten the inoculations the day after Abie first came home at the ripe age of one day old, and then had taken him for all his subsequent vaccines. By the age of two, he was considered to be "developmentally delayed."

Abie was born on January 25, 1999. In March 1998, ten months prior to his birth and a month before his conception, I had made the decision I would not see autistic and developmentally delayed patients any longer. Looking back, it's clear that God had a specific plan for me, but I was moving away from the right path. Now I understand that this experience was nothing more than God upping the ante, sending me a clear message: "You're going to do what you were meant to do, what you were created to do!" It was obvious to me that Abie's loss of speech was more than a transient delay in his development. As time passed, the pediatricians kept saying the same thing. "Oh well, there's probably nothing there. Just wait. Maybe he's a late developer." But I knew there was something wrong because he had lost his ability to speak. It wasn't that he never acquired it. He had lost it! A twelve-to-fifteen-word vocabulary isn't much, but it's still something! And now those words were all gone.

I didn't know what to do. Although I had treated hundreds of patients with mercury and lead toxicity, I hadn't treated a child this young. I knew from having treated autistic children in the past that his behavior was the same, with the toe walking, hand flapping and stimming—repetitive stereotypic behavior commonly found in developmental delays indicative of decreased sensory input—and that terrified me. I knew my son was not supposed to be like this. I subsequently spent thousands of hours—many if not most of them late at night, sometimes all night—studying, researching, learning, crying and praying that my son would be returned to me. I pleaded, begged and threatened God. I bartered with the Creator, negotiating my arms or my legs in exchange for the return of my son. Throughout this ordeal, Abie always looked at me with his gentle, milk-chocolate-colored eyes that would say, "Don't worry, Dad, I know you'll figure it out."

Eventually I did. Realizing that mercury was the most likely culprit, I tested Abie four times before his challenge test finally came back positive for mercury. As a result, I developed an innovative detoxification method for him, which up until then had never been contemplated. Five months after I began his detoxification, Abie went from no language to a vocabulary of five-hundred-plus words. He was nearly three and a half years old. And, as I shared with you in chapter 2, on May 6, 2004, at the age of five, Abie became the youngest formal witness to appear before the U.S. Congress, testifying in front of the U.S. Congressional Sub-Committee on Human Rights and Wellness regarding innovative methods to treat neurological injuries and the dangers of mercury in vaccines.

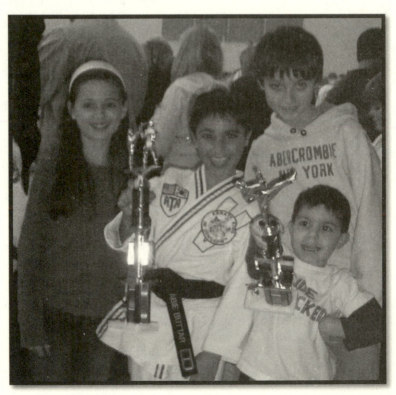

Today, people ask me if he's "normal." It makes me smile to think about it, because he's anything but normal. He's extraordinary, exceptionally handsome, surprisingly gentle, ahead of his peers in school in all subjects and two to three grade levels ahead in math and English, an incredible athlete in every sport he tries, a gifted martial artist who is a triple-crown state champion and ranked among the top ten in the world in both forms and sparring two years in a row and now working on his second-degree black belt in Taekwondo. He touches everyone who meets him, and to know him is to truly love him. Even the parents of the children he competes against come to me to remark on his style, grace and sportsmanship. It is, without any exaggeration whatsoever, truly one of my greatest life blessings to be his father. At the risk of sounding overly sentimental, I have at times literally felt such terrible sadness for the rest of world because they will never know the incredible and indescribable feeling of being Abie's father.

One point about heavy metals I believe is crucial to understand is the synergistically destructive nature of this first category of toxins. In science, a lethal dose (LD) of any substance is measured as the amount needed to kill 1 person out of 100. This measurement is known as LD1. A substance with an LD17 would be sufficient to kill 17 people out of a 100. If you took an LD1 of mercury (sufficient mercury to kill 1 out of a 100) and you took an LD1 of lead (sufficient lead to kill 1 out of a 100) and put these amounts in the same 100 people, you would kill all 100 people! That's how synergistically dangerous heavy metals are, and virtually everyone is walking around with more than one of these toxins in their bodies.

There is just one study of which I'm aware that has been conducted to assess the synergistic destructive nature of heavy metals. Done in the 1970s, it looked at only mercury, lead and cadmium. So we really don't know how destructive some of these other metals are when combined with other metals within the same individual. However, all these substances are removable through the proper detoxification protocols. In time, the body can completely be cleaned, rebound and rebuild itself, leaving no room for chronic disease to begin, as long as you maintain your body's lowered burden of toxins.

More than thirty-five hundred doctors in the United States address the issue of chronic heavy-metal toxicity. However, most of these doctors don't have any training in addressing this crucial issue of heavy metals and fewer than two hundred of them are board certified through the American Board of Clinical Metal Toxicology (ABCMT) in heavy metal toxicology. I strongly suggest you find one of these board-certified or board-eligible doctors at www.ABCMT.org, the board's official website. Remember that the medical hierarchy does not *recognize chronic metal toxicity as an issue that should be addressed and also does not recognize ABCMT, an organization founded almost thirty years ago. At the time of this writing, I serve as the chairman of ABCMT.* **99**

MORE ON VACCINATIONS

Dr. Archie Kalokerinos was a physician who began routinely vaccinating aboriginal children in Australia during the late 1960s. Shortly after he began vaccinations, he noticed that extremely high numbers of these children became very ill or died. He also noticed that children who were sick at the time of vaccination were more likely to experience adverse reactions. In his book Every Second Child, Dr. Kalokerinos also noted that children experiencing adverse reactions would recover after receiving large doses of vitamin C and the numbers of children who suffered adverse reactions declined dramatically when only healthy children who had taken large doses of vitamin C received vaccinations.

*"One would have expected, of course, that the authorities would take an interest in these observations that resulted in a dramatic drop in the death rate of infants in the area under my control. But instead of taking an interest, their reaction was one of extreme hostility. This forced me to look into the question of vaccination further and the further I looked the more shocked I became. **I found that the whole vaccine business was a hoax**. Most doctors are convinced that they are useful, but if you look at the proper statistics and study the instance of these diseases you will realize that this is not so."* - Interview of Dr. Archie Kalokerinos in the *International Vaccination Newsletter*, June 1995.

One study found that 3,000 children die within four days of vaccination each year in America. Another researcher's studies concluded that half of American SIDS cases (between 2,500 and 5,000 infant deaths annually) are **caused** by vaccinations. (Viera Scheibner, Ph.D., Vaccination: 100 Years of Orthodox Research Shows that Vaccines Represent a Medical Assault on the Immune System) It is amazing how much medical literature that exists which documents the failure of vaccinations. In 1989, the Center for Disease Control *(CDC)* reported, *"Among school-aged children, [measles] outbreaks have occurred in schools with vaccination levels of greater than 98 percent. (Morbidity and Mortality Weekly Report (MMWR), 38 (8-9), 12/29/89)*

The parallels between childhood vaccines and chemotherapy are astonishing but not surprising given that it's the same industry and the same manufacturers who are responsible for both.

> ➢ Both vaccines and chemotherapy are shown to be "effective" by scientists whom the manufacturer is paying.
> ➢ Both have resulted in injury and death.
> ➢ Both are extremely profitable.
> ➢ Both are considered sacred and won't be seriously challenged.
> ➢ Both represent a paradigm that the body can only be healed or made whole by the use of dangerous extrinsic chemicals.

I know we are all brought up to blindly trust our doctors. But the fact is that they no longer deserve that kind of blind trust. Physicians take an oath to *"First, do no harm,"* but today, what gets injected into your child is being decided not by physicians but by Big Pharma which has a financial incentive to inject as many vaccinations as possible. Only by keeping people in the dark can Big Pharma continue its absurd profiteering from the vaccination industry. We assume that because vaccinations are mandated by American law that the government is verifying to their safety and effectiveness. Nothing could be further from the truth.

"SACRED" QUACKERY

As I mentioned previously, I am well aware that vaccinations are considered "sacred" to most conventional doctors. As a matter of fact, questioning them is tantamount to blasphemy. I can assure you that I would not challenge the efficacy and safety of something as "holy" as vaccinations unless I were certain, beyond a shadow of a doubt, that I am accurate when I state that vaccinations are **not** safe and they are **not** effective in preventing the spread of disease.

Over the past 60 years, as the cornerstone of public health policy, vaccinations have **caused**, not prevented the spread of disease. If you are able to look at this subject with "objective spectacles," you will easily be able to see that mass vaccinations are linked to global epidemics of neurological and behavioral problems as well as world-wide proliferation of autoimmune diseases. Unfortunately, it's likely that you will dismiss me as a "quack" or "idiot," put your head back into the sand, and take your children back to the doctor for more **poison injections.**

You see, most Americans will do whatever they are told. From the cradle, we are encouraged **not** to think for ourselves. We are programmed to place blind faith in our physician and the Medical Mafia. We are taught **not** to ask questions. The poignant fact is that most Americans simply believe in vaccinations, although it is likely that they have no idea what is in them. Decades of studies published in the world's leading medical journals have documented serious adverse effects (including death) from vaccinations.

Hundreds of published medical studies and dozens of books written by doctors and researchers have documented vaccine failure, adverse effects, and serious flaws in practice and theory. Yet, incredibly, most pediatricians and parents are unaware of these findings. Inexcusably, most pediatricians don't even know what's in the vaccinations they are administering. Don't believe me? Just ask them...and be prepared to see a perplexed look on their face...right before they get mad at you for daring to ask questions or threaten you if you don't submit to their policy of "mandatory" vaccinations! Sadly, most pediatricians have staked their reputations on the presumed safety and effectiveness of vaccinations, so they are not exactly "open" to hearing any information to the contrary.

For example, when our eldest daughter, Brianna, was about 18 months old, we took her to the doctor's office for a checkup. The doctor told us that it was time for her vaccinations, among them the MMR vaccine. We had been doing a little research on vaccinations and were a bit concerned that they may not be quite as safe as they are reported to be. So, we told the doctor that we were concerned and did not want Brianna to be vaccinated, thinking that he would honor our wishes.

His response was staggering. *"If you choose not to have her vaccinated, then she can no longer be a part of our practice here. You will have to go elsewhere. We are not buying into or promoting all that hype (on autism). Vaccinations do not cause autism. Eating kids' fish sticks is more of a risk at causing autism than these vaccinations."* **What arrogance!** What a pompous hypocrite. We should have walked out of his office immediately, but like thousands of other parents, we caved to the pressure and allowed that doctor to inject our little girl with poison.

POISONING OUR CHILDREN

Every day, millions of children are lined up and injected with toxic, putrid substances called vaccinations. Before they begin first grade, children can get as many as 36 vaccinations! There are about 200 more vaccinations in the pipeline. Scenarios for the future even include consuming vaccines in nose sprays, ointments and fruits and vegetables. This *"Vaccination Obsession"* has gone beyond what anyone can possibly defend on scientific grounds. Pumping more vaccinations into our precious children borders on the criminal.

With every child on the planet a potential "required recipient" of multiple vaccinations, and with every healthcare system and government a potential buyer, it is little wonder that billions of dollars are spent nurturing the vaccination industry. Without public outcry, we will see more and more new vaccines required of us and our children. And while profits are readily calculable, the real human costs are being ignored. Dr. James R. Shannon (former director of the National Institute of Health) reported in December 2003 that *"the only safe vaccine is one that is never used."*

Remember, vaccinations are mandated but they are **not** mandatory! Besides certain laws that apply only to government medical specialists, **THERE IS NO LAW** that enforces the mandatory use of any vaccine in the United States. Waiver forms for personal or religious exemptions are freely available. Enforced medical treatment is an assault and a violation of the 14th amendment.

In the December 1994 Medical Post, Canadian author of the best-seller <u>Medical Mafia</u>, Dr. Guylaine Lanctot stated, *"The medical authorities keep lying. Vaccination has been a disaster on the immune system. It actually causes a lot of illnesses. We are actually changing our genetic code through vaccination...Ten years from now we will know that the biggest crime against humanity was vaccines."*

EMAIL EXCHANGE WITH A PEDIATRICIAN

After I initially published the first edition of this book in August 2006, I had an interesting email discussion with a pediatrician regarding vaccinations, specifically the DPT. He accused me of being "irresponsible" for claiming that vaccinations are poison to our children. Below is the entire email thread...

Pediatrician: *On an emotional level, I just have to add that it only takes seeing one unimmunized child die of pertussis (whooping cough) to make one question those who decry immunizations and claim we are "poisoning our children with vaccinations."*

My response: Over 11,000 annual cases of adverse reactions to vaccinations are reported to the VAERS (*Vaccine Adverse Effects*

Reporting System), a branch of the FDA, of which 1% result in death. (National Technical Information Service - Springfield, VA - 703.487.4650) The lion's share (over 100 per year) of deaths are attributed to reactions to the pertussis vaccine (the "P" in DPT). It is unknown exactly how many deaths have occurred from the pertussis vaccine, because doctors underreport all vaccine adverse events. In New York State, for example, the National Vaccine Information Center (NVIC) recently found that only one out of 40 doctor's offices (2.5%) confirmed that they report a death or injury following vaccination. (National Vaccine Information Center (NVIC), 512 Maple Ave. W. #206, Vienna, VA 22180, 703-938-0342; *"Investigative Report on the Vaccine Adverse Event Reporting System"*)

The truth is that the number of vaccine-related deaths dwarfs the number of deaths caused by the disease, which have averaged around **10** annually for the past 2 decades, according to the CDC. As the FDA estimates that only approximately 10% of adverse reactions are reported, we can estimate that the chances of dying from the pertussis vaccine are **100 times greater** than the chances of dying from pertussis itself.

Simply put, **the vaccine is 100 times more deadly than the disease**. Given the many instances in which highly vaccinated populations have contracted pertussis and the fact that the disease was on the decline well before mandatory vaccinations (pertussis deaths declined 79% **prior to** vaccines), the enormous number of vaccine casualties can hardly be considered a necessary sacrifice for the benefit of a disease-free society.

In the USA in 1986, 90% of 1,300 pertussis cases in Kansas were "adequately vaccinated." (Neil Miller, *Vaccines: Are They Safe and Effective?* p 33) In 1993, 72% of pertussis cases in the Chicago outbreak were fully up to date with their vaccinations. (Chicago Dept. of Health) Sadly, the vaccine-related-deaths story doesn't end here. Both national and international studies have shown vaccination to be a cause of SIDS (Viera Scheibner, Ph.D., *"Vaccination: 100 Years of Orthodox Research Shows that Vaccines Represent a Medical Assault on the Immune System"* and W.C. Torch, *"Diphtheria-pertussis-tetanus (DPT) immunization: A potential cause of the sudden infant death syndrome (SIDS),"* (Amer. Academy of Neurology, 34th Annual Meeting, Apr 25 - May 1, 1982).

The Torch study found the peak incidence of SIDS occurred at the ages of 2 and 4 months in the United States, precisely when the first two routine immunizations are given. It also found that 3,000 children die within 4 days of vaccination each year, and concluded that half of SIDS cases (approximately 2,500 to 5,000 infant deaths in the United States per year) are caused by vaccines.

Interestingly, on November 26, 2005, the Bush administration asked a federal claims court to seal documents relating to hundreds of cases of autism allegedly caused by thimerosal, one of the toxic ingredients used in many childhood vaccines. The government's legal action comes on the heels of an insertion into the Homeland Security bill that protects Eli Lilly, the drug company giant that developed thimerosal, from lawsuits involving the additive. **The bill removes all liability from the pharmaceutical industry and health officials for the injuries and death resulting from the preservative.** This is sickening! Yet another instance of Big Pharma and governmental corruption.

Pediatrician: *You point out that there are only 10 deaths from pertussis each year. I wonder why that is. In 1934 there were around 8000 deaths attributed to pertussis in the US. The pertussis vaccine was developed around that time and became used wide-spread about 20 years later. So the 10 deaths each year from pertussis is actually a vaccine success story.*

My response: It is common knowledge that whooping cough, like measles, scarlet fever and diphtheria, is a very much less severe disease than in times past, and it is the generally accepted idea in the medical community that vaccination has been mainly responsible for this. In fact nothing could be further from the truth. Scarlet fever declined dramatically in both morbidity and mortality without vaccination and for the most part prior to the advent of antibiotics. Measles declined in a similar fashion prior to the introduction of vaccination and, since it is a "viral disease," it is not affected by antibiotics. Diphtheria also declined prior to the advent of immunization. As I mentioned in an earlier email, whooping cough also had declined by 79% **BEFORE** immunizations.

The evidence indicates that the decline in severity in these diseases was due to **improved sanitation, better nutrition, better housing, and improved hygiene** rather than to any specific immunizations. The truth be told, England actually saw a drop in pertussis deaths when vaccination rates dropped from 80% to 30% in the mid 1970s.

Swedish epidemiologist B. Trollfors' study of pertussis vaccine efficacy and toxicity around the world found that *"pertussis-associated mortality is currently very low in industrialized countries, and no difference can be discerned when countries with high, low and zero immunization rates were compared."* He also found that England, Wales, and West Germany had more pertussis fatalities in 1970 when the immunization rate was high, than during the last half of 1980 when rates had fallen. I know you don't like statistics from 20 or 30 years ago, but facts do **not** change.

The truth does **not** change. The laws of physics do **not** change.

Pediatrician: *Just for full disclosure, you might want to point out that the National Vaccine Information Center, the group that put out the paper you quote, is an anti-vaccination organization. They've got a nice link to "lawyer referral" on their website.*

My response: What difference does that make? Should I ask you to point out that the groups that you cite are pro-vaccination groups? C'mon, what's good for the goose is good for the gander. Let's just be realistic and admit that much of the literature which I cite is from groups that oppose vaccinations, while much of the studies which you will cite are from pro-vaccination groups. The trick is to find out who (if anyone) is manipulating the data, and why....$$$...

Pediatrician: *Why are the papers you're quoting from the early 80s? I've not read them, but that's an eternity in medical literature. Surely you have some newer data (last 5 years) to support these claims. Right?*

My response: As I mentioned earlier, the truth does **not** change. Have the laws of physics changed over the past 2 decades? If so, I wasn't aware of it. And the papers I quoted were just examples of pertussis epidemics that broke out in vaccinated populations, thus demonstrating that the DPT is not near as effective as Big Medicine would have us to believe. The dates are what they are. If I wanted to demonstrate that the Nazi party committed genocide, then I would refer you to the German death camps of the 1940s. I doubt that you would ask for **newer data**, rejecting the fact that millions of innocent people were murdered by Nazis, since, after all, it did happen over 60 years ago...an "eternity in medical literature"...

But since you asked...the *New England Journal of Medicine* documents that the pertussis epidemic in Cincinnati (1993) was in a fully vaccinated population. The authors assert that the proportion of cases in fully vaccinated children provides evidence of *"the failure of the whole-cell pertussis vaccine."* (11/24/94 *NEJM*)

The CDC's own website indicates that a sudden increase in cases reflecting a pertussis outbreak in the Netherlands in 1996 **could not be explained by a decrease in vaccination coverage**, which remained stable at 96% for at least three vaccinations in the first year of life. www.cdc.gov/ncidod/eid/vol6no4/demelker.htm.

I could list many more studies conducted within the last decade, but you get my point, right?

Pediatrician: *The autism question: The Cochrane database did a systematic review (very statistically-powerful paper that combines the results of many studies over a long period of time) this year looking at MMR and autism. They reviewed one hundred thirty-nine studies and found no link.*

 My response: The Cochrane Study is oftentimes cited in an effort to support vaccinations (*specifically the MMR*), show that there is no link to autism, demonstrate that the anti-vaccination wackos' fears are unfounded, and give the MMR the "all's clear ahead." But this is a load of bologna. Most of these people should start by reading the **actual study** rather than regurgitating the press release.

The study didn't say anything like this at all. The press release said: *"There was no credible evidence behind claims of harm from the MMR vaccination."* **But the study did not say that**. What the study **did say** (but was not mentioned in the press release) was: *"The design and reporting of safety outcomes in MMR vaccine studies ... are largely inadequate."* The study also stated: *"We found only* **limited evidence** *of the safety of MMR compared to its single component vaccines."*

In other words, far from saying MMR was safe, the study said **explicitly** that the evidence for its safety was ***not good enough***. Now, I'm not saying that the study didn't say that the evidence it looked at did not support any association between MMR and autism. It did say that. But that does not equate to stating that the MMR is safe. It means that the study did not find anything to suggest that it was not safe. Kind of like in a trial when you find a person "**not guilty**"...rather than "**innocent**." What was the reason that they said the evidence didn't support a link between the MMR and autism? Well, you know that epidemiological studies are intrinsically **un**likely to reveal the truth about the effects of MMR. Here's why: **they rely on medical records.** But the fact is that most doctors quickly dismiss parents' concerns about autism *(I know first hand about this);* thus, they never enter anything out of the ordinary on their medical records.

The authors of the Cochrane Study were far from "independent." Did you know that Dr. Tom Jefferson one of the Cochrane study's authors, acknowledged that in 1999, he acted as a consultant for a legal team advising the MMR vaccine manufacturers? Can anyone say "*Conflict of Interest?*" And this is not the only instance of the "incest factor." A number of epidemiological studies which the FDA has used to state that MMR is safe have been written by researchers with links to Big Pharma companies. Remarkably, the Cochran Study concluded that the safety studies into MMR were so poor that *"the safety record of MMR is probably best attested by almost universal use."* In other words, because the vaccine is so widely used, it must be safe. **Talk about**

circular reasoning!! This is a dangerous and extremely **un**scientific assumption.

Pediatrician: *The most damning piece of evidence for the autism-MMR question is the fact that the vaccine companies completely removed the traces of mercury from the vaccine in 1999, yet the rates of autism continue to rise. Why autism is increasing is an interesting question, but the answer is not in vaccines.*

My response: This is not true. In 2004, after much public controversy surrounding the mercury content of childhood vaccinations, Health Advocacy in the Public Interest (HAPI) tested 4 vaccines for heavy metal content. The vials were sent to Doctor's Data, an independent lab which specializes in heavy metal testing. Many manufacturers voluntarily began producing supposed "mercury free" vaccines in 1999. Some product inserts currently claim that a "trace" amount of mercury still exists in the final product but that the amount has been greatly reduced. Others claim to be producing completely mercury free products.

During an investigation into the mercury issue, HAPI learned that thimerosal, a 50% mercury compound, is still being used to produce most vaccines and that the manufacturers are simply "filtering it out" of the final product. However, according to Boyd Haley, PhD, Chemistry Department Chair, University of Kentucky, mercury binds to the antigenic protein in the vaccine and cannot be completely, 100% filtered out.

All 4 vaccine vials tested contained mercury despite manufacturer claims that two of the vials were completely mercury free. All four vials also contained aluminum (one had 9 times more than the other 3), which tremendously enhances the toxicity of mercury causing neuronal death in the brain. www.whale.to/a/mercury7.html

Conclusion of Debate: After this thread of emails, the pediatrician disengaged from the conversation and would not respond to my emails. I guess he was too busy poisoning children…

THE "BOTTOM LINE"

Vaccine mythology is medical fascism based on "voodoo" science and fraudulent data. It is a "medical house of cards" that is collapsing right before our very eyes. Vaccines cause disease, disability, and even death. Hygiene and sanitation, **not** vaccinations, have resulted in the decrease of nearly every infectious disease over the past century.

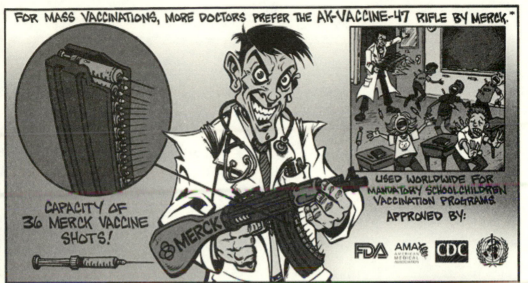

Thanks to Mike Adams and *www.NaturalNews.com* for the cartoon above.

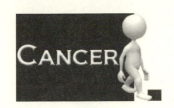
CHAPTER 18
MERCURY & ALZHEIMER'S

> ### FRAUD:
> AMALGAM DENTAL FILLINGS HAVE BEEN SHOWN TO BE 100% SAFE. THERE IS NO RELATIONSHIP BETWEEN FILLINGS, MERCURY, AND ALZHEIMER'S DISEASE.
>
> ### FACT:
> AMALGAM DENTAL FILLINGS CREATE "TOXIC TEETH." FOR SEVERAL DECADES, IT HAS BEEN KNOWN THAT HEAVY METALS, INCLUDING MERCURY, ARE A CAUSE OF ALZHEIMER'S DISEASE AND MULTIPLE OTHER CHRONIC HEALTH PROBLEMS.

For decades, most people have seen a visit to the dentist and subsequent cavity filling as a necessary and regular procedure. Side effects have not routinely been brought to light, so few have challenged the status quo. Evidence suggests, however, that such an apparently harmless procedure can have serious detrimental effects.

Did you know that dental amalgam fillings (popularly called "silver fillings") are actually 50% mercury, which is a **deadly poison** that wreaks havoc with the human body? The mercury contained in dental amalgam would be hazardous waste in a river, yet it's sitting in your mouth, slowly leaking mercury into your system. A fairly large mercury filling contains enough mercury to kill a child if given as a single dose!

What is wrong with this picture?

In this chapter, we will look closely at the relationship between "silver" amalgam (*i.e.,* mercury) dental fillings and Alzheimer's disease.

Mercury Madness

Have you ever read <u>Alice in Wonderland</u>? Do you remember the "Mad Hatter?" Did you know that the term "mad as a hatter" originated from a disease peculiar to the hat making industry in the 1800s? A complicated set of processes was needed to turn the fur into a finished hat. With the cheaper sorts of fur, an early step was to brush a solution of a mercury compound on the fur to roughen the fibers. This caused the hatters to breathe in the fumes of this highly toxic metal, leading to an accumulation of mercury in the hatter's bodies. This resulted in symptoms such as trembling (known as "hatters' shakes"), slurred speech, loss of coordination, anxiety, personality changes, depression, and memory loss. This eventually became known as "Mad Hatter Syndrome" and is still used today to describe mercury poisoning.

The ADA continues to remain in denial about the toxicity of mercury. In an ADA news release on June 13, 2001, ADA President Robert Anderton stated, *"There is no sound scientific evidence supporting a link between amalgam fillings and systemic diseases or chronic illness."* Shame on you Dr. Anderton! This is a blatant lie. All evidence indicates that "silver" amalgam fillings (which typically contain close to 50% mercury) are extremely toxic to the human body.

The late Dr. Patrick Störtebecker, world renowned neurologist and writer from Stockholm, Sweden, wrote in his book <u>Mercury Poisoning from Dental Amalgam – a Hazard to Human Brain</u>, *"Dental amalgam is a highly unstable metal that easily gives off mercury vapor. The most dangerous route for transport of mercury vapor, being released from dental amalgams, is from the mucous membranes of the upper nasal cavity and directly upwards to the brain where mercury vapor easily penetrates the dura mater (i.e., blood-brain barrier). Mercury (vapor) can act in a much stronger concentra-tion straight on the brain cells."*

You wouldn't take a leaky thermometer, put it in your mouth, and leave it there 24 hours a day, would you? But, according to Dr. Michael Ziff, executive director of the International Academy of Oral Medicine and Toxicology (*IAOMT*), that is *"exactly what happens when an amalgam filling is installed in your mouth."* According to Tom Warren, *"Worldwide there are over 4,000 research papers indicating mercury is a highly toxic substance. How can dentists be so thoughtless as to place one of the **deadliest toxins** in existence two inches from our brain?"* www.whale.to/a/toxic_dentistry.html

Evidence now demonstrates that amalgam fillings are constantly being broken down and then are released into the mouth. These minute particles of mercury filling are then acted upon by oral and intestinal bacteria to produce methyl mercury (an even more toxic form of mercury than elemental mercury) with target areas being primarily the pituitary gland, thyroid gland, and the brain. That's right, the brain! After the fillings have been inserted into the mouth, subtle changes in blood chemistry have been observed that point to specific chronic disease, e.g., cancer, multiple sclerosis (MS), and Alzheimer's. The difficulty in recognizing the "amalgam connection" to chronic disease is that clinical symptoms are not present until the patient's immune system collapses, which may be in 40 or 50 years.

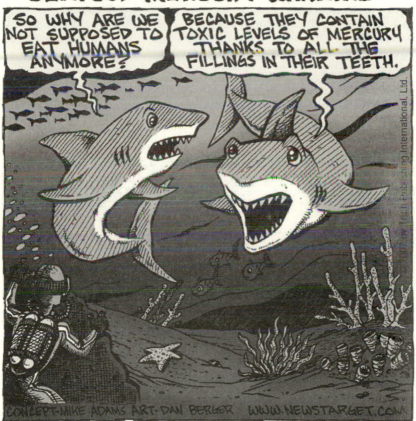

Thanks to Mike Adams and *www.NaturalNews.com* for the cartoon above.

So how much mercury is in your mouth? There is approximately ½ gram of mercury in each dental filling. You may think that since you only have a couple of mercury fillings it's not a big deal. Think again. According to Dr. Richard Fischer, past president of the IAOMT, *"Dental amalgam ('silver') fillings contribute more mercury to the body burden in humans than all other sources (dietary, air, water, vaccines, etc.) combined. These fillings contain 50% mercury – which is more neurotoxic than lead, cadmium, or even arsenic."* To put this in perspective, the amount of mercury contained in one average size filling exceeds the EPA standard for human exposure for over one hundred years. Put in other terms, it takes only ½ gram of mercury (the amount in one filling) to contaminate all fish in a ten acre lake.

According to Pam Floener, former spokesperson for the IAOMT, *"The metallic mercury used by dentists to manufacture dental amalgam is shipped as a **hazardous material** to the dental office. When amalgams are removed, for whatever reason, they are treated as **hazardous waste** and are required to be disposed of in accordance with OSHA regulations, and it is inconceivable that the mouth could be considered a safe storage container for this toxic material."* www.mercola.com/2001/apr/21/mercury.htm

So, let me get this straight...if a dentist were to dump some mercury amalgam in a lake, he'd be breaking the law. But if this same dentist dumps some mercury in your mouth (via dental amalgam fillings), then it's completely legal and would no longer be considered a threat to the environment. *"I don't feel comfortable using a substance designated by the Environmental Protection Agency to be a waste disposal hazard. I can't throw it in the trash, bury it in the ground, or put it in a landfill, but they say it is OK to put it in people's mouths. **That doesn't make sense**."* - Richard Fischer, D.D.S.

Dr. Dietrich Klinghardt, mercury toxicity expert at the American Academy of Neural Therapy, states, *"As soon as anybody has any type of medical illness or symptom, whether medical or emotional, the amalgam fillings should be removed, and the mercury residues should be eliminated from the body, especially the brain. ... Most – if not all – chronic infectious diseases are not caused by a failure of the immune system but are a conscious adaptation of the immune system to an otherwise lethal heavy metal environment."*

But don't expect your dentist to jump on board with you if you ask to have your fillings removed. According to the ADA's code of ethics, a dentist who acknowledges that mercury amalgam fillings are toxic and recommends their removal has acted unethically. According to ADA Resolution 42H-1986, *"The removal of amalgam restorations from the non-allergic patient for the alleged purpose of removing toxic substances from the body when such treatment is performed solely at the recommendation of the dentist is **improper and unethical**...."*

What? Unethical to remove toxic poison from your mouth? Yet more proof that the ADA is still in the Dark Ages...

Did you know that dentists have the highest rate of suicide of any profession? They also suffer a high incidence of depression and memory disorders. Two of the effects of mercury poisoning are loss of memory and depression. Do you think the high rate of suicide (*due to depression*) and memory disorders in dentists has anything to do with low-level mercury exposure over several years? **This is mercury toxicity**, plain and simple.

The Alzheimer's Connection

You may have heard that lead poisoning is suspected to cause Alzheimer's, but according to Dr. Marcia Basciano, "*The maximum amount of mercury that the Environment Protection Agency allows people to be exposed to is 5,000 times smaller than the permissible amount of lead exposure; in other words the EPA apparently considers mercury to be 5,000 times more toxic than lead.*" It is likely that the most common cause of Alzheimer's disease is due to toxic mercury that leaches from amalgam dental fillings.

In the words of Dr. Charles Williamson, co-director of the Toxic Studies Institute and outstpoken critic of mercury amalgams: "*there are studies from world renowned institutions that categorically show a cause-and-effect relationship between mercury and disease; **this is particularly true of Alzheimer's**. Mercury is a cytotoxin (i.e., it poisons cells). Why wouldn't it make you sick?*" www.lef.org/magazine/mag2001/may2001_report_mercury_1.html.

According to Dr. Murray Vimy, a researcher from the University of Calgary, Canada, and member of the WHO: "*On March 9, 1995, a friend faxed to me her mother's autopsy report from Mayo Clinic. Her mother died of AD (Alzheimer's Disease). The poor woman had 53 times more mercury in her brain than people who die of other causes.*" In 1991, Dr. Boyd Haley, a research toxicologist at the University of Kentucky, discovered some hard evidence that changed the mercury debate for good. "*It was almost accidental...I found out how damaging mercury amalgam is to the brain while studying tissue affected by Alzheimer's disease...I did an experiment. I put mercury amalgam in water. Then, I placed a sample of brain tissue in that water and checked on it over time. After a period of several weeks, I noticed that the exposure to mercury had suppressed the secretion from the brain tissue of tubulin—a major enzyme that performs critical functions in the brain. This finding was consistent both with mercury toxicity and with brain tissue as affected by Alzheimer's disease. From that, I* *concluded that there's clearly leakage from mercury amalgam—and that there's a strong probability that people who have such fillings in their teeth are being exposed to chronic, low-dose mercury leakage...(Dentists) insist mercury amalgam is safe, non-toxic and that it doesn't leak ... (but) mercury is a neurotoxin. It leeches out of dental fillings, of that there is no doubt. ...It heightens the risk of Alzheimer's and Parkinson's disease as well as other neurological disorders. Dentists defend their use of mercury amalgam, but it's unjustifiable. I feel like I've been arguing with the town drunk for eight or nine years. My conclusion is simple and direct: **mercury is the toxicant behind Alzheimer's**."* www.lef.org/magazine/mag2001

Other scientists have shown that trace amounts of mercury can cause the type of nerve damage that is characteristic of the damage found in Alzheimer's disease. The level of mercury exposure used in the test was well below those levels found in many humans with mercury/amalgam dental fillings. The research was conducted at the University of Calgary Faculty of Medicine by professors Fritz Lorscheider and Naweed Syed. The professors found that exposure to mercury caused the formation of "neurofibrillar tangles," which are one of the two diagnostic markers for Alzheimer's disease. Previous research has shown that mercury can cause the formation of the other Alzheimer's disease marker, "amyloid plaques."

Dr. Lorsheider and Dr. Syed noted that no other material or metal tested, including aluminum, has ever produced even remotely similar reactions. They also produced the visual documentation of the biochemical mechanism by which the introduction of mercury induces hallmark diagnostic markers indistinguishable from those seen in the Alzheimer's diseased brain. When Dr. Lorscheider submitted the paper to the British journal *NeuroReport*, which eventually published it, he added the video as an accompanying document, making it one of the few times that a piece of animation was subjected to the peer-review process. View the video here: http://commons.ucalgary.ca/mercury

Get Rid of the Mercury & Reverse Alzheimer's

According to Dr. H. Richard Casdorph, *"In large measure, those martyred by dementia are showing the results of toxicity from mercury, aluminum, lead, cadmium, arsenic and other heavy metals. **Their neurons have been poisoned.** They are turned into Alzheimer's victims directly through the efforts of dentists who blindly follow the party line of their trade union organisation, the ADA. Since 1952 the medical profession has had the means to reduce or **reverse** the signs and symptoms of Alzheimer's disease."* I recommend you read the report by Tom Warren entitled "Reversing Alzheimer's Disease."

Chelation therapy is the means to reduce or reverse the signs of Alzheimer's disease. Taken from the Greek word *"chele"* meaning *"claw,"* the word chelation refers to the way the therapy binds heavy metals, toxins, and metabolic wastes in the bloodstream. According to Doctors H. Richard Casdorph and Morton Walker, authors of <u>Toxic Metal Syndrome: How Metal Poisoning Can Affect Your Brain</u>, chelation therapy has been shown to help at least 50% of elderly people with Alzheimer's who have tried it. They are documented as showing greater mental clarity, increased IQ, and improved memory. In their book, the authors state that the Alzheimer's patients *"were observed by loved ones to have returned to normal, or near normal, functioning. It was a gratifying experience for everyone involved with the testing and treatment: diagnosticians, clinicians, health care technicians, the patients, plus their family and friends."*

The first step in removing the mercury from your system is to get rid of your amalgam fillings! However, there are safe ways to do this and there are unsafe ways. If you get your fillings removed by a dentist who doesn't take precautions, then the end result will be that you are worse off than before. Careless removal of amalgam fillings can release even more mercury into your system than what was leaking before the fillings were removed.

When we lived in Dallas, my dentist was Dr. Ellis Ramsey. He has been aware of the dangers of mercury for almost three decades. In 2007, he removed all of my mercury fillings. He is an expert at safe mercury removal, and I highly recommend him if you are in the North Texas (DFW) area. If you live elsewhere, be sure that you seek out a "biological dentist," preferably a member of the IAOMT, who understands the issues surrounding amalgam fillings.

Two safety precautions: 1) Request oxygen during the procedure – this will insure that you breathe clean oxygen rather than toxic mercury vapor when the fillings are drilled out. 2) Request a rubber dam – this keeps pieces of the filling from falling down your throat or onto your tongue.

After you have had your fillings removed, the next step is to chelate the heavy metals. The quickest and most potent chelation method available today is intravenous EDTA chelation therapy. The chelating agent, EDTA, is an amino acid which has negative charges associated with it. Once inside the body it looks for positively charged molecules such as lead, iron, mercury, and cadmium. The number of IV EDTA treatments necessary is generally between twenty and fifty sessions, depending on your condition. This will cost between $2,000 and $5,000.

According to Webster Kehr, *"This treatment has been known about for decades, but because EDTA chelation is **not profitable enough** for orthodox medicine the treatment has been buried. It is not that EDTA chelation is not expensive, it is expensive. The problem is that it **cures the patient too quickly**, and it does not treat the symptoms of Alzheimer's. In short, it is not profitable enough for Big Pharma and it is not "sophisticated" enough, meaning it is too simple, for Big Medicine. Big Pharma and Big Medicine like to treat symptoms, not causes."* www.cancertutor.com

Oral EDTA costs significantly less than IV EDTA, between $20 and $50 per month, depending on your intake. Clinical experience suggests that oral EDTA chelation provides many, but not all, of the benefits of IV therapy. Only between five and ten percent of an oral dose of EDTA is absorbed into the bloodstream (compared with one hundred percent of an IV dose). Yet, due to continuous daily intake, the amounts add up and can achieve similar benefits. Overall, the differences in benefits are more those of degree, convenience, speed, and cost per dose than of quality.

Another weapon in our "chelation arsenal" is **chlorella**. High doses of chlorella (10 to 20 grams) have been found to be very effective for mercury elimination. This is an important part of a good systemic mercury elimination program, because approximately 90% of the mercury is eliminated through the stool, and chlorella helps fecal excretion. And remember, chlorella is a food, so you cannot eat too much of it! However, you will need to work up to 20 grams since it can cause diarrhea.

Chlorella should be used in conjunction with **cilantro.** Dr. Omura, a Japanese researcher, discovered that cilantro could mobilize mercury and other toxic metals rapidly from the central nervous system. However, cilantro alone often does not remove mercury from the body. It often only displaces the metals from deeper body stores to more superficial structures. Cilantro will help mobilize mercury out of the tissue so the chlorella can bind to it and allow it to be excreted from the body. Along with chlorella and cilantro, you should start eating fresh **garlic** every day. This will enhance sulfur stores. Between two and three cloves a day is an excellent idea. Make sure you crush the garlic to release its active ingredients. Jon Barron has a fantastic product called "Metal Magic" which contains both chlorella and cilantro. You can purchase it at www.baselinenutritionals.com.

Also, I suggest taking **MSM** as well. MSM, which we discussed in the cancer treatments chapter, is a form of sulfur which acts on cell membranes and which will help your body eliminate the mercury. Here is Karl Loren's explanation of how MSM chelates toxins and metals:

"*The brain is made up of billions of nerve cells, intricately connected with each other like electrons in an electrical circuit. When you think - you send electrical impulses throughout your brain. Alzheimer's disease is a condition where the many of these cells are coated with aluminum, causing them to short circuit and sends brain impulses to the wrong synapse creating confusion. MSM opens the membrane that contains the aluminum and allows the unwanted deposits to be flushed into the blood stream. The hot bath with Clorox makes the body sweat and release the aluminum. Then the Clorox leeches it right off your body.*" www.bulkmsm.com/research/msm/msm6.htm#alzheimer

According to Dr. Andrew H. Cutler, "*Amalgam illness is analogous to a war. Your enemy, mercury, captured a beachhead in your teeth and fortified it with amalgam. Then it launched an attack. House to house. Organ to organ. Cell to cell. Slowly capturing your body. You win the war with a surgical strike. Dental surgery. Drill out those fillings. Removing your amalgam declares an armistice. Fighting stops, but the mercury atoms are still dug in wherever they reached. Chelation sends clean up squads off to round up the enemy and escort them out. Meanwhile the surviving cells in your body get to work and to repair the war damage.*" www.noamalgam.com

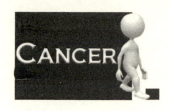
CHAPTER 19
ROOT CANALS

FICTION:
ROOT CANALS ARE SAFE AND OFTENTIMES
NECESSARY TO PREVENT A TOOTH FROM BEING
EXTRACTED.

FACT:
A ROOT CANAL TOOTH IS ALWAYS INFECTED
REGARDLESS OF ITS APPEARANCE AND LACK OF
SYMPTOMS.

You probably thought that mercury was the only "toxic teeth" issue and that you're home free! Well, not if you have had a **root canal**. Approximately 20,000,000 root canal operations are performed annually in the United States. Nearly every dentist is oblivious to the serious health risks this operation produces. While many intelligent dentists refuse to put mercury fillings into the mouths of their patients, these same dentists will go right ahead and gladly perform a root canal, without any idea that these procedures cause horrific damage to their patients. According to Dr. James Howenstine, *"Many chronic diseases, perhaps most, are a result of root canal surgery."*

A root canal treatment is done to save a tooth which otherwise would have needed to be extracted. They are usually done when severe infection has spread to the roots of the tooth. The root canal is a narrow canal that runs from the middle of the tooth down to the roots, which are buried in the jawbone. In the root canal procedure, a hole is drilled in the tooth to gain access to the root canal, the dead or infected nerves and tissue are removed, and the root canal area is cleaned, sterilized, and disinfected. Then the inside of the tooth is filled, and the hole is typically sealed with a crown.

Each year, millions of root canals are done with an apparent success rate of over 90%. In other words, there is no pain, and the x-rays indicate that the tooth has been "healed." Unfortunately, this masks a problem which can still be occurring. Many dentists now recognize that it is **impossible** to clean out all of the dead tissue or to completely sterilize a tooth. There are over 3 miles of tubules (tiny channels) in every tooth, and only an arrogant (or insane) dentist would claim to be able to clean or sterilize 100% of the 3 miles of tubules. This then leaves areas of necrotic (dead) tissue in the tooth to continue decomposing and being infected. Our immune system's white blood cells don't travel into tubules nor do antibiotics filter into these areas. Thus, the tubules become a "safe haven" for microbes (viruses, yeasts, fungi, molds, bacteria, etc). And since the nerve tissue, blood vessels, and living tissue inside the tooth have been removed, it is now **dead**.

In 1993, Dr. Hal Huggins gave a lecture to the Cancer Control Society. In an almost comical fashion, Dr. Huggins stated, "*Then we get into the root canal business, and that is the most tragic of all. Isn't there something you can put in the centre of the canal that is safe? Yeah, there probably is, but that is not where the problem is. **The problem with a root canal is that it is dead**. Let's equate that. Let's say you have got a ruptured appendix, so you go to the phone book, and who do you look up? Let's see, we have a surgeon and a taxidermist, who do you call? You going to get it bronzed? That is all we do to a dead tooth. We put a gold crown on it, looks like it has been bronzed. It doesn't really matter what you embalm the dead tooth with, it is still dead, and within that dead tooth we have bacteria, and these bacteria are in the absence of oxygen. In the absence of oxygen most things die except bacteria. They undergo something called a **pleomorphic** change...like a mutation ...they learn to live in the absence of oxygen...now produce **thio-ethers**, some of the strongest poisons on the planet that are not radioactive.*" www.whale.to/d/root2.html

Remember that cancer and a host of other diseases have links to **microbes**. To cure cancer, the microbes must be killed throughout the body so the immune system can restore the body to its normal state. However, a root canal is the perfect "breeding ground" for microbes. As Dr. Huggins stated above, some of the most dangerous of these microbes are the thio-ethers, including dimethyl sulfate. A German oncologist named Josef Issels was able to confirm that the thio-ethers released from these root canal microbes are very closely related to the chemicals used by the Germans in World War I to create mustard gas. According to the EPA, dimethyl sulfate has been classified as a Group B2 human carcinogen. Tumors have been observed in the nasal passages, lungs, and thorax of animals exposed to dimethyl sulfate. www.epa.gov/ttn/atw/hlthef/di-sulfa.html

According to Dr. Karen Shrimplin, the thio-ethers are so toxic because they are fat soluble and therefore concentrate in the lipid (fat) framework of the cell, especially the mitochondria. The mitochondria are the "cellular power plants" and are responsible for the production of energy. If the mitochondria are damaged, then the cells can no longer make energy via aerobic respiration, and they are forced to switch to fermentation (**an**aerobic respiration) to produce energy. Remember, all cancer cells use fermentation as their means of energy production.

Basically, what Dr. Shrimplin is saying is that the pleomorphic microbes which inhabit the tubules in a root canal began as normal aerobic bacteria, but when they are sealed into the tooth their environment changes and they become anaerobic and produce toxins such as thio-ethers. These thio-ethers then are released into the rest of our body and damage the mitochondria of our cells, thus causing them to become anaerobic. **It's a vicious cycle, all started by the root canal!** These anaerobic microbes, which thrive inside root canals, excrete toxicity from digesting necrotic tissue, and this leads to chronic infection and degenerative disease. Think about it...if an organ or limb dies in our body, we would remove it. Not so with **dead teeth**!

If you went to the doctor and told him that your appendix hurts and he told you that he was going to cut the nerve to the appendix so you won't feel the pain and then rip the artery off the appendix so it will die, I think you would probably find another doctor. To my knowledge, dentists are the only physicians that purposely leave **dead** tissue in the body. Dentist Frank Jerome stated: "*The idea of keeping a dead, infected organ in the body is only thought to be a good idea by dentists. **A root canal-treated tooth always negatively affects your immune system.***" Using the example above, if your appendix dies and you don't remove it, you will die from peritonitis. The medical fact is this: **ALL DEAD TISSUE GETS INFECTED**.

In the following image, you can see a study published in the Endodontists Journal. (Endodontists are root canal specialists.) In the study, they took people that were going to have wisdom teeth removed and performed a root canal on one side and then removed both wisdom teeth in three months. As you can see, the tooth that didn't have anything done had only 1.1% of the tubules infected (i.e. 98.9% healthy). However, the tooth that had a root canal three months earlier had 39% of the tubules infected and only 61% healthy.

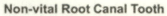

Nagaoka, et al. (1995). Bacterial invasion into dentinal tubules of human vital and non-vital teeth.
J. Endodon. **21: 70-73**

Vital Tooth   Non-vital Root Canal Tooth

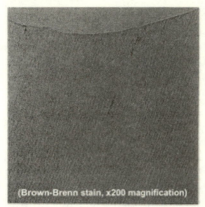 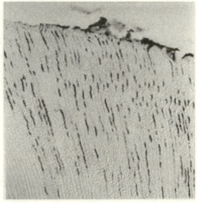

(Brown-Brenn stain, x200 magnification)

% Invaded Tubules: 1.1% vs. 39.0%

Way back in the 1920s, Dr. Weston A. Price performed experiments which at first were hailed by the American Dental Association, but which were later ignored. Dr. Price suspected that bacterial infection accompanied many degenerative diseases. He suspected that these infections arose from the teeth. He decided to implant an extracted root-filled tooth under the skin of an animal. He found that by implanting the root-filled tooth, the disease of the patient was transferred to animals. Whatever disease the patient had, the animal with the extracted tooth under its skin developed the same disease as the patient. He also observed that when root-filled teeth were taken out using correct techniques then a variety of health problems improved, from arthritis to kidney problems to cancer. This was done with hundreds of patients.

Dr. Price had found that none of 100 disinfectants was able to penetrate and sterilize the dentin, which makes up 95% of the structure of the teeth. Neither are any antibiotics capable of sterilizing root canals. Very few dentists are aware of or willing to admit that dentin tubules are always infected after root canal surgery. These bacteria escape into the blood and proceed to initiate a vast number of degenerative diseases. Most dentists believe that the disinfecting substances used to pack the root canal after surgery effectively sterilize the root canal site which is unfortunately not true. What Dr. Price reported and what he found with the tests which involved some 5,000 animals over the 25-year period was that "root canal teeth," no matter how good they looked, or how free they were from symptoms, always remained infected. Dr. Price documented his findings in two monumental volumes entitled <u>Dental</u>

<u>Infections Oral & Systemic</u> and <u>Dental Infections and the Degenerative Diseases</u>. Not surprisingly, the books were effectively suppressed for 50 years until Dr. George Meinig, a retired endodontist, discovered these books. He republished a shortened version of these books called <u>Root Canal Cover-up</u>. Meinig, who actually invented the root canal procedure, spent the last years of his career trying to get dentists to stop doing the procedure which he invented.

If you have a root canal, you may need to see a specialized type of dentist called a "biological dentist" or a "holistic dentist." These dentists are sometimes persecuted by the ADA, so don't expect to find one in the local telephone book. They can be difficult to find. Bill Henderson may have the only major alternative cancer treatment that requires the removal of root canals. He will work with his patients to find a biological dentist. His website is <u>www.beating-cancer-gently.com</u>.

Let's look at the work of Josef Issels in Germany, who treated terminal cancer patients for over 40 years. The immune systems of these patients had already been destroyed by the "Big 3" conventional treatments. They already had three strikes against them. However, Dr. Issels cured 24% of his 16,000 terminal patients during that 40 year period. What was the first thing he did? He had a dentist take out the root canal teeth!

However, if you get your root canal teeth pulled, then you may create another problem. A cavitation is a hole in the bone (because of a pulled tooth) which has not healed correctly. The tissue in the cavitation (such as the ligaments which once held the tooth) becomes infected. The highly toxic bacteria produced can cause osteonecrosis (bone death), weaken overall health, and lead to degenerative diseases such as cancer ... oftentimes without any obvious pain in the jaw area!

If you have a root canal, cavitations, or periodontal (gum) disease, I suggest the following supplements:

> **ORAL GUARD** – This is by far, the best single product on the market to treat periodontal disease. With an impressive and powerful list of ingredients like St. John's Wort, CoQ-10, folic acid, green tea extract, lipoic acid, and Vitamin K1, ORAL GUARD is simply the most potent protection against gum disease available. We use this product daily and purchase it at the following website: <u>www.naturalhealthteam.info</u>

> **DMSO** – *"DMSO, 25% in water (optional). Take one teaspoon as a mouthwash, twice daily. Swish slowly over gums. Hold several minutes. Swallow for maximum effectiveness. This "pushes" your supplements into your tissues. It also helps to*

draw toxins out of cavitations. You may add wintergreen drops to the mouthwash. 50% DMSO is preferred, if available. Must be medical grade DMSO." (taken from <u>Cure for All Advanced Cancer</u>, page 198)

> **Co-enzyme Q10** – This supplement exerts its protective and strengthening action in all tissues. Working from the cellular level, it strengthens the gums as well as the heart muscle. Many scientists believe that periodontal disease is a good indicator of low levels of co-enzyme Q10 in other tissues.

> **Vitamin C** – I know a fellow that lives in Waco, Texas who had periodontal disease. He took 15,000 mg of vitamin C each day (5,000 mg with each meal) and his periodontal disease literally disappeared!

Obviously, many people appear to be able to handle root canals with no ill effects. The problem is that we have no way of knowing if or when our toxic threshold will be reached or how much it will damage the immune system. When our immune systems are at a low point, the microorganisms or toxins produced by the bacteria more readily move toward a target organ in the body based on acupuncture meridians. If you are healthy and strong, the better the odds that the toxins from the root canal will be quarantined and not have a systemic effect.

The bottom line is that alternative cancer treatments may still fail if a patient continues to harbor infection in his/her mouth. The infection that has chronically compromised the immune system may come from root canals as discussed above, but also from infected teeth, cavitations, and periodontal (gum) disease. **It is crucial for the cancer patient to be diligent to treat potential infections arising from the mouth.** If you are interested in treating your root canal teeth and/or treating cancer that may have resulted from dental problems, I recommend that you visit their website: <u>www.breastcancercured.com</u>.

I end this chapter with a quote from one of my Facebook fans, who posted this comment after my daily health tip (which happened to be on root canals): *"I refused to have a root canal on the first tooth that needed it. I chose instead to have the tooth pulled and I thought my dentist was going to lose his mind. He had a total 'tooth nazi' break down and got hostile about my decision. I was in shock watching him have a 'man-child' fit. Guess he forgot he worked for me; I then fired him and went somewhere else."*

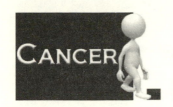
CHAPTER 20
SOY: THE "MAGIC BEAN"?

> **FRAUD:**
> SOY IS A "WONDER-FOOD" THAT PROTECTS AGAINST
> BREAST CANCER & OSTEOPOROSIS. SOY IS A COMPLETE
> PROTEIN.
>
> **FACT:**
> UNFERMENTED SOY PRODUCTS ARE INDIGESTIBLE. SOY
> IS NOT A COMPLETE PROTEIN, IS NOT A NATURAL
> FOOD, CONTAINS SEVERAL HARMFUL CARCINOGENS,
> AND MOST SOYBEANS IN THE UNITED STATES HAVE
> BEEN GENETICALLY MODIFIED.

According to most mainstream and "alternative living" media, soy beans are the most versatile, natural, heart-friendly, health-improving, fat-preventing, growth-promoting and generally "*all-around good for you*" food ever grown on God's green earth. With food aisles brimming with hundreds of soy products, including soy protein, soy breakfast bars, soy burgers, soy ice cream, and an endless array of soy beverages, is soy beer soon to follow?

Actually, it's already here! Doctors, athletes, nutritionists, farmers, government officials, and respected companies all make a point of telling us how safe and wonderful soy is for us and about soy's myriad of health benefits. They tell us that it is so excellent and so safe that it doesn't even need to be listed as an ingredient in many processed foods. But we don't mind, do we? I mean, **everyone knows** it's safe, right?

Along with being the new health food, soy has also become the latest cash cow for companies like Monsanto. Across the globe, billions of acres are earmarked for soybean cultivation, thus providing a secure cash crop for millions of farmers who gladly disburse a "tariff" to Monsanto, the developers of their genetically modified soybeans. What is the modern gospel of food production? *"**Soy is Good For** You."*

Or is it? Sadly, for several decades, corporations have been aware of (and suppressed) the evidence that ingestion of soy causes cancer, destroys bones, and creates havoc with our hormonal systems. The truth behind the blatantly commercial integration of soybeans into our diet is a distressing tale of fraud, greed, propaganda, suppression, corporate irresponsibility, corruption, bad science, and political opportunism.

Have you ever seen the "soy cows" that soy milk comes from? Not sure if you're aware of this, but you can't milk a soy bean! According to Elaine Hollingsworth in her book <u>Soy – The Abominable Bean</u>, *"In order to obtain that pure-looking, inviting stream of white liquid pictured so appealingly in the ads, many processes are needed. It is necessary to grind the beans at high temperature, and then extract the remaining oils with dangerous solvents, some of which remain in the meal. Then the meal is mixed with an alkaline solution and sugars, in a separation process designed to remove fiber. Then it is precipitated and separated, using an acid wash. At each stage of processing a tiny amount of poison remains within the soy."*

She continues, *"Regulators say it's so small an amount that it doesn't count. I wonder who told them that? And why don't they take notice of the scientists who say it does count, due to its accumulation in the body over long periods of soy ingestion? Are you really happy to accept the manufacturer's assurance that it's safe to eat a tiny amount of poison each day, perhaps several times a day, until you have a serious health problem?"* <u>www.doctorsaredangerous.com</u>

One of the many marketing ploys for soy is that it contains isoflavones, which are basically plant hormones (aka "phytoestrogens"). Despite the fact that he/she has no idea what an isoflavone is, your typical soy milk drinker will repeat the mantra they hear on the nightly news about isoflavones. What you won't hear on the news is that scientists have known for years that isoflavones in soy products can depress thyroid function, causing autoimmune thyroid disease and even cancer of the thyroid. Scientists have known for over half a century that soy negatively impacts the thyroid gland.

Research in Japan concluded that daily consumption of only one ounce of soybeans over the course of ninety days caused enlargement of the thyroid and suppressed thyroid function. Some subjects even developed goiter. The subjects returned to normal when they quit eating soy. (Y. Ishisuki et al, "The effects on the thyroid gland of soybeans administered experimentally in healthy subjects", 1991) The soy isoflavone genistein inhibits thyroid function more effectively than prescription drugs which control hyperthyroidism. According to a 1996 NIH/NCI report, the Japanese (and Asians in general) have much higher rates of cancer of the esophagus, stomach, pancreas, thyroid, and liver. This makes sense in light of the fact of the above facts, doesn't it?

As far back as the 1950s, **phytoestrogens** were being linked to increased cases of cancer, infertility, and leukemia. According to Dr. William Wong, *"Soy is poison, period!"* In his article entitled "Soy: The Poison Seed," Dr. Wong describes several reasons why soy is poison. Two of soy's isoflavone phytoestrogens (genistein and daidzein) are basically built in insecticides for the soybean. He asks, *"If they kill bugs, are they good for humans?"* www.totalityofbeing.com/ArchivedSoyPoison.html

Dr. Mike Fitzpatrick, a respected toxicologist who is at the forefront of the New Zealand campaign against soy, wrote a paper in 1998 citing much of the published work on the dangers of soy isoflavones, which he submitted to the FDA. This paper was also published as an article in the February 2000 *New Zealand Medical Journal* entitled "Soy Formulas and the Effect on the Thyroid." In this paper, Dr. Fitzpatrick states, *"The toxicity of isoflavones to animals first raised the awareness of the scientific community to the fact that soy isoflavones are endocrine disruptors... There have been profound negative endocrine effects in all animal species studied to date... Soy isoflavones increase the risk of breast cancer... Soy isoflavone disrupts the menstrual cycle during, and for up to three months after, administration... Dietary concentration of genistein may stimulate breast cells to enter the cell cycle... Concern was expressed that women fed soy protein isolate have an increased incidence of epithelial hyperplasia."*

Charlotte Gerson, of the Gerson Cancer Clinic, has published detailed research proving that genistein is more carcinogenic than DES, a synthetic estrogen drug that was given to millions of pregnant women primarily between the years 1938 and 1971. (*Gerson Clinic: Cancer Research*, June 1, 2001 - 61) DES inflicted death and misery on countless women and their daughters during this period. In an article entitled "Dietary estrogens stimulate human breast cells to enter the cell cycle" published in the 1997 issue of *Environmental Health Perspectives*, Dr. Craig Dees found that soy isoflavones cause breast cancer cells to grow!

As if we need more damning evidence, soy also contains **phytic acid**. The presence of phytic acid in soy totally destroys the credibility of the manufacturers' claims that soy is a good source of calcium and helps prevent osteoporosis. Here's why: phytic acid blocks the uptake of essential minerals (calcium, magnesium, copper, iron, and zinc) in the intestinal tract. Since soy contains more phytic acid than any other grain, it literally sucks the nutrients right out of your body! Only a long period of fermentation will significantly reduce the phytic acid content in soy. Scientists are in general agreement that diets high in phytic acid contribute to widespread mineral deficiencies in third world countries.

Soy is not a complete protein, as it lacks the essential amino acids methionine and cystine. And soy protein is difficult to digest because it contains substantial amounts of **trypsin inhibitors**. Remember, trypsin is essential in protein digestion, and cancer cells are protected by a protein coating which makes them "invisible" to the immune system. Soy also contains hemagglutinin, a clot-promoting substance that causes red blood cells to clump together. These clustered blood cells are unable to properly absorb oxygen for distribution to the body's tissues, which can damage the heart and lead to cancer. We all know about the relationship between oxygen and cancer, don't we?

According to Dr. Tim O'Shea, *"Yet another toxin found in some processed soy products is **aluminum**, which is said to be 10 times higher in infant soy formulas than in milk-based formulas--and 100 times higher than in unprocessed milk. Levels are even higher when soy products are hydrogenated. Aluminum, a cause of Alzheimer's, can also damage the newly forming kidneys of an infant who drinks soy formula. Worse yet, aluminum can directly damage the infant brain because the blood-brain barrier has not formed yet. Processed soy can also contain a known carcinogen called lysinoalanine. It is a by-product of a processing step called alkaline soaking, which is done to attempt to eliminate enzyme inhibitors. Even though the beans are thoroughly rinsed, the lysinoalanine by-product can remain from the interaction of the soybeans with the alkaline solution."*

And just when you thought it couldn't get any worse, a recent study of Japanese men (living in Hawaii) found that consuming 2 or more weekly servings of tofu was linked to the development of dementia! (L.R. White, et al, "Brain aging and midlife tofu consumption," *Journal of American College of Nutrition*, April 2000) But don't the Chinese and Japanese eat lots of soy? The answer is *"no, they don't."* And the majority of the soy products which they do eat are fermented (tempeh, tamari, natto, and miso). Long ago, they discovered that fermentation caused the protein to be more easily digested, and the phytic acid, toxins, and "anti-nutrients" to be destroyed. This being so, fermented soy products are acceptable, but only in small amounts.

Concerning soy, other countries are light years ahead of the USA. In July of 1996, the *British Department of Health* issued a warning that the phytoestrogens found in soy-based infant formulas could adversely affect infant health. The warning was clear, indicating that soy formula should only be given to babies on the advice of a health professional. They advised that babies who cannot be breastfed or who have allergies to other formulas be given alternatives to soy-based formulas.

With their cash cow at stake, the market for soy must be maintained. American soy farmers "contribute" almost $80 million each year to help fund what must be considered one of the most effective brainwashing campaigns in history. The resultant high-powered media blitz ensures that "news" stories about soy's myriad of benefits abound, from radio to TV to the internet. But don't fall for the labyrinth of lies! Soybeans are not a complete protein, are not a natural food, contain several harmful carcinogens, and most soybeans in the USA are genetically modified.

And just in case you need one more reason to stay away from soy, "natural" food manufacturers are now using a toxic chemical called hexane to process soy in their products. Yes, hexane is the same substance in glue that gets you high and in gasoline that makes it explode. The fumes from hexane go straight to your brain and cause damage almost instantaneously. Hexane is so toxic that the EPA has it listed as a hazardous chemical that causes cancer and birth defects and even Parkinson's disease.

In 2009, an independent lab found levels of hexane residue as high as 21 parts per million in soy oil and soy meal which is used in soy infant formula and protein bars (www.naturalnews.com/026303.html). But everyone is *"hush hush"* about this dirtly little secret because the soy industry is powerful and the FDA doesn't require testing for hexane in food or baby formula. Soy formula is one of the worst foods that you could feed your child. Not only does it have profoundly adverse hormonal effects as discussed above as well as dangerously high levels of hexane, but it also has over 1000% more aluminum than conventional milk based formulas.

But that's not all! According to GMO Compass, an online mecca of genetically modified ("GMO") industry information, 91% of soybeans grown in the USA are GMO. In a recent Russian study, researchers found that GMO soy caused sterility in 3rd generation hamsters! In 2005, Dr. Irina Ermakova reported that over 50% of the babies from mother rats that were fed GMO soy died within three weeks. When she wanted to further investigate, her documents were burned.

Conscious of the public's growing awareness of the dangers of GMO and displaying the kind of "creative duplicity" which even Prince Machiavelli would applaud; Monsanto Corporation has almost 50 million acres of GMO soybeans growing in the USA.

Here's the catch: American law permits these crops to be mixed with a small amount of organic soybeans, and the resultant combination may then be labeled "organic"! And you still think the government wouldn't let them lie to you? This deadly "food" belongs in the toxic waste dump, but the multinational corporations like Monsanto are disposing of it in you, your family, and in baby formulas! For those who ask if organic soy is safe, I say, *"Would you eat **organic anthrax**?"*

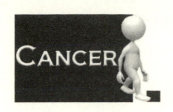
CHAPTER 21

CODEX ALIMENTARIUS

FRAUD:
THE PURPOSE FOR CODEX ALIMENTARIUS IS TO "HARMONIZE"
MANUFACTURE AND DISTRIBUTION OF NUTRITIONAL
SUPPLEMENTS TO PROTECT CONSUMERS.

FACT:
CODEX WILL TAKE AWAY ALL REMNANTS OF HEALTH FREEDOM
AND PUT US FURTHER UNDER TYRANNICAL RULE.....

Codex Alimentarius (Latin for *"food code"*) is the proposed set of international guidelines for nutritional supplements, food handling, production, and trade which is now gradually being ratified in countries around the world, starting in the European Union (EU). Codex is a joint project of the United Nations (UN), World Health Organization (WHO), and the Food and Agricultural Organization (FAO). The **"official line"** is that some "harmonization" on safety, trade, manufacture, and distribution of nutritional supplements would help the world in so many ways. The **truth** is that Codex is one more step toward total **health tyranny**.

Codex is made up of thousands of standards and guidelines. One of them, the Vitamin and Mineral Guideline (VMG), is designed to permit only ultra- low doses of vitamins and minerals, essentially making supplements illegal. Vitamin C, for example, at any dosage higher than two hundred milligrams per day will be illegal. A gram of Vitamin C will be an illegal substance! The dose of coenzyme Q10 which has been shown to resolve breast cancer in some patients (400 mg per day) will be illegal because coenzyme Q10 will be totally illegal at any dose following the European Supplements Directive model. Only 28 nutrients will be allowed, but the maximum upper limits have been set so low that they have little or no clinical impact in keeping us healthy and none at all in returning us to a state of health if we are ill. And those which are available will be exorbitantly priced.

One of the committees within Codex, the Codex Committee on Nutrition and Foods for Special Dietary Uses (CCNFSDU), is chaired by Dr. Rolf Grossklaus, a German physician who believes that nutrition has no role in health. Yes, the "top-guy" for Codex nutritional policy has publicly declared that *"nutrition is not relevant to health."* As crazy as it may sound, Dr. Grossklaus actually declared nutrients to be **toxins** in 1994.

Codex also stipulates which conditions may be treated using herbs. Only minor, self-limited conditions may be treated by herbal means. Treating any other conditions with herbal remedies will constitute a crime. Codex sets permissible upper limits for pesticide residues, toxic chemicals in the environment, hormones in food and other environmental contaminants which are many times higher than levels advocated by chemical and pesticide industry lobbying groups. Current toxic levels are already responsible for most of the cancers, heart disease, autism, chronic degenerative conditions, and organ failures which are killing people at increasing rates around the globe. Making permissible toxic levels higher will accelerate this destructive world-wide trend.

The Stockholm Convention, signed by 176 countries including the USA (May 2005), commits the signatories to eliminate world's twelve most dangerous "persistent organic pollutants" (POP's). Codex allows **seven of the twelve** agreed upon killer POPs to be used in the production of foods!! This is insane. The seven restricted POP's banned by both the Stockholm Convention and United States law but permitted by Codex are Hexachlorobenzene, Mirex, Aldrin, Chlordane, Dieldrin, Endrin, and Heptachlor.

Codex makes irradiation of food legal and even mandatory under certain circumstances. Under the guise of *"protecting us from food borne illness,"* the irradiation of food is by no means agreed to be a safe procedure since there is considerable scientific evidence that protein structures are modified in unhealthy ways by introducing ionizing radiation into food before it is consumed. Codex makes the non-labeled use of GMO legal in all foods under all circumstances. Many GMO have been genetically engineered so that seeds will not germinate without the use of specific pesticides. In fact, mounting scientific evidence makes it clear that birth defects, chemical sensitivity, chronic fatigue syndrome, asthma, severe allergies and a host of other conditions are caused by pesticide exposure (which these crops will require).

Using their multi-billion-dollar marketing budgets, Big Pharma has launched a massive media propaganda campaign to paint Codex as a benevolent tool of "consumer protection," as well as to negatively taint the image of natural health options and mislead people to fear them as "dangerous," so they will take more drugs. Contrary to the propaganda you may have heard about Codex, it has nothing to do with consumer protection. Nothing! Codex is about protecting the cash cow -- prescription drugs.

And here is the kicker – Codex is based in the Napoleonic Code, not Common Law. That means that under Codex, anything not explicitly permitted is forbidden. Under Common Law, we hold that anything not explicitly forbidden is permitted. **The difference is the difference between health freedom and health tyranny.**

CounterThink

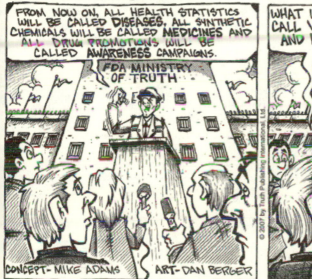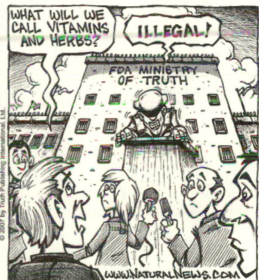

Thanks to Mike Adams and *www.NaturalNews.com* for the cartoon above.

The Dietary Supplement Health and Education Act (DSHEA) is an American law classifying our supplements and herbs as foods (which can have no upper limit set on their use) and was passed by unanimous Congressional consent in 1994. DSHEA is the only law which currently protects us from Codex's deadly VMG. But DSHEA is under significant legislative attack right now. There are many members of Congress who want to overturn this law. They have sold out like cheap harlots. I suggest that you write your Congressman and let them know that if they ever vote against your health freedom, that you will vote them out of office. Tell your representatives that you want to make sure that DSHEA is vigorously protected here in the USA and that you expect to continue to have access to any kind of dietary supplement that you wish at any potency and level of dosage.

We are witnessing the end of America as a nation-state right now, and with these changes, none of our domestic laws or constitutional rights are secure. All of our laws and institutions of government are subject to "harmonization" to international standards. Globalization is right around the corner. We are facing a frightening future, not to mention the fact that children born after 1990 have no clue about their food, water, vaccinations, or anything else. It's by design. We are being slowly "starved to death" from lack of nutrition. This too is by design... irradiated food, pasteurized milk and juice, viruses sprayed on our meat, chemicals sprayed on fruit and vegetables, now we're being forced without our consent to eat genetically modified foods. Codex is nothing more than Big Pharma's worldwide "control" agenda (as well as a genocide agenda). It is an enormous assault on humanity and health freedom. Sadly, much of the "dumbed down" populace sees it as a "good thing" that the benevolent government "cares enough to protect us." You know the old saying, *A nation of sheep results in a government of wolves.*"

To learn more about Codex, please visit www.healthfreedomusa.org – the website of Major General Albert (Bert) N. Stubblebine III (*US Army, Retired*) and Rima E. Laibow, M.D. If Codex becomes the "law of the land" here in the USA, stories like the one that follows will be commonplace.

THE STOWERS FAMILY "MANNA STOREHOUSE"

The Stowers family has run a very large, well-known food cooperative called Manna Storehouse, just outside Cleveland for many years. On Monday, December 1, 2008, a SWAT team of eleven agents armed with semi-automatic rifles entered their private home in La Grange, Ohio, herded the family into the living room, and kept guns pointed at the parents, children, infants and toddlers, for approximately nine hours! The SWAT team was aggressive and belligerent. Needless to say, the children were quite traumatized.

Agents began rifling through all of the family's possessions, a task that lasted hours and resulted in a complete upheaval of every private area in the home. Many items were taken that were not listed on the search warrant. In direct violation of the United States Constitution, the family was not permitted a phone call, and they were not told what crime they had allegedly committed, they were not read their rights. Additionally, over $10,000 of food was "confiscated" (stolen) including their personal food storage for the upcoming year. All of their computers and all of their cell phones were taken, as well as phone and contact records.

What was their crime? Presumably Manna Storehouse might eventually be charged with running a retail establishment without a license. Why then the "Gestapo" style interrogation for a third degree misdemeanor charge? Is there some rabid new interpretation (of existing drug laws) that considers food a controlled substance worthy of a SWAT raid?

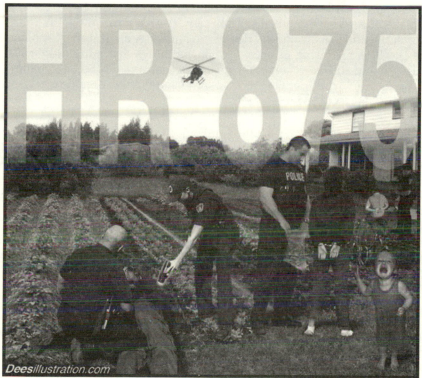

Thanks to David Dees and *www.DeesIllustration.com* for the picture above.

RAWESOME FOODS RAID

On August 3, 2011, Rawesome Foods (*a private California buying club offering raw milk and cheese*) was raided in blitzkrieg style by SWAT-style armed agents from the FDA, CDC, LA County Sheriff's Office, and the Department of Agriculture. What was their crime? "*Producing Milk Without a License*" and "*Mislabeling Cheese*" and "*Conspiracy to Commit a Crime*" were 3 of the 13 charges. Law enforcement demanded that all customers of the store vacate the premises, and then they demanded to know how much cash the owner had at the store. The LA County Sheriff proceeded to "confiscate" over $4,000 of cash, arrest the owner, and destroy the inventory of the store (*pouring the milk down the drain and confiscating the cheese and vegetables*).

Thank God for those "brave" government agents. Risking their lives to "protect" us from those "evil" raw food **terrorists**! How dare they raise cows without injecting them with *recombinant bovine growth hormone* (*rBGH*)! How dare they sell beef that is from grass-fed cows and vegetables that are organic! We should all feel better that the FDA Gestapo destroyed those "dangerous" eggs produced by free range chickens! And we should all say a hearty "**thank you**" to the LA Sheriff for "protecting" us from that deadly raw milk! A big round of applause to the FDA for giving us access to all the things that admittedly cause disease and kill us (*chemotherapy, toxic vaccines, MSG, aspartame, and fluoride*) while denying us access to healthy, raw, organic foods. Of course ... **SARCASM** intended!

Folks, this was an **illegal** raid conducted by government **thugs** who engaged in acts of **terrorism** against small farmers and honest raw foods retailers. The LA County Sheriff, the Department of Agriculture, the CDC, and the FDA represent a "*clear and present danger*" to the lives and safety of the American people. They are terrorists and should **ALL** be arrested and charged with the crimes they have committed (i.e. *destruction of property, conspiracy to commit a felony, trespassing, theft, and kidnapping*). This is a declaration of **war** by the rogue US government against people who try to promote healthy raw and living foods. The FDA once again proves that it is nothing more than the "leg-breakers" for the Medical Mafia.

These "Nazi-esque" raids raise the disturbing possibility that it could become a crime to raise your own food, milk your own cows, buy eggs from the farmer down the road, or butcher your own chickens for family and friends. Will Americans retain the right to purchase food that is uncontaminated by pesticides, herbicides, antibiotics, hormones, allergens, additives, dyes, preservatives, MSG, GMOs, radiation, etc.? Honestly, I'm waiting for people to have to get "permits" to grow gardens in the USA. I can foresee police raiding homes and pulling up gardens in backyards as whole families have guns pointed at their heads...for the "crime" of not having the required permit.

The bottom line is this: If we don't take a stand against this type of "Nazi-esque" thuggish behavior by our government, we may as well lie down, curl up in a fetal position, suck our thumbs, and wait for our next serving of soylent green...

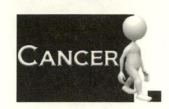

CONCLUSION

I trust that this book has made it abundantly clear that you **do** have natural alternatives to the "Big 3," although these alternatives may not have the "stamp of approval" from the Cancer Industry or the Medical Mafia. Hopefully, you now realize that you do **not** have to poison, slash, or burn your body. Neither are you limited to the alternative cancer treatments which I have addressed in this book. While the treatments included in this book have been deemed to have the best track records and have shown the great merit with cancer patients, there are literally hundreds of other alternative cancer treatments which work better than the "Big 3."

Beware of wolves in sheep's clothing! Hospitals and other providers that offer so-called "nutrition-based" or "holistic" or "integrated" programs oftentimes are only paying lip-service to patients' requests for alternative cancer treatments, just to get them in the door. However, once you're there, they frequently will try to convince you that the "Big 3" is your only hope. Don't fall for this lie. You know better. How you treat **your** cancer is **your** choice. If the doctor tells you that your cancer is terminal, what he really means is that it's terminal if you use the "Big 3."

It's sad that money rather than altruism is what drives Big Pharma and Big Medicine, but that's reality. And it always will be, since if alternative cancer treatments were to become mainstream, millions of pharmaceutical salespeople and researchers would immediately be looking for a job, shareholder profits would plummet, and CEOs would lose their golden parachutes. Let's face it folks, Big Pharma runs the show. They want you to remain ignorant and "*in the dark.*" Those that profit from cancer are like the slave owners 200 years ago. If you ran a plantation back in the slave days, you wanted to make sure that your slaves remained obedient, submissive, and illiterate. If a slave had the nerve to disobey "the master," then he was beaten within an inch of his life. Books weren't allowed, thus slaves were unable to learn to read. These steps were taken to insure that they would never have the boldness to venture off the plantation and the master would have a "slave for life." In the Cancer Industry, patients are like slaves, and the slave owners want to make sure that they remain enslaved by suppressing information about alternative treatments and persecuting those who dare to question their authority and use an alternative treatment. *"Keep 'em dumb"* seems to be their slogan. So I say, *"Don't donate!"*

The next time you are asked to donate to a cancer charity, please keep in mind that your money will be used to sustain an industry which has been deemed by many eminent scientists as a qualified failure and by others as a complete fraud. If you would like to make a difference, please consider donating money to the Independent Cancer Research Foundation (ICRF). This non-profit organization's goal is to develop highly potent alternative cancer treatments that work quickly and are very effective on advanced cancer patients. Visit their website at www.new-cancer-treatments.org.

Thank you for reading this book. I sincerely hope that it has given you both ammunition and hope. God willing, the day will come when the general public has free access to all alternative cancer therapies. But until then, perhaps this book will be a source of information for you and your loved ones who desperately need assistance navigating through the cancer jungle and "stepping outside the box."

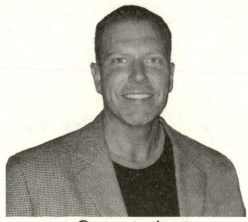

ty@cancertruth.net

MAY GOD BLESS YOU WITH A LONG AND HEALTHY LIFE!

APPENDICES

CANCER CLINICS

SPIRITUAL CANCER

EXERCISE ESSENTIALS

&

DAVID VS. GOLIATH: "JASON VALE AND THE CANCER MAFIA"

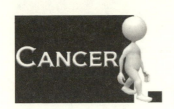

APPENDIX 1
RECOMMENDED CANCER CLINICS

WHILE MANY ALTERNATIVE CANCER TREATMENTS CAN BE EFFECTIVELY ADMINISTERED AT HOME, SOME CANCER PATIENTS (*AND THEIR FAMILIES*) MAY FEEL MORE COMFORTABLE IF TREATMENT IS ADMINISTERED BY A MEDICAL PROFESSIONAL IN A CLINICAL ENVIRONMENT. THE CANCER CLINICS MENTIONED IN THIS SECTION ALL USE FANTASTIC CANCER TREATMENT PROTOCOLS, AND THEY ARE ALL OPERATED BY PEOPLE WITH A LONG HISTORY OF SUCCESSFULLY TREATING CANCER PATIENTS. THEY ARE IN ALPHABETICAL ORDER.

ARIZONA INTEGRATIVE MEDICAL CENTER

Location: Scottsdale, Arizona
Phone: (480) 214-3922
Website: *www.drstallone.com*

Arizona Integrative Medical Center is run by Dr. Paul Stallone. He currently practices in Scottsdale where his patients seek assistance with a variety of ailments ranging from the common cold to Stage IV cancer.

His main focus is to listen and understand the underlying cause of an individual's illness. His belief is that oftentimes, the underlying cause is a combination of nutritional, structural, emotional, chemical, and lifestyle factors. He uses a vast array of modalities including

Nutrition/Supplements, Homeopathy, Detoxification, Acupuncture, Oxygen/Ozone Therapy, and Intravenous Nutritional-Vitamin Therapy to effectively treat diseases such as cancer.

BIO-MEDICAL CENTER

Location: Tijuana, B.C. Mexico
Phone: 011-52-664-684-9011
E-mail: biomedicalcenter@prodigy.net.mx
Address: 3170 General Ferreira Ave, Colonia Madero Sur
                Tijuana, B.C. Mexico 22180

Since 1963, this clinic has provided Hoxsey therapy. It was one of the first alternative cancer facilities in Mexico. Mildred Nelson, who was Harry Hoxsey's chief nurse at the Hoxsey Clinic in Dallas until he left clinical practice, carried on the therapy in Mexico until her death in 1999. Her sister now runs the clinic.

In addition to the Hoxsey treatment, comprised of a liquid elixir containing a mixture of herbs and several topical salves, the clinic may also use other supplements, diet, nutrition, and chelation therapy. They treat most types of malignancies, but it is said to be especially effective with skin cancer (including melanoma), breast cancer, and has been successful with some recurrent cancers and even with patients who've had radiation and/or chemotherapy. Often what people will do is combine Hoxsey treatment with other approaches, like laetrile (B17).

CAMELOT CANCER CARE

Location: Tulsa, Oklahoma
Phone: (918) 493-1011
Website: *www.camelotcancercare.com*

At Camelot Cancer Care, no "toxic treatments" are on the menu! They utilize gentle but powerful natural alternatives to try to mitigate the damage caused by the "Big 3." According to their website, "*Mainstream medicine treats the symptoms of disease, and sometimes eradicates it. We in Complementary or Alternative Medicine also try to treat the underlying cause. Orthodox medicine 'swats mosquitoes' —and sometimes puts out citronella repellant. Alternative, progressive medicine issues quinine, and tries to 'drain the swamp.'*"

Camelot is one of a very few dedicated DMSO clinics operating in the USA which accepts cancer patients. They use only pure, pharmaceutical grade DMSO. Camelot also offers a full range of supplemental support treatments. They also have a proven track record of success in treating brain cancer, colon cancer, and many sarcomas. I suggest you read the FAQ's on their website.

CENTER FOR ADVANCED MEDICINE & CLINICAL RESEARCH (CFAMCR)

Location: Huntersville, North Carolina
Phone: (704) 895-9355
Website: *www.drbuttar.com*

At the Center for Advanced Medicine & Clinical Research, their mission statement has always been "*not only to extend our patients lives, but to improve the quality of that extended life.*" They have achieved this mission by effectively addressing the toxicities that are the cause of all chronic disease and have been the guiding principals and the foundation of Dr. Rashid Buttar's clinical work. Dr. Buttar is one of the top physicians in the USA and is unsurpassed in his knowledge of detoxification, nutrition, and heavy metal chelation.

According to their website, they "*offer 39 different IV Therapies oriented towards the principles of detoxification and immune modulation including heavy metal chelation, hyperbaric oxygen therapy, nutritional IV's, and many other treatments that detoxify and enhance the immune system. None of the IV therapies done at our clinic have ever caused any harm to any patient in our practice and we have now administered well over 200,000 IV treatments over the last 11 years.*"

I know Dr. Buttar personally and I highly recommend this clinic.

CLINIC OF BIOMEDICINE

Location: Toronto, Ontario, Canada
Phone: (416) 255-3325
Website: *www.biomedici.ca/index.html*

For more than a decade, the Clinic of Biomedicine has been utilizing a combination of different non-toxic cancer protocols to treat malignancies.

The "Basic Metabolic Cancer" program is frequently recommended and involves an initial 60 day therapy including the following procedures: detoxification, chelation, enzyme therapy, IV laetrile, cancer vaccines, biological response modifiers, iscador, colostrum, stress management, nutritional guidance, and other individualized protocols.

Their treatment plan is almost identical to treatments utilized at the Oasis of Hope in Tijuana, Mexico.

GERMAN CANCER CLINICS

Only a small number of German cancer clinics use alternative medicine, such as hyperthermia, oxygen therapy, & mistletoe therapy, but these clinics are excellent. The book German Cancer Breakthrough, by Andrew Scholberg, is an excellent place to learn about seven of the major German alternative cancer clinics. The big advantage to the German cancer clinics is that they are run by Medical Doctors who have small clinics (by American standards) and who have a great deal of interaction with the patients. In other words, the German Cancer Clinics are more like a "*bed and breakfast*" than a hospital. If you think you may be interested in traveling to Germany for treatment, please visit www.germancancerbreakthrough.com.

DR. NICHOLAS GONZALEZ

Location: New York City
Phone: (212) 213-3337
Website: *www.dr-gonzalez.com*

Dr. Nicholas Gonzalez has been investigating nutritional approaches to cancer and other degenerative diseases since 1981 and has been in practice in New York since 1987. Dr. Linda Isaacs has been working with Dr. Gonzalez in his research and practice since 1985. Doctors Gonzalez and Isaacs share their concept of treating cancer with Robert Beard (*a Scottish embryologist*) and William Donald Kelley (*a Texas orthodontist*) who developed a remarkably successful metabolic approach to treat cancer.

They use an individualized aggressive nutritional protocol to work with many types of cancer, specializing in pancreatic cancer. The Gonzalez program requires an aggressive number of daily supplements (*130-160 capsules*). The pancreatic enzymes (*central to the treatment*), vitamins, minerals, amino acids, and antioxidants are normally taken for 15 days, then flushed from the system for 5 days, and then started anew. Coffee enemas, liver flushes, and a whole-body purge with psyllium husks, which Dr. Gonzalez calls *"the clean sweep,"* are essential to the success of the program. I know Dr. Gonzalez and Dr. Isaacs personally and **highly** recommend them.

HAWAII NATUROPATHIC RETREAT CENTER

Location: Hawaii
Phone: (808) 933-4400
Website: *http://alternativecancertreatmentgerson.com/*

Maya Nicole Baylac N.D. (Founder and Director of the Hawaii Naturopathic Retreat Center) has been treating cancer and conducting Gerson therapy programs for over ten years. Through her practice she came to understand that it is necessary to use more than one approach to conquer cancer.

Hawaii Naturopathic Retreat focuses on Gerson therapy along with detoxification, nutrition, supplementation (*therapeutic doses of melatonin, artemisinin, B17/Laetrile, curcumin, enzymes, & vitamin D*), coffee enemas, oxygenation, IV therapy, iscador therapy, and meditation.

HEALTH*QUARTERS* MINISTRIES

Location: Colorado Springs, Colorado
Phone: (719) 593-8694
Website: *www.healthquarters.org*

Health*Quarters* is run by Dr. David Frahm, who wrote the book <u>A Cancer Battle Plan</u>. They offer a 10 day detox retreat, as they believe proper nutrition heals the body at the cellular level, but before nutritional changes can be effective, detoxing the system must take place.

Health*Quarters* is a Christian organization and there is a very strong spiritual aspect to their program. Their "heartbeat" is to help God's people be healthy, both physically and spiritually, in order that they may more effectively serve Jesus Christ in His world. This is an awesome clinic, and Dr. Frahm is a wonderful Christian man. I highly recommend Health*Quarters*.

HOLISTIC MEDICAL CLINIC OF THE CAROLINAS

Location: Wilkesboro, North Carolina
Phone: (336) 667-6464
Website: *www.holisticmedclinic.com*

Holistic Medical Clinic of the Carolinas (*HMCC*) began offering holistic care in June of 1978 under the direction of Dr. R. Ernest Cohn who has been practicing medicine for over 30 years.

Dr. Cohn's professional team of medical, chiropractic, and naturopathic physicians offers a wider array of services ranging from alternative chemotherapy, holistic oncology, heavy metal and cardiovascular chelation, acupuncture, colonic irrigation, live cell analysis, and yeast/fungal treatments.

At HMCC, they focus on removing their patients from unnecessary drugs, and their chief emphasis is to "*get people well.*" I know Dr. Cohn personally and I highly recommend this clinic.

HOPE4CANCER INSTITUTE

Location: Jamul, California
Phone: (888) 544-5993
Website: *http://www.hope4cancer.com/*

At Hope4Cancer Institute, their motto is, "*No chemo, no radiation, no side effects.*" The institute provides patients with the highest quality medical care combined with some of the best and most successful alternative cancer treatments such as Sono-Photo Dynamic Therapy, BX Protocol, Indiba Hyperthermia, and their exclusive biological vaccine AARSOTA and more. Hope4Cancer Institute also offers many well established natural treatment protocols such as Whole Body and Local Hyperthermia, PolyMVA, Laetrile, Vitamin C, Coffee Enema, and Juice Fasting.

Dr. Antonio Jimenez, M.D. has over 25 years of experience as an oncology expert and clinical researcher. He has developed a unique combination of therapies and medicines that continue to have consistent successful results.

LEIGH ERIN CONNEALY, MD

Location: Irvine, California
Phone: (949) 581-4673 and (949) 680-1880
Websites: *www.cfnmedicine.com/* and
                  http://cancercenterforhope.com/

I met Dr. Connealy at the 2012 CCS convention in Los Angeles (where we were both speakers) and had a chance to eat lunch with her. She impressed me. She treats the whole person with integrative therapies and is open to all potential treatment possibilities. Dr. Connealy has over 27 years of experience in finding the "root cause" of an illness. Impressively, she has taken numerous advanced courses, including homeopathic, nutritional and lifestyle approaches, while studying disease, chronic illness, and cancer treatments. Dr. Connealy serves as the Medical Director of *Center For New Medicine* and *Cancer Center For Hope* in Irvine, California.

Dr. Connealy's medical centers offer a vast array of services including the latest in cancer therapies, detoxification, holistic dentistry, nutrition, pain management, allergy therapy, acupuncture, massage therapy, hyperbaric oxygen therapy, sleep disorders, and much more. Some of the chronic conditions treated at the clinics include all types of cancer, heart disease, diabetes, and neurological and auto-immune disorders.

NATURAL HEALING CENTER OF MYRTLE BEACH

Location: Myrtle Beach, South Carolina
Phone: (843) 839-9996
Website: *www.naturalhealingcentermb.com/*

Combining 30 years of experience in the medical field and alternative health, Dr. Jin Li Dong has made it a priority to educate patients about their health and preventive care as well as treating patients with their illnesses and problems. Natural Healing Center offers multiple electronic medical devices to build your body's immune system, kill unwanted microbes, improve circulation, increase energy level, and more. Dr. Brian Brown recently joined Dr. Dong and the rest of the team at the Natural Healing Center of Myrtle Beach.

The doctors at the Natural Healing Center believe in a "whole person approach" while caring for their patients, combining the most effective hands-on techniques, physiotherapy procedures, natural vitamin and mineral supplements.

Protocols include juicing, coffee enemas, LifeOne, hyperbaric oxygen, acupuncture, laser therapy, Budwig Diet, and chiropractic. Diagnostic tools include the AMAS test, hCG test, live blood analysis, and the biophotonic scanner.

NEVADA CENTER OF ALTERNATIVE & ANTI-AGING MEDICINE

Location: Carson City, Nevada
Phone: (775) 884-3990
Website: *www.antiagingmedicine.com*

The Nevada Center is a unique, state of the art, full service medical clinic, offering individualized cancer treatment programs. Dr. Frank Shallenberger has been practicing medicine for 27 years. He is one of only 16 physicians in Nevada that are licensed both in conventional medicine and in alternative and homeopathic medicine. This allows him to integrate the best of these approaches for optimal results.

Dr. Shallenberger uses dietary manipulation, herbs, vitamins and minerals, homeopathy, detoxification, chelation therapy, ozone therapy, hydrogen peroxide, state-of-the-art IPT, and natural hormonal replacement in order to optimize the body's innate ability to heal itself. He is internationally recognized as a leading expert in the use of ozone therapy.

NEW HOPE MEDICAL CENTER

Location: Scottsdale, Arizona
Phone: (480) 473-9808
Website: *www.newhopemedicalcenter.com*

New Hope uses alternative methods to treat immune deficient illnesses such as cancer. Dr. Fredda Branyon, Dr. Mario Galaburri, and Dr. Ronald Peters all agree that a physician should never just treat the **symptoms** of the illness, but treat the individual as a whole. This is a wonderful philosophy of healing.

At New Hope, they focus on strengthening the immune system, since it is our first line of defense. They offer nutritional therapy, enzyme therapy, intravenous Vitamin C, ozone therapy, oxygen therapies, and colon therapy, just to name a few. New Hope is an outpatient facility. Please call them and their complimentary concierge service will help you with your travel arrangements and hotel reservations.

Reno Integrative Medical Center

Location: Reno, Nevada
Phone: (775) 829-1009
Website: *www.renointegrative.com*

Reno Integrative Medical Center is a treatment center for alternative medicine and research in cancer. Dr. Douglas Brodie used to run this clinic, but he died in 2005. Currently, Dr. Bob Eslinger, and Dr. David Holt are the managing doctors.

At RIMC, they believe that cancer research, with some notable recent exceptions, has continued in the same basic direction for the last half century or more, seeking that elusive "magic bullet" through development of ever more toxic synthetic chemicals. They focus on restoring your body's natural innate ability to defend itself. This is done by assisting your body in healing itself using alternative medicine and other therapies without attacking your body with harmful toxins. Their cancer treatment protocols include homeopathy, oxidation therapy, heavy metal chelation therapy, German "new medicine," and vitamin-mineral infusions.

Their philosophy is to embrace many different treatment modalities, offering the best of both traditional and alternative approaches to health care.

Rhythm of Life Comprehensive Cancer Care

Location: Mesa, Arizona
Phone: (480) 668-1448, (877) 668-1448
Website: *www.rhythmoflife.com*

Dr. Charles Schwengel is licensed as an Osteopathic Physician and Surgeon, as well as a Homeopathic Medical Doctor. This additional license is available in Arizona to physicians who wish to add the extra dimension of holistic medical treatments to their practices.

Being licensed as a Homeopathic Physician allows him to incorporate a much wider variety of advanced medical therapies that are commonly used around the world, but are less available in the USA. Their cancer treatment protocols include IPT, heavy metal chelation therapy, detox, live cell analysis, and many more. Personally, they are a bit too *"new age"* for my taste, but they do offer excellent cancer treatments.

RIORDAN CLINIC

Location: Wichita, Kansas
Phone: (316) 682-3100
Website: *http://riordanclinic.org*

The Riordan Clinic is run by Dr. Ron Hunninghake and a staff of doctors, all of whom are involved in orthomolecular research and other cancer research. Orthomolecular medicine describes the practice of preventing and treating disease by providing the body with optimal amounts of substances which are natural to the body. The key idea in orthomolecular medicine is that genetic factors affect not only to the physical characteristics of individuals, but also to their biochemical environment.

At Riordan Clinic, their goal is to find and correct the underlying reasons for disease by evaluating the patients "biochemically," which includes measuring nutrient levels. They are specialists in certain alternative approaches, including intravenous vitamins and nutrition, nutritional medicine, acupuncture, heavy metal chelation, chiropractic, detecting adverse food reactions and hidden parasites, and therapeutic massage.

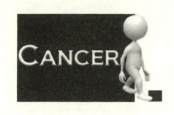

APPENDIX 2
SPIRITUAL CANCER

> "FOR GOD SO LOVED THE WORLD THAT HE GAVE
> HIS ONLY SON, THAT WHOEVER BELIEVES IN HIM
> SHALL NOT PERISH BUT HAVE ETERNAL LIFE."
> *JOHN 3:16*

This book has been focused on *physical* cancer and the ways to cure it. I trust that the information contained herein will help you in your quest to get healthy, stay healthy, fend off cancer, and even cure your cancer. But even if you are able to cure your cancer and live a long, full life, the fact of the matter is that one day you will die. I know that is an uncomfortable subject with many people, but that is reality. **We will all die.** We are all *"terminal."* There are **no exceptions**. The probability of death is 100%.

You see, *physical* cancer is not our biggest foe. The fact is that we were all born with *"spiritual cancer."* Similar to physical cancer, if it is left untreated, spiritual cancer will certainly result in death. Not physical death but spiritual death...eternal death. But, *"What is spiritual cancer?"* you may ask. Spiritual cancer is **sin**. The Bible tells us that humanity became separated from God when Adam and Eve sinned by disobeying Him and eating of the fruit of the Tree of the Knowledge of Good and Evil (*the tree from which God had forbidden them to eat*). Humanity became separated from God because all people are descended from Adam. As a result, the sinful nature Adam acquired through his disobedience was passed down to all people, including you and me.

Because of this inherited *"sin nature,"* everyone sins. It comes naturally. It is part of the fabric of being human. I never had to teach any of my children to sin or to be selfish – it came naturally. The book of Romans tells us that because of our sin, we are under God's condemnation. The effect of sin on humans is that it extends to every part of our personality, our thinking, our emotions, and our will. This does **not** mean that we are as evil as we possibly can be, but it *does* mean that sin has extended to our entire being. The Bible tells us that we are born "*dead in our sins.*" I know that sin is not a popular concept today. It is considered old-fashioned and passé to say that someone is a sinner. But the Bible is clear – we are **ALL** sinners.

Sin is a cancer that infects all of us. And you either get the cancer, or the cancer will get you! The good news is that there is a cure for the spiritual cancer of sin! There is an antidote to sin and its deadly effects. You have probably seen it when you watch NFL football games on TV. You know, the "*wacko Christian*" dude in the end zone with the "**John 3:16**" sign. Have you ever read John 3:16? It states, "*For God so loved the world that He gave his only Son, that whoever believes in Him shall not perish but have eternal life.*"

Jesus provided the cure for our spiritual cancer by His atoning death on the cross for our sins. You see, Jesus was unique because He was born of a virgin by the Holy Spirit. He was not born of Adam's seed as all other human beings are, thus He did not inherit a sinful nature. In other words, He did not have the tendency to sin as we all do. The Bible teaches that the payment for sin is death, and it also teaches that without the shedding of blood there can be no forgiveness of sin.

Jesus Christ died an excruciatingly terrible death on the cross. He was the perfect, unblemished Lamb of God, who paid the price for sin in order to end the separation between humanity and God. *He provided the cure for our spiritual cancer*. The **ONLY** cure. Unlike physical cancer, for which there are many cures, spiritual cancer has only one cure. Jesus says it Himself in John 14:6: "*I am the way, the truth, and the life. No man comes to the Father but through me.*"

Truth is by nature exclusive.

Consider the truth that 1 plus 1 equals only 2 and not any other number. The same exclusivity applies to Jesus. All religions do **not** lead to God. If someone tells you that all roads lead to heaven, they are sadly mistaken. Trusting in Jesus Christ, the God-Man, as He is proclaimed in the Bible, is the *ONLY* way to inherit eternal life and to cure our spiritual sickness. It's not just me saying it...*Jesus said it Himself!*

Modern religions teach that Jesus' death on the cross was not enough to pay for all of our sins. They say that you must perform certain good works, certain rituals like water baptism, belong to a particular church, observe certain religious days, or make pilgrimages to "holy cities" in order to be saved. However, this is contrary to what the Bible teaches. Jesus, before He died said, *"It is finished."* The Greek text uses the word *"tetelestai,"* which means *"paid in full."* Jesus did all the works necessary to secure salvation for sinners **without their help**. He didn't pay for some sins and then require sinners to pay the remaining balance with certain rituals or with good works. Ephesians 2:8-9 says, *"For by grace you have been saved through faith; and that not of yourselves, it is the gift of God; not as a result of works, so that no one may boast."*

When you confess your sins to God and trust in Jesus as your Savior and Lord, He forgives you eagerly, instantly, and completely. Romans 10:9-10 says: *"That if you confess with your mouth Jesus as Lord, and believe in your heart that God raised Him from the dead, you will be saved; for with the heart a person believes, resulting in righteousness, and with the mouth he confesses, resulting in salvation."* Right now, Jesus is holding out His hands to you in invitation. **All are invited to come to Him. All are invited to repent and believe.** Jesus is the **ONLY** cure to your spiritual disease. You do not need to go to eternal punishment in hell for your sins. No matter where you have been or what you have done, come to Him and He will welcome you with open arms.

But make no mistake, time is of the essence. Do not say, *"Tomorrow I will come to Him."* **Tomorrow may never come.** Isaiah 55:6-7 says, *"Seek the LORD while He may be found; call upon Him while He is near. Let the wicked forsake his way and the unrighteous man his thoughts; and let him return to the LORD, and He will have compassion on him, and to our God, for He will abundantly pardon."* Do not postpone coming to Christ for what you think is a more convenient time, but honestly confess your sins, repent of your sins, and believe in Christ **NOW**.

This next section is entitled "He Died For His Patients." It was written by William Plumer in 1867.

"The whole head is hurt, and the whole heart is sick. You are sick from head to foot – covered with bruises, welts, and infected wounds!" (Isaiah 1:5-6) Often in Scripture, sin is spoken of as a disease, a sickness, a hurt. Christ, as the great Physician, has the only sovereign balm.

Sin is a **dreadful** disease! Yes, it is the very **worst** disease! It was the **first**, and so is the **oldest** malady. It infected man very soon after his creation. For six thousand years sin has committed its ravages and been gaining inveteracy. No other disease is so old. Sin is also a **universal** disease! Other maladies have slain their thousands; but sin has slain its millions! The whole world is a graveyard, full of death and corruption. No person ever lived without sin. As soon as we begin to live, we begin to transgress.

Sin makes men spiritually blind, and deaf, and dumb, and lame, and lethargic. Sin is a terrible compilation of diseases. It is rottenness in the bones. It is a maddening fever, a wasting consumption, a paralysis of all the powers. Human nature is wholly corrupt! Sin is a **perpetual** disease. It rages day and night; on the sea and on the land; in the house of mirth and in the house of God. Sin is a **hereditary** disease. We are conceived in sin and brought forth in iniquity. Sin is also **contagious**. Sinners are enticers, seducers, corrupters.

Sin is also the most **deceitful** and **flattering** disease. One of its strong delusions is, *"You shall not die!"* See the throng of ungodly people marching to perdition – the slaves of Satan, the servants of corruption, the enemies of God! Their mirth would make one think them to be the happiest of people – and not, as they really are – condemned criminals, on their way to the eternal prison-house of inflexible justice! Sin has its delusive dreams. The worse a man is, the better he thinks himself to be.

Sin is the **worst** disease, because it is the parent of all other diseases. But for sin, we would never have seen a human being in pain, or sick, or die. Suffering and agony have one parent – sin! Other diseases are calamities – but sin is a **wickedness**! Sin is not a misfortune – sin is a crime! It is a wicked thing to be a sinner. Transgression brings guilt. God is angry with the wicked every day. The more sinful anyone is – the more is God displeased with him.

Sin is the most **loathsome** of all diseases. Pride is the worst kind of malady. No heart is so vile as a hard heart. No vileness compares with an evil heart of unbelief. No sight is so appalling as a sight of vile affections. Sin is horrible and abominable to God! Sin is also the most **dolorous** disease. They multiply their sorrows – who hasten after transgression. The most bitter cries that ever were heard – were extorted by sin.

Other diseases do but kill the body – but sin **kills soul and body in hell forever!** Sin will rage more violently beyond the tomb than on earth. It will be followed by eternal regrets and reproaches, eternal weeping and wailing, eternal wrath and anguish!

Sin **cannot be cured** by any means of human devising. All reformations can never cure the heart. *"I fast twice in the week; I give tithes of all that I possess,"* said the Pharisee – while spiritual wickedness reigned within. We may weep and lament over our sins – but that will neither dethrone sin nor atone for it! Our tears are nothing; our works are nothing; all our righteous deeds are as filthy rags; they are of no avail.

The **only remedy for sin** is found only in Jesus! He is the **Physician of souls**. None but He can cure a sin-sick soul. He makes no charge for all His cures! **He died for His patients!** His blood cleanses from all sin. With His stripes we are healed. Christ's death atones. By His sufferings we have remission of sin. In all cases where it is applied, **the gospel remedy** is sovereign and effectual. It availed for the dying thief, for the bloody Saul of Tarsus, for the cruel jailor, and for millions and millions who once esteemed themselves as vile, and as worthy of everlasting death!

And now, poor, sin-sick, dying soul – flee to this Physician, submit your case to Him, and seek for the healing remedy! If you stay away, you must die! *"The wages of sin is death."*

"The blood of Jesus cleanses us from every sin!" 1 John 1:7

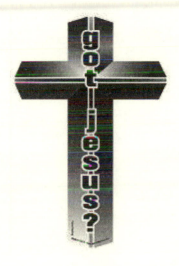

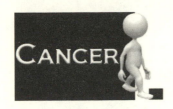

APPENDIX 3
EXERCISE ESSENTIALS

> "EXERCISE HAS BEEN SHOWN TO REDUCE THE RISK OF MANY TYPES OF CANCER."   -DR. JOSEPH MERCOLA

Back in the late 1980s and early 1990s, I competed in and won numerous bodybuilding contests. At competition, my normal contest weight was around 220 pounds and my body fat measured around three percent. I "looked" like the picture of health. However, as the saying goes, *"Looks can be deceiving."* The reality was that due to years of steroid use, my liver and kidneys were on their "last legs."

I recall visiting my doctor when I was about 25 years old, and he said that if I didn't get "off the juice" (*i.e.,* steroids), that I wouldn't make it to age 30. Well, that was certainly a wake up call for me. **Thank God** that He saved me and I became a Christian a couple of years later. I now lift weights as part of an exercise program aimed at overall health.

I include this information about my experience as a competitive bodybuilder for a couple of reasons. First, I want to emphasize that "looking healthy" is not necessarily equivalent to actually "being healthy." Our society puts far too much emphasis on the **external** (how we look) and not enough emphasis on the **internal** (how we feel) or the **spiritual** (where we are going when we die).

You can see from my picture on the next page that I **looked like** I was very healthy. Today, many people will do what ever it takes to have a "killer body," but the truth is that many of them are awfully **un**healthy people and don't feel very good.

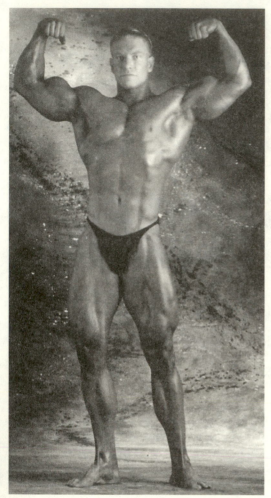

For example, one of my good bodybuilder friends died at age 34 from a stroke caused by years of steroid use. He **looked** like he was as healthy as a horse. But as I said, looks can be deceiving. Now, don't get me wrong. Appearance is important. That's why I take a shower every day, make sure my clothes match, and check that I don't have anything green stuck in my teeth. But I worry that we've gotten so obsessed with how we **look** that we no longer care about how we **feel.**

Secondly, since I am very familiar with the concepts of weight training and cardiovascular (aerobic) training, I have some valuable insights into how to incorporate these activities into a "healthy" exercise regimen. Regular exercise also has been shown to increase quality of life and improve the maximal oxygen uptake during exertion, sleep patterns, and cognition. For a cancer patient, a healthy exercise regimen is a vital part of your "get well and stay well lifestyle." It is not just good for you. **It is essential**.

AEROBICS

What is aerobic exercise?   Remember, the term aerobic means "with oxygen." During an aerobic workout, the cardiovascular system, which includes the heart, lungs and blood vessels, responds to physical activity by increasing the oxygen that is available to the body's working muscles. This sounds like a good thing for a cancer patient, doesn't it? The goal of aerobic exercise is to increase your heart's capacity to pump blood, thus increasing oxygen delivery to the tissues. The American College of Sports Medicine recommends aerobic exercise done for a minimum of 20 minutes, three times a week at 60% of the maximum heart rate.

Many activities can give you an aerobic workout. Some examples include biking, running, walking, jumping rope, swimming, playing basketball, roller skating, and dancing. In addition to these activities, you can get an aerobic workout through stationary exercise machines such as cycles, treadmills, stair steppers, and rowing machines. These can be found at a local gym or health club. Most of these machines can also be used at home.

A "warm up" and a "cool down" period, both of which should incorporate stretching exercises, are essential parts of aerobic exercise. Warming up helps your body prepare for exercise by slowly raising your heart rate and muscle temperature. This also decreases the likelihood of injury. Cooling down allows your heart rate to slowly return to normal and to get the blood circulating freely back to the heart.

General Guidelines for **Aerobic Exercise**:

> **Keep it simple**. If you're confused about what to do, start with the basics. You need at least 20 minutes per workout to get your heart pumping, so start there. Get out your calendar, find 20 minutes of time on 3 different days and do something, whether it be walking, jogging, going to the gym, working in the yard, swimming, playing basketball, etc.
> **Mix It Up**. The nice thing about aerobic exercise is that you can choose any activity that raises your heart rate. You don't have to do the same workout all the time. If you are bored with your workout, change it up.
> **Drink plenty of water** before, during, and after your workout.

The key to aerobic workouts is the "aerobic" part, *i.e.*, the part that deals with **oxygen**. Oxygen nourishes cells, creates energy, combats fatigue, breaks down waste products and toxins, provides energy needed to metabolize carbohydrates, regulates body pH balance, strengthens immune system defense, and fights off invading hostile organisms.

The importance of oxygen therapy through regular aerobic exercise cannot be stressed enough. It's a matter of health or disease and sometimes (as in the medical studies of cancer) life or death. Remember, **cancer cannot live in the presence of oxygen**. So, instead of "zoning out" on the couch and watching television, get up and do some jumping jacks or take a jog around the block. In addition to helping prevent cancer, remember that a program of regular aerobic exercise can also help you avoid chronic diseases such as heart disease, hypertension, stroke, and diabetes, too.

REBOUNDING

What is rebounding? One excellent choice of exercise is rebounding (jumping) on the mini-trampoline. You can rebound several times a day while listening to the radio or watching TV.

Research has led many scientists to conclude that jumping on a mini-trampoline is possibly the most effective exercise yet devised by man, especially because of the effect rebounding has on the lymph system. **The human body needs to move**. The lymph system bathes every cell and carries nutrients to the cell while removing toxins such as dead and cancerous cells, heavy metals, infectious viruses, and other assorted wastes. But unlike the blood (which is pumped by the heart), the lymph is totally dependent on physical exercise to move.

Lymphocytes (the primary cells of the lymph system) make up roughly 25% of all white blood cells in the body. Like other white blood cells, they are produced in the red bone marrow. Lymphocytes constantly travel throughout the body, moving through tissues or through the blood or lymph vessels. There are three major subtypes of lymphocytes: T-cells, B-cells, and NK cells. The letter "T" refers to the thymus, where those lymphocytes mature. The letter "B" refers to the bone marrow, where that group of lymphocytes matures. The "NK" is an acronym for "natural killer" cells.

T-cells carry out two main defensive functions: they kill invaders and orchestrate or control the actions of other lymphocytes involved in the immune process or response. In addition, T-cells recognize and destroy any abnormal body cells, such as those that have become cancerous.

Like T-cells, B-cells are also programmed to recognize specific antigens on foreign cells. When stimulated during an immune response (such as when foreign cells enter the body), B-cells undergo a change in structure. They then produce antibodies, which are protein compounds. These compounds bind with specific antigens of foreign cells, labeling those cells for destruction.

NK cells are the most aggressive lymphocytes in the immune system. They make up about 5% to 15% of the total lymphocyte circulating population. They target tumor cell and protect against a wide variety of infectious microbes. NK cells are known to differentiate and mature in the bone marrow, lymph nodes, spleen, thymus, and tonsils where they then enter into the circulation.

You can see that B-cells, T-cells, and NK cells are key players in our immune response. But without muscular contraction, adequate exercise, and movement, these lymphocytes are not able to do their job, because the lymph doesn't flow. Thus, the body's cells are left stewing in their own waste products and starving for nutrients, a situation which contributes to cancer and other degenerative diseases, as well as premature aging. **<u>Rebounding has been shown to increase lymph flow by up to 30 times!</u>**

Also, all of the body's cells become stronger in response to the increased "G forces" during rebounding, and this cellular exercise results in the self-propelled lymphocytes being up to five times more active!

Rebounding on a mini-trampoline directly strengthens the immune system, increases lymph flow, and oxygenates the blood. Unlike jogging on hard surfaces which puts extreme stress on certain joints such as the ankles and knees eventually damaging them, rebounding affects every joint and cell in the body equally. Plus, there are no cars, dogs, and bad weather to worry about.

CIRCUIT WEIGHTS

In order to stimulate the muscle cells, I recommend doing "circuit weight" training.

Circuit weight training is a combination of aerobics and resistance training designed to be easy to follow, give you a great workout, and target fat loss, muscle building, and heart-lung fitness. Typically, in a gym, there will be several weight machines strategically placed in a certain order which makes up what is called a circuit. You just go from one machine to the next until you complete the circuit. Circuit weight training will help you to tone your muscles, strengthen your tendons and ligaments, and if done at a fast pace, can also have an aerobic effect.

General Guidelines for Circuit Weight Training:

> **Keep it light**. Don't try to show off. Lift light weights for at least twenty repetitions per set. And if you feel pain of any kind (other than a "burn" in your muscles), then **STOP**. The pain is warning you that you are overdoing whatever you are doing. Decrease the weight until you can achieve 20 repetitions.

> **Exercise slowly.** Specific exercises should be performed very slowly, with emphasis on the "negative" portion of the movement.
> **Keep it quick.** Your entire workout should not last more than 45 minutes. Rest only enough time between sets to walk from one machine to the next. This will allow you to get both a muscle building workout and an aerobic workout at the same time.
> **Breathe properly.** Don't hold your breath when lifting weights. Be sure to intake plenty of oxygen, inhaling and exhaling regularly.

I won't go into details about the specifics of weight training in this book. Any good personal trainer will be able to assist you with a personalized weight lifting program.

BEWARE: From the viewpoint of immune function, the optimal exercise regimen is one of **low volume**, reports Dr. Roy Shephard and colleagues at the University of Toronto in Canada. Their findings are published in a recent issue of the *Journal of Sports Medicine and Physical Fitness*. Previous studies have shown that while exercise enhances the immune system, an **excess** of exercise can actually depress immune function. During intense exercise, free radical production is greatly increased which is associated with oxidative damage to the muscles, liver, blood, and other tissues.

One of the world's leading authorities on antioxidants and free radical research, Dr. Ken Cooper, stated in his book titled, <u>Antioxidant Revolution</u>, *"When you exercise **intensely**, the blood flow in your body is shunted away from the organs that are not actively involved in the exercise process, such as the liver, kidneys, stomach, and intestines. Instead, the blood is diverted to the working muscles, including the heart and legs. During the shifting of blood flow, a part or all of the body regions or organs not involved in exercise will experience an acute lack of oxygen (known as hypoxia)."*

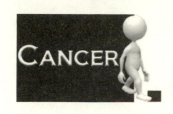

APPENDIX 4
DAVID VS. GOLIATH:

> "THE FDA AND THE FTC ARE THE LEG-BREAKERS FOR THE PHARMACEUTICAL CARTELS."   –DR. GARY GLUM

"JASON VALE & THE CANCER MAFIA"

My first experience with alternative cancer treatments was in 1997. My father had recently died, and I was determined to learn all I could about alternative treatments. I don't remember exactly how, but I stumbled across some information about vitamin B$_{17}$ and ordered a video from Jason Vale, an arm wrestler who had cured his terminal cancer through eating apple seeds and apricot seeds.

After my wife and I watched the video, we were flabbergasted. The video contained the "Extra" TV show interview that spotlighted Jason's miraculous recovery from cancer, and it also contained voluminous amounts of data about vitamin B17 and its effects on cancer cells. This was the genesis of my crusade to learn and spread the word about alternative cancer treatments. It's only fitting that twelve years later, I would finally get the opportunity to interview Jason. This entire chapter is the synopsis of a phone interview I did with Jason Vale on January 24, 2009.

Jason Vale, a highly articulate New Yorker, was diagnosed with terminal cancer when he was only eighteen. *"I had a rare type of cancer called Askin's tumor. At that time, there were only twenty recorded cases of this type of cancer, and no one had ever recovered. The death rate was 100%."*

See the actual letter to Dr. Rabinowitz below.

BOOTH MEMORIAL RADIATION THERAPY ASSOC.
Booth Memorial Medical Center
Flushing, New York 11355
(718) 670-1500

JOHN T FAZEKAS, M.D.
DIRECTOR

DAVID VEGA, M.D
RADIATION ONCOLOGIST

NIKITAS KESSARIS M C.
RADIATION PHYSICIST

October 6, 1986

Dr. Sidney Rabinowitz
43-70 Kissena Blvd.
Flushing, N.Y. 11355

Re: <u>Jason Vale</u>

Dear Dr. Rabinowitz:

I had the pleasure of seeing this 18-year-old high school graduate
soon to enter Stony Brook University, suffering from a "neuroepithelioma of chest wall". His history began in the early summer
of 1986 when he developed pain in the left chest with unexpected
loss of weight, approximately 20 lbs. over a period of 10 weeks.
He denies cough and hemoptysis which led to a chest X-ray, showing
a density at the left lung base. This was felt to represent
pneumonia and he received a course of antibiotics with subsequent
chest X-ray showing no improvement of the basilar density. This
led to a CT of the thorax on 8/8 showing a combination of fluid
and atelectasis. A clinical diagnosis of empyema was made and it
was recommended that this be surgically drained with a left
thoracotomy done on 8/11/86. Review of this operative report indicates the presence of a large tumor mass, approximately 18 cm in
width and 25 cm in length adherent to the chest wall and involving
the anterior, mid, lateral, and part of the posterior wall. The
mass was removed totally and the tissue was seen by several pathologists including Dr. Hadju of Memorial Sloan Kettering as well as
Dr. Dickerson of Massachusettes General Hospital. The final diagnosis is a neuroepithelioma, certainly a very rare tumor, which in this
case shows numerous mitoses, necrosis, and other signs of malignancy.
I will perform a library research of the so-called Askin tumor with
special emphasis on the possible role of radiotherapy. This patient
was also seen in consultation by Dr. Sordillo of Memorial Sloan
Kettering and I will speak with him personally as well as to obtain
the return of Booth CAT scan and other pertinent X-rays. The patient
has recovered well and I believe there are plans for chemotherapy
following irradiation.

Past medical history is totally negative, except the patient states
he has been having pain in his upper left back for about 2 years.
Since he also plays hockey and is involved in frequent violent
contact, this symptom has been attributed to trauma. He has regained

Continued......

Page 2
Re: Jason Vale

his weight and has no symptoms of bone pain, cough, or malaise,
consistent with complete work-up including CT of abdomen, ultrasound
of his testicles, bone scan, and laboratory evaluations, all of
which are negative (with the exception of LDH elevated to 1091).
Both alpha-fetoprotein and HCG determinations are also negative.

Physical exam reveals a pleasant and very healthy-appearing lad
who looks his stated age of 18 and is in no apparent distress,
totally recovered from his recent thoracotomy. His incision is
beautifully healed and lung exam is normal, no nodes are palpable
in the neck, and heart sounds are normal. A somewhat tender 1.5
cm left axillary node is appreciated today but this is probably
of no clinical significance. On abdominal exam, the liver and
spleen are nonpalpable and no masses are felt. No boney tenderness
could be elicited except for some slight discomfort on palpating
along his thoracotomy incision (as expected, the bone scan showed
increased uptake along the site of thoracotomy).

IMPRESSION: Neuroepithelioma of chest wall (Askin tumor) with
outside confirmation by Drs. Hadju and Dickerson.

RECOMMENDATION: I will continue to perform a search of the medical
literature in order to define the potential role of radiotherapy in
preventing local recurrence of this large neuroectodermal tumor
and will adjust the dose and fields according to the total plan
including whether he will be receiving Adriamycin or not. If long-
term survival is a strong likelihood, then clearly the treatment
regimen must be delivered in such a way as to avoid disabling
complications related to the heart and underlying pulmonary tissues.
Details as to exact plan, fields, and dosage will be forthcoming
in a separate note. I have discovered several articles, including
a section of the textbook by Dr. Nelly published in 1979 by the
publisher Lee and Farber. The premier article appeared in Cancer,
Vol. 43, #6, p. 2438, 1979 with 20 cases presented, most of whom
received both radiotherapy and chemotherapy but with a uniform
poor outcome and with essentially 100% mortality.

With kind regards,

John T. Fazekas, M.D.
Director of Radiation Therapy

JTF/sn

cc: Dr. Peter Sordillo   Dr. Fouad Lajam
    55 E. 34 St.   87-10 37 Avenue
    New York, N.Y. 10016   Jackson Heights, N.Y. 11372

Jason said that his mother didn't even show him the doctor's letter for a
couple of months, since she was afraid of his reaction. But Jason told
me that when he finally did see the letter, he wasn't afraid. He didn't
worry. God had given him the peace that passes all understanding.
"That alone was the victory" says Jason.

Jason had a huge tumor the size of a grapefruit between his back and ribs which was causing fluid in his lungs to build up. The surgeons removed the tumor. Although they recommended chemo and radiation, Jason decided not to undergo these treatments.

Jason said he immediately began to play hockey and handball again. However, within a year, he began to feel the same back pains he felt when he was first diagnosed. The cancer was back. Jason could hardly walk, as the tumor had now invaded his spinal cord. After a CAT scan revealed that the tumor was *"bigger and better than ever,"* they operated immediately.

Jason then opted to do both chemo and radiation, despite the fact that the doctors were a little hesitant to do so because the toxicity level from the chemo would be multiplied by the radiation. Within a couple of months, he had lost 40 pounds and was near death. If it weren't for the fact that he was such a physical specimen, he would have died from the treatments. However, with his background as an arm wrestler and also with his young age (only nineteen), Jason survived.

He knew that something needed to be done. According to Jason, *"...it was then that I changed all of the foods that I ate without even realizing it. The chemotherapy made me so sick that I would nearly throw up at the smell of my old favorites, like Chinese food, Kentucky Fried Chicken, and pizza."* So Jason began to "clean up" his diet.

When Jason was about 25 years old, it was discovered that he had a malignant tumor in his kidney. Jason said he felt like *"it was about to start all over again."* When he went to the kidney specialist, he was told that he needed to have his kidney removed. The more questions Jason asked him, the more aggravated he became. Jason walked out of his office right before he was scheduled to have surgery, and he never went back.

Through God's providence, a friend from church, Bill DePap, gave Jason the videotape *"World Without Cancer"* by G. Edward Griffin. When the pastor told him to *"take it with a grain of salt"* since the man was a bit *"eccentric,"* this made Jason even more intrigued. This video documents the fact that Vitamin B_{17} kills cancer cells. Jason said that when the video ended, he was dumbfounded and knew this was the answer. That very night, he went to the grocery store to buy peaches and get their pits. He began to buy cases and cases of apples just to get to their seeds. The seeds, filled with vitamin B_{17}, were curing his cancer. At one point, Jason was eating the seeds of 20 to 30 apples per day. According to Jason, *"I would take out the seeds and throw away the apples. Mom would get the apples out of the trash and make apple pie.*" What a great mother!

He also believes in the power of prayer. "*My church began a one month prayer chain where every half hour someone new was praying for victory in the situation. Every half hour 24 hours a day someone new in my congregation was praying.*"

If you look back at chapter 6, you will be able to refresh yourself on the actual cancer killing mechanism of vitamin B_{17}, which is truly remarkable. According to Jason, "*As I ate cyanide filled seeds, the cancer dissipated from my body.*" The effectiveness of vitamin B_{17} in curing cancer is astonishing! According to Dr. Dean Burk, former head of the National Cancer Institute's cell chemistry section, "*When we add vitamin B_{17} to a cancer culture under the microscope (providing the enzyme glucosidase also is present), we can see the cancer cells dying off like flies!*"

Jason reached national prominence when he appeared on the television show "Extra" as the arm wrestler self-cured of cancer with apricot kernels, provoking a response so great that the episode was run a second time. Immediately, Jason set up a website (www.apricotsfromGod.info) and began to supply people with apricot seeds and an information video through his company, Christian Brothers. Over the next few years, literally thousands of cancer

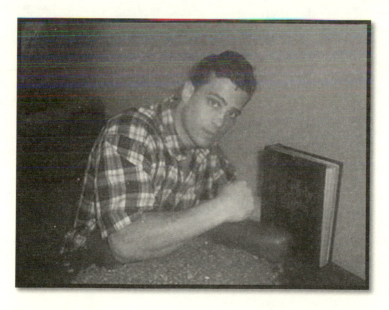

survivors emailed Jason with their B_{17} success stories.

Now, we all know that the FDA is nothing more than a den of thieves, legalized mobsters, a gang of thugs, who don't care about people's health but only care about protecting Big Pharma's cash cow. Jason was quickly becoming a threat to the Cancer Industry. Since Big Pharma is unable to patent or claim exclusive rights to vitamin B_{17} (as it is derived from a natural source), they have launched attacks of unprecedented vicious propaganda against B_{17} despite the overwhelming proof of its effectiveness in controlling all forms of cancer.

Jason's problems began October 28, 1998, when the FDA sent him a three-page "warning letter" concerning his *"promotion and distribution of the unapproved drug Laetrile in the form of ... 'apricot seeds', 'vitamin B_{17} tablets' and 'amygdalina' ampoules."* The letter stated that the *"labeling for these products make[s] therapeutic claims which cause the products to be drugs as defined in Section 201 (g) of the Federal Food, Drug and Act ..."*

Jason eventually signed an injunction that he wouldn't promote apricot seeds as a cancer *"cure."* He <u>never</u> signed any document stating he would quit selling apricot seeds altogether. All in all, Jason had over 28,000 customers worldwide. In the midst of all this turmoil, Jason went on to become the arm wrestling World Champion in 1999.

Eventually, without even one customer complaint in ten years, the FDA came in and seized apricot seeds and computers and brought Jason to criminal court for promoting this natural answer to cancer. The Cancer Mafia was doing their best to make an example of Jason. Bail was set at ... not $5,000 ... not $25,000 ... not even $100,000. **Jason's bail was $800,000!** In the summer of 2002, Jason's family had to put liens on their properties to pay the bail that was placed on him pending his trial.

The judge at his trial was John Gleeson, who was the prosecutor at the John Gotti trial. Being a competitor through and through, a *"rule-oriented"* guy (*in his own words*), and being principled on honesty and integrity, Jason said that he thought the judge would be fair. *"I trusted the judge since I thought he was smart...I thought he would go against the grain...but I was wrong. He sold out...he cheated...he wasn't fair."* At the trial, Gleeson arrogantly declared that the injunction stipulated that Jason couldn't sell apricot seeds, despite the fact that is NOT what the injunction said. When Jason tried to explain to Gleeson what the injunction stipulated, Gleeson said, *"Take it to the appeals court."*

On July 14, 2003, Jason lost his Constitutional Rights to be able to continue to tell his story of how he defeated cancer with apricot and apple seeds. He was sentenced to 63 months in the New York State Penn. This is truly amazing if you think about it. We have pedophiles, rapists, murderers, and drug dealers walking the streets, but if you sell a natural cure for cancer, you're going to jail. Is this America?

While in prison, Jason said that he spent almost a year in *"the hole"* (*i.e., solitary confinement*) for *"silly stuff"* ... like not making his bed properly or having too many booklets of stamps. He said he spent four months in the hole for getting into a fight with three inmates who wanted to watch "rap" videos on TV, but Jason wanted to watch American Idol. Let's just say the three inmates ended up in the infirmary. I guess they didn't realize Jason is a martial arts expert.

And his mother (God bless her) would sneak him apricot seeds when she came to visit. She would put them in mixed nuts bags, since they look just like almonds. He said he would sit there talking to his mom and eating the "*contraband*" apricot seeds, helping to keep his cancer at bay, right in front of the guards.

After almost five years in prison, Jason was released from prison on April 15, 2008. According to Jason, *"It was the greatest day of my life."* Jason is currently petitioning FDA to allow him to sell apricot seeds without any "claims." It's a sad state of affairs when you must get official FDA "approval" to sell apricot seeds, isn't it?

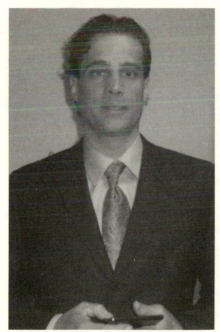

Of course, vitamin B_{17} is only "*dangerous*" to the parasitic FDA officials whose salaries are funded by American taxpayers and to Big Pharma who hires and plants FDA officials and makes billions of dollars every year killing over **one hundred thousand** Americans with their man-made poisons.

Let's be honest here. The FDA is nothing more than a bunch of "*hit men*" for the Medical Mafia and is in a state of treason toward "*we the people.*" When it comes to health fraud, the FDA is the biggest culprit.

Nevertheless, Jason is a free man! When I asked him what he was going to do now that he's free, Jason said that Brooklyn Queens Experiment (a production company) has purchased the movie rights for the "Jason Vale Story" – a major motion picture based on Jason's life. I don't know about you, but I can't wait to see the movie!!

Best wishes Jason! Fighting the FDA might have seemed like David vs. Goliath, but you're a **GIANT** in my book!

Jason's website is www.ApricotsfromGod.info.

Update:

In the fall of 2013, Jason won the New York "Empire State" arm-wrestling championship, not only winning his class, but then defeating the superheavyweight opponent for the overall title. Nice job Jason!

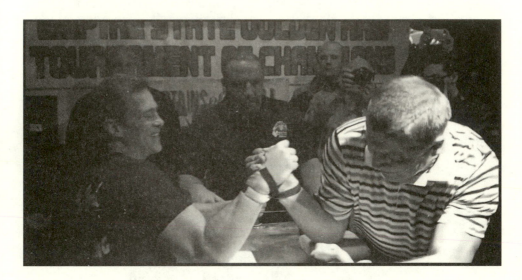

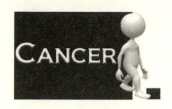

GLOSSARY

Acetogenins – long chains of carbon atoms which reduce the growth of blood vessels that nourish cancer cells and inhibit the growth of MDR cells.

Acidic – having a low pH.

Acrylamides – carcinogenic chemical formed by the heating of starches.

Adaptogenic – the ability to enhance the body's ability to resist a stressor.

Adenosine Triphosphate (ATP) – the "energy currency" of cells.

Adrenal Glands – a pair of glands located above the kidneys; produce hormones such as epinephrine, corticosteroids, and androgens.

Aerobic – "with oxygen" (contrasted with anaerobic – "without oxygen")

Alkaline – having a high pH.

AMAS test – "*Anti-Malignin Antibody in Serum*" test. The most accurate diagnostic test to detect cancer.

Amylase – digestive enzyme that breaks down carbohydrates.

Anaerobic Respiration – the process of creating energy "without oxygen"; also referred to as "anaerobic metabolism."

Anemia – a condition in which a decreased number of red blood cells may cause symptoms including tiredness, shortness of breath, and weakness.

Angiogenesis – the physiological process involving the growth of new blood vessels from pre-existing vessels.

Antibiotics – drugs that fight infections.

Antibody – a protein produced by plasma cells when they encounter foreign invaders; specific antibodies bind to specific invaders (antigens).

Antioxidants – chemical compounds or substances that inhibit oxidation.

Antineoplastic – preventing the growth or development of cancer cells.

Apoptosis – programmed cell death.

Autoimmune Response – a condition in which a person's immune system produces antibodies that attack the body's own tissues.

Bacterium (plural Bacteria) – a simple single-celled microorganism.

Benign – a non-cancerous tumor; antonym of malignant.

Beta Carotene – precursor to vitamin A; the most well-known carotenoid.

Bile – a yellowish-green fluid produced by the liver that aids in digestion of fats and the excretion of toxins.

Biopsy – the surgical removal of tissue for microscopic examination.

Blood Cells – minute structures produced in the bone marrow; consist of erythrocytes (red blood cells), leukocytes (white blood cells), and platelets.

Bone Marrow – spongy material found inside the bones.

Cachexia – the "wasting" cycle of many cancer patients.

Capillaries – tiny blood vessels that deliver oxygen and nutrients to and remove waste products from cells.

Carcinogen – a cancer-causing substance or agent.

Carcinoma – cancer that starts in the skin or the lining of organs.

    Adenocarcinoma – malignant tumor arising from glandular tissue.
    Basal cell carcinoma – most common type of skin cancer.
    Bronchogenic carcinoma – cancer originating in the lungs or airways.
    Cervical carcinoma – cancer of the cervix.
    Endometrial carcinoma – cancer of the lining of the uterus.
    Squamous cell carcinoma – cancer arising from the skin or the surfaces of other structures, such as the mouth, cervix, or lungs.

CAT scan – a test using x-rays to creat images of various body parts.

CEA (carcinoembryonic antigen) – a blood tumor marker.

Cell Fibers – the "muscles" of our cells.

Cell Membrane – the "skin" of our cells.

Chelation – the process of removing a heavy metal from the bloodstream by means of a chelating agent (such as chlorella or cilantro).

Chlorophyll – a group of related green pigments that convert light energy into ATP and other forms of energy needed for biochemical processes; found in green plants, brown and red algae, and certain aerobic and anaerobic bacteria.

Cirrhosis – a type of liver damage in which normal liver cells are replaced with fibrous scar tissue.

Co-Enzymes – an organic substance that usually contains a vitamin or mineral and combines with a specific protein to form an active enzyme system.

Collagen – the fibrous protein "cement" that holds our bones, cartilage, tendons, and connective tissue, and cells together.

Conjugated Linoleic Acid (CLA) – naturally occurring free fatty acid found mainly in grass-fed meats and dairy products; builds muscle and reduces body fat; classified as an omega-6 fatty acid.

Cytokines – "messenger cells" such as interferons and interleukins which set off a cascade reaction of positive changes throughout the immune system.

Cytopenia – low levels of blood cells.

Cytoplasm – the jelly-like part of a cell.

Deoxyribonucleic acid (DNA) – carries the cell's genetic information and hereditary characteristics via its nucleotides and their sequence; capable of self-replication and RNA synthesis.

Dimethyl sulfoxide (DMSO) – a non-toxic, 100% natural product that comes from the wood industry.

Dioxin – any of several carcinogenic chemicals that occur as impurities in petroleum-derived herbicides.

Disaccharide – a chain of two sugar molecules (*like lactose which is composed of glucose and galactose*).

EDTA – a therapy by which repeated administrations of a weak synthetic amino acid (*EDTA, ethylenediamine tetra-acetic acid*) gradually reduce atherosclerotic plaque and other heavy metal deposits throughout the cardiovascular system by literally dissolving them away.

Electron – an elementary particle with a negative charge.

Electron Transport Chain – the final stage of the Krebs Cycle.

Enzymes – any of numerous proteins produced by living organisms and functioning as biochemical catalysts.

Epidermis – the outer layer of skin.

Erythrocyte – see "Red Blood Cells."

Eukaryotic Cell – a cell with a nucleus and organelles.

Excitotoxins – substances, usually amino acids, that react with specialized receptors (neurons) in the brain in such a way as to lead to destruction of certain types of brain cells.

Fasciolopsis Buski – a fluke that is parasitic on humans and swine.

Free Radical – an atom or group of atoms that has at least one unpaired electron and is, therefore, unstable and highly reactive; damages cells and accelerates the progression of cancer and other diseases.

Glioblastoma Multiforme – the most common and most aggressive type of primary brain tumor in humans, involving glial cells.

Gluconeogenesis – the formation of glucose, especially by the liver, from noncarbohydrate sources, such as amino acids and the glycerol portion of fats.

Glucose – A monosaccharide sugar the blood that serves as the major energy source of the body; it occurs in most plant and animal tissue. Also called *blood sugar*.

Glutathione – the master antioxidant.

Glycan – a chain of saccharides.

Glyconutrients – around 200 naturally occurring biologically active plant monosaccharide sugars; researchers have identified a small group of 8 essential glyconutrients, which includes *glucose, galactose, mannose, fucose, xylose, N-acetylglucosamine, N-acetylgalactosamine, and N-acetylneuraminic acid.*

Golgi Body – a net-like structure in the cell's cytoplasm which stores ATP.

Glycogen - a polysaccharide that is the main form of carbohydrate storage in animals and occurs mainly in liver and muscle tissue; it is readily converted to glucose; also called *animal starch.*

Granulocytes – white blood cells filled with granules of toxic chemicals that enable them to digest microbes by a process called phagocytosis (literally "cell-eating"). Three types of granulocytes are neutrophils (which kill bacteria), eosinophils (which kill parasites), and basophils.

Hemoglobin – the protein pigment in red blood cells that contains iron and transports oxygen to the tissues and carbon dioxide from them.

Heterocyclic amines (HCA) – carcinogenic substances formed by cooking any meat (*beef, lamb, pork, fowl, or fish*) at high temperatures.

Human chronic gonadotropin (HCG) – a hormone produced by the placenta that maintains the corpus luteum during pregnancy.

Hydrogen – the most abundant chemical element; constitutes 75% of the universe.

Hydrogenation – the addition of hydrogen to a compound, especially to solidify an unsaturated fat or fatty acid.

Hydrolysis – the decomposition of a chemical compound by reaction with water.

Hypoxia – lack of oxygen – one of the prime causes of cancer.

Immune System – the bodily system that protects the body from foreign substances, cells, and tissues by producing the immune response and that includes the thymus, spleen, lymph nodes, lymphocytes, and antibodies.

Insulin – a hormone secreted by the pancreas which regulates the metabolism of carbohydrates and fats, especially the conversion of glucose to glycogen, which lowers the blood glucose level.

Interferon – a naturally produced chemical released by the body in response to viral infections.

Interleukin – a naturally produced chemical released by the body.

Krebs Cycle – cycle of creating energy w/in our cells; aka *citric acid cycle*.

Lauric Acid – a fatty acid obtained chiefly from coconut oil.

Leukemia – cancer of the blood cells.

Leukocytes – see "White Blood Cells."

Lymphocytes – white blood cells found in the lymphatic system; includes T-cells, B-cells, and NK cells.

Lymphoma – cancer of the lymphatic system which originates in the lymphocytes; two types are Hodgkin's (includes the presence of a Reed-Sternberg cell) and non-Hodgkin's (Reed-Sternberg cell is not present).

Lipids – group of molecules including fats, oils, and cholesterol.

Lipase – digestive enzyme that breaks down lipids.

Macrophages – a type of white blood cell that ingests foreign material; key players in the immune response to foreign invaders such as infectious microbes, antigens, and other foreign substances.

Malignancy – a cancer, neoplasm, or tumor that grows in an uncontrolled manner, and may invade nearby tissue and metastasize (spread) to other areas of the body.

Mammogram – x-ray of the breast.

Melanocytes – cells that produce the pigment melanin that colors our skin, hair, and eyes and is heavily concentrated in most moles.

Melanoma – the most serious form of skin cancer; a malignant tumor that originates in melanocytes.

Melatonin – a hormone produced from the amino acid tryptophan by the pineal gland; causes you to get sleepy when it's dark.

Microbe – a microorganism, especially a bacterium that causes disease.

Mineral – an inorganic element that promotes chemical reactions within the body and is necessary for proper cellular metabolism.

Mitochondria – "cellular power plant;" an organelle in the cytoplasm of nearly all eukaryotic cells containing genetic material.

Monosaccharide – any of several carbohydrates that cannot be broken down to simpler sugars.

Monocytes – white blood cells that ingest dead or damaged cells and provide immunological defenses against many infectious organisms; eventually develop into macrophages.

Monosodium glutamate (MSG) – food additive made from glutamic acid; an extitotoxin.

Monounsaturated – containing only one double or triple bond per mole-cule; monounsaturated fats decrease the amount of LDL cholesterol in the blood and include olive and avocado oils.

Methyl sulfonyl methane (MSM) – basically DMSO with an additional oxygen atom attached to the sulfur atom.

Mycotoxins – fungal toxins.

Myeloma – malignant tumor of the bone marrow.

Neoplasm – an abnormal new growth of tissue; a tumor.

Neurons – nerve cells; conduct electric impulses.

Nitrosamines – carcinogenic substances which result from the digestion of sodium nitrate and/or sodium nitrite.

Nucleotide – the basic component of DNA and RNA.

Nucleus – the "control center" of the cell; includes the DNA of the cell.

Oligosaccharide – a chain of sugars that is from 3 to 20 molecules long.

Omega-3 fatty acids – polyunsaturated fatty acids that are found especially in fish, fish oils, vegetable oils, and green leafy vegetables; omega-3 fats include alpha-linolenic acid (ALA), eicosapentaenoic acid (EPA), docosahex-aenoic acid (DHA), and docosapentaenoic acid (DPA).

Omega-6 fatty acids – polyunsaturated fatty acids that are found especially in nuts and grains; omega-6 fats include linoleic acid (LA), conjugated linoleic acid (CLA), gamma linolenic acid (GLA), dihomo-gamma linolenic acid (DGLA), and arachidonic acid (AA).

Omega-9 fatty acids – found in olive oil and avocados; also known as oleic acids.

Oncologist – physician specializing in cancer.

Organelle – a differentiated structure within a cell that performs a specific function.

Orthomolecular – the theory that diseases can be cured by restoring the optimum amounts of substances normally present in the body.

Osteosarcoma – most common type of bone cancer.

Oxidation – the addition of oxygen to a compound with a loss of electrons.

P53 – protein that is the product of a tumor suppressor gene, regulates cell growth and proliferation, and prevents unrestrained cell division after chromosomal damage.

Pathogenic – capable of causing disease.

pH Balance – the acid/alkaline balance in our body; pH = potential hydrogen.

Phagocytosis – the process the human body uses to destroy bacteria by surrounding and digesting them with digestive enzymes; macrophages are the scavenger cells that are part of this process; literally "cell eating."

Plasma – the yellow-colored liquid component of blood, in which blood cells are suspended; part of the immune system.

Platelets – the smallest of the three types of blood cells; also called thrombocytes; principal function is to prevent bleeding.

Pleomorphic – having many forms.

Polysaccharide – any of a class of carbohydrates whose molecules contain chains of 10 or more monosaccharides.

Probiotics – "good bacteria;" live microbial supplements which improve intestinal balance.

Prokaryotic cell – a cell (*such as bacteria*) which lacks a nucleus.

Protease – digestive enzyme that breaks down proteins.

Proton – an elementary particle with a positive charge.

Protoplasm – the complex substance that constitutes the living matter of plant and animal cells; composed of proteins and fats; includes the nucleus and cytoplasm.

PSA (prostate specific antigen) – test used to diagnose prostate cancer.

Recombinant bovine growth hormone (rBGH) – genetically engineered hormone injected into cows to increase milk production; manufactured by Monsanto; sold under the trade name Posilac.

Red blood cells (erythrocytes) – blood cells that deliver oxygen to tissues and take carbon dioxide from them.

Resveratrol – a compound found in grapes, red wine, and purple grape juice which inhibits the growth of cancer cells.

Ribonucleic acid (RNA) – transmits genetic information from DNA to the cytoplasm and controls certain chemical processes in the cell.

Saccharide – a sugar molecule.

Sarcoma – malignant tumor of the muscles or connective tissue such as bone and cartilage.

Seizure – a burst of abnormal electrical activity in the brain.

Selenium – trace mineral that acts as an antioxidant.

Sesquioxide – an oxide containing three atoms of oxygen with two atoms (or radicals) of some other substance.

Sodium Bicarbonate – baking soda; NAHCO3

Sodium Nitrite – carcinogenic substance used to preserve and color food especially in meat and fish products.

Stroke – interruption of the normal flow of blood to the brain due to a blood clot or hemorrhage.

Superoxide Dismutase (SOD) – enzyme that destroys free radicals.

Thrombopoietin (TPO) – cytokine that stimulates production of platelets.

Thrombosis – development of blood clots within blood vessels or the heart.

Thyroid Gland – organ at the base of the neck that produces thyroxin and other hormones involved in regulating metabolism.

Trans-Fats – "pseudo-fats" produced by the partial hydrogenation of vegetable oils; present in hardened vegetable oils, most margarines, commercial baked foods, and fried foods; increase the risk of cancer.

Trophoblasts – cells that attach the fertilized ovum to the uterine wall and serve as a nutritive pathway for the embryo.

Tumor – abnormal growth of cells.

Turmeric – spice that contains curcumin; has multiple anti-carcinogenic effects when consumed.

Vitamin – an organic substance that acts as a co-enzyme or regulator of metabolic processes.

White blood cells (leukocytes) – blood cells that engulf and digest bacteria and fungi; an important part of the body's immune system; specific white blood cells include lymphocytes, granulocytes, and monocytes.

Xenoestrogens – "foreign" estrogens; have been "altered" and act like free radicals in the body; shown to cause various types of cancer.

X-ray – electromagnetic radiation used to diagnose disease.

Zeolites – natural volcanic minerals with a unique, complex crystalline structure.

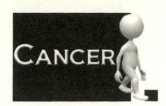

INDEX

D

E

F

G

Q

R

S

y

Z

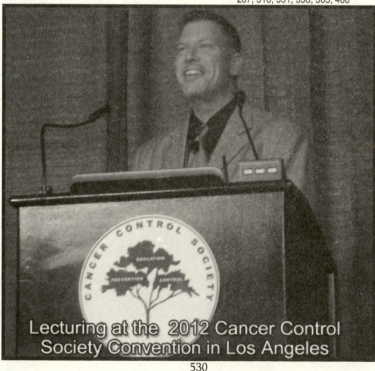

Lecturing at the 2012 Cancer Control Society Convention in Los Angeles

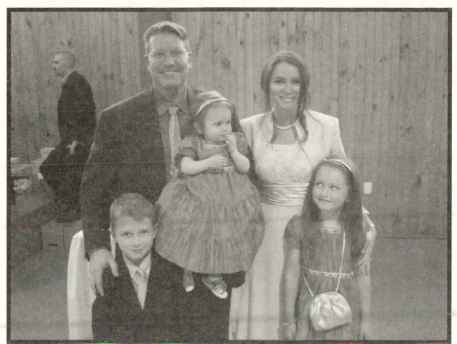

Above – February 2008 at the wedding of Pete & Genevieve de Deugd in Palmerston North, New Zealand   **Below** – with our friends the Rivicre family at Le Mont in Pittsburgh, Pennsylvania in April 2008 (celebrating 3 birthdays!)

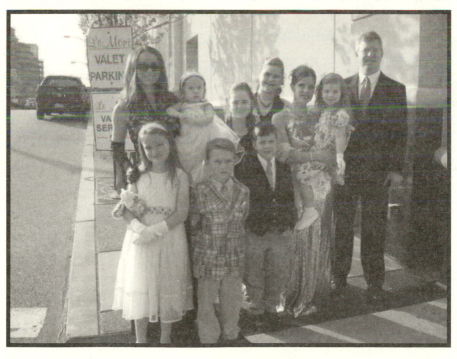

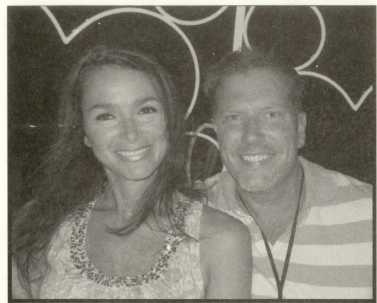

Above – Charlene and me on a carriage ride in downtown St. Louis (2011)
Below – At the home of my good friend, Dr. Irvin Sahni, MD in May of 2013

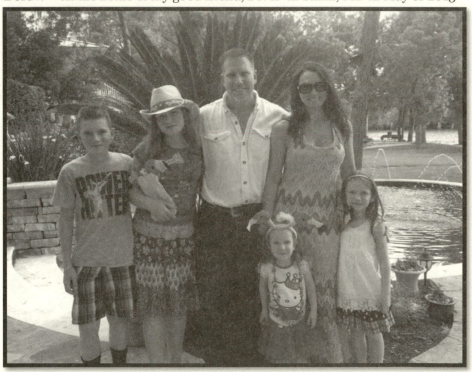

For more books by Ty Bollinger
(published by Infinity 510² Partners):
http://www.Infinity510Partners.com

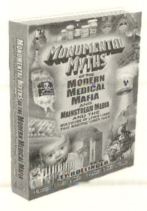

Monumental Myths of the Modern Medical
Mafia and Mainstream Media and the Multitude
of Lying Liars that Manufactured Them
http://www.MythBustersBook.com

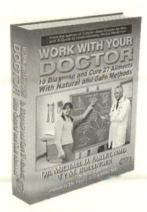

Work With Your Doctor To
Diagnose and Cure 27 Ailments With
Natural and Safe Methods
http://www.MedicalDreamTeam.com

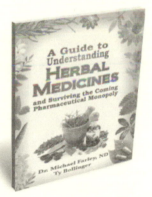

A Guide to Understanding Herbal Medicines and
Surviving the Coming Pharmaceutical Monopoly
http://www.SurvivalHerbs.com

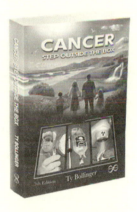

Cancer-Step Outside the Box
http://www.CancerTruth.net